ROUTLEDGE LIBRARY EDITIONS:
MARRIAGE

Volume 10

SEXUAL ADJUSTMENT IN MARRIAGE

SEXUAL ADJUSTMENT IN MARRIAGE

HENRY OLSEN

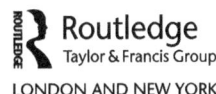

LONDON AND NEW YORK

First published in 1954 by George Allen & Unwin Ltd

This edition first published in 2023
by Routledge
4 Park Square, Milton Park, Abingdon, Oxon OX14 4RN

and by Routledge
605 Third Avenue, New York, NY 10158

Routledge is an imprint of the Taylor & Francis Group, an informa business

© 1954 Henry Olsen

All rights reserved. No part of this book may be reprinted or reproduced or utilised in any form or by any electronic, mechanical, or other means, now known or hereafter invented, including photocopying and recording, or in any information storage or retrieval system, without permission in writing from the publishers.

Trademark notice: Product or corporate names may be trademarks or registered trademarks, and are used only for identification and explanation without intent to infringe.

British Library Cataloguing in Publication Data
A catalogue record for this book is available from the British Library

ISBN: 978-1-032-46071-0 (Set)
ISBN: 978-1-032-48465-5 (Volume 10) (hbk)
ISBN: 978-1-032-48480-8 (Volume 10) (pbk)
ISBN: 978-1-003-38928-6 (Volume 10) (ebk)

DOI: 10.4324/9781003389286

Publisher's Note
The publisher has gone to great lengths to ensure the quality of this reprint but points out that some imperfections in the original copies may be apparent.

Disclaimer
The publisher has made every effort to trace copyright holders and would welcome correspondence from those they have been unable to trace.

Language Disclaimer
This book is a re-issue originally published in 1954.
The language used and views portrayed are a reflection of its era and no offence is meant by the Publishers to any reader by this re-publication.

SEXUAL ADJUSTMENT IN MARRIAGE

HENRY OLSEN
M.D.

LONDON
GEORGE ALLEN & UNWIN LTD
RUSKIN HOUSE MUSEUM STREET

FIRST PUBLISHED IN GREAT BRITAIN
IN 1954

Copyright in the U.S.A.

This book is copyright under the Berne Convention. Apart from any fair dealing for the purposes of private study, research, criticism or review, as permitted under the Copyright Act, 1911, no portion may be reproduced by any process without written permission. Enquiry should be made to the Publishers.

PRINTED IN GREAT BRITAIN BY
BRADFORD AND DICKENS
LONDON W.C.1

*To Karen-Margrethe
my wife*

PREFACE

How This Book Came to be Written

When I was a big boy of fifteen I considered myself a man. I had reached the period of life in which one becomes an adult person, physiologically, at least. I do not mean, of course, that you are an adult as soon as you have passed the age of fifteen. Some people contend that you are not really grown-up or mature until you are fifty. But I was, in fact, at the age when biologically you undergo a thorough change that makes you feel adult. And it is a period which in many respects represents the best of one's abilities. My ingenuity has never been greater, nor my initiative more vigilant, my unselfishness more genuine, my good intentions better, or my strivings more confident.

With regard to the other sex, however, the situation was this: my knowledge of sexual matters I had acquired—as most other children do—through older boys on stairways and playgrounds and, during the years I lived in the country, through observing the sexual behaviour of the domestic animals. This, unfortunately common, patch-work pattern of information sharpened my curiosity toward the sexual behaviour of older "adults" about me. And this led to an ever-increasing wonderment and scanning of articles and illustrations on the subject in our big encyclopedia when I was at home alone. The knowledge I had thus acquired had made the whole problem mysterious, exciting, stimulating. For me, sex had become to a certain degree dangerous, to a certain degree abominable, yet all the same attractive and most desirable to delve into.

As the years went by, I came to realize the great importance of sex in the life of man. I was fortunate in being able to avoid any difficulties during my early years, guarded by a sincere faith and a firm resolution that my sexual life should at all times help to make my existence richer and not poorer. And my medical study, in connection with sociological studies, quickly gave me a sure conviction. I was convinced that many different factors of a physical, psychological, ethical, and sociological nature determine whether the individual's sex life was to be happy or not. I found that society, in fact, assumed one sexual moral code but practised another. The most conspicuous cause of the numerous disappointments I witnessed in this field, was that people simply *did not know* the most elementary laws of life. There is another, a deeper cause, which is considered later in this book.

In 1937, just after passing the medical examination, I was fortunate enough to be appointed by the city of Copenhagen as organizer and director of instruction in sexual hygiene for the students of the Continuation Course and the Voluntary Youth School of the Copenhagen Municipality. The course almost immediately achieved a great measure of popular success. During the past thirteen years instruction has been given to about 50,000 in Copenhagen proper (the total population of Greater Copenhagen is 758,000 of which 127,000 are of the ages between 15 and 25), and in numerous municipalities throughout the country similar courses have been organized.

Sexual instruction has also been adopted by most Danish colleges, and in 1945-1946 it was introduced in all Copenhagen public schools and high schools and in many corresponding schools all over the country. In 1946 all but three of the 1,232 public libraries in Denmark were provided with—from one to more than 100—copies of my *Textbook on Sexual Hygiene*. A further public move was taken on local initiative through the organization of truly local study circles on sexual hygiene which have established a constructive national framework.

The actual results of sexual information activities in Denmark during the past fifteen years are difficult to express in figures alone. During this period we experienced a war and a military occupation with a resultant increase in the number of venereal diseases and divorces. But these figures are rapidly going down. The most important result is this:

Twenty years ago sexual life was something which "decent" people in Denmark as a rule would not speak of. The children and the youngsters especially were kept in what was considered healthy splendid isolation. One quite graphic result of this attitude could be found on the walls of the public lavatories which were full of pornographic drawings. Whenever sexual difficulties asserted themselves there was never anyone to consult except Catholic priests and a few well-meaning physicians and interested educators. A constructive guidance system for preventing the disasters of sexual life and the *preparation* for its happiness were nowhere to be found.

The situation to be found in Denmark today is almost entirely different. The taboo placed on sex is shattered. In the homes the parents no longer shrink from giving the children their first sexual instruction. The whole country is, in fact, sexually instructed. Consulting sexual clinics have been established. Any practising physician, teacher, and clergyman are now capable of offering guidance which may also be valuable biologically and psychologically. The radio is now open as another channel for sexual instruction. In 1947 a new act designed to combat venereal diseases became the national law. It provides for free but compulsory treatment and for compulsory investigation of the source of infection. The number of venereal cases is rapidly decreasing. Throughout the country, in good public, advertising spots, some of the extensive publicity in the fight against venereal disease is to be found. One can find the address of the closest free consulting clinics on the many street-corner posters. The lavatory drawings have now practically disappeared.

I am quite aware of the fact that information and knowledge alone cannot prevent all disasters in the difficult field of sexual life. This would only be possible through a universal alteration of the human traits of character. Although many forces might work together with this goal in view, and no matter how luckily or skilfully they might acquit themselves in their task these forces would never be able to make the human beings—all of them!— *good* and kind, unselfish and responsible, and forgiving.

Information is needed, there is no doubt about that. There is much to consider. Think of the high level of sexual neurosis among women, think of the great spread of venereal diseases, think of the unhappy masturbants, and think of the numerous women who destroy their lives and health in attempted abortions. Think of the diseases which are due to the neglect of sexual physical care, think of the unhappy married couples, the problems of pregnancy, the great problems of sexual compatability and birth control. The tasks must therefore be: *to educate* people to unselfishness and unconditional sense of responsibility; *and to inform* them of the sexual life, its laws, its possibilities, and its dangers.

In order to lead a conscious sex life, young men and women—and middle-aged men and women, too—must have the correct knowledge regarding sex at the right time so that none will run the risk of having acted unwisely. How each individual person will act depends upon his or her inborn character and its development. But all of them should know about the most elementary laws of life so that there will be a possibility for them to act with a sense of responsibility. It is our duty to give them this information. *We who are in the know* are responsible.

I am very much indebted to the publications of numerous physicians, educators, sociologists, lawyers, clergymen, journalists, and private persons for the comprehensive knowledge they have given me of conditions elsewhere than in Denmark. Especially I wish to thank J. Labon Linard, an American journalist and sociologist, who gave invaluable assistance to the preparation of the material, and Gerda M. Andersen, who assisted in the original translation of the book.

HENRY OLSEN

CONTENTS

	PAGE
PREFACE	vii

1 *The Human Organism*

Chapter 1: THE LIVING BEING — 1

1. THE HUMAN ORGANISM — 1
2. STRUCTURE AND FUNCTIONS OF THE HUMAN ORGANISM — 2
3. THE ORGANS — 3
4. THE CELL — 3
5. THE SINGLE-CELLED ORGANISM — 3
6. DIVISION OF THE CELL — 4

Chapter 2: GLANDS AND SEX LIFE — 4

7. GLANDULAR CELLS AND GLANDS — 4
8. OPEN GLANDS — 4
9. DUCTLESS GLANDS — 5
10. SEX GLANDS AND SEX CELLS — 5
11. FUNCTIONS OF THE SEX ORGANS — 5

2 *The Sex Organs*

Chapter 3: THE MALE SEX ORGANS — 6

12. GENERAL FUNCTION OF THE MALE SEX ORGANS — 6
13. THE MALE SEX GLANDS: THE TESTES — 6
14. SEX GLANDS INITIALLY BISEXUAL — 6
15. DESCENT OF THE TESTES — 6
16. THE SCROTUM — 7
17. IMPERFECT DESCENT OF THE TESTES — 7
18. SENSITIVITY OF THE TESTES — 7
19. STRUCTURE OF THE TESTES — 8
20. SEMINAL CELLS — 8

21. THE SPERMATOZOA	8
22. NUMBER OF SPERMS	8
23. LIFE EXPECTANCY OF THE SPERMS	9
24. THE CHROMOSOMES	9
25. THE EPIDIDYMIS	10
26. VAS DEFERENS	10
27. PSEUDO-CRYPTORCHISM AND HERNIA	10
28. VESICAL GLANDS	12
29. URETHRAL CREST	12
30. THE PROSTATE	12
31. THE URETHRA IN THE MALE	13
32. CLOSING OF THE BLADDER DURING EJACULATION	13
33. BULBO-URETHRAL GLANDS	13
34. WHAT IS A REFLEX?	14
35. VARIOUS TYPES OF REFLEXES	14
36. THE MALE ORGAN, THE PENIS	15
37. PUBIC HAIR, PUBES	15
38. ERECTION OF THE PENIS	15
39. THE ERECTILE SYSTEM	16
40. PURPOSE OF ERECTION	16
41. ERECTION WITHOUT ANY SEXUAL PURPOSE	16
42. THE PENIS HEAD	17
43. THE FORESKIN, PREPUCE	17
44. STRICTURE OF THE PREPUCE (PHIMOSIS)	17
45. NORMAL ENLARGEMENT OF THE PREPUCE	18
46. CIRCUMCISION	18
47. CIRCUMCISION AS A SHIELD AGAINST VENEREAL DISEASE	18
48. SIGNIFICANCE OF CIRCUMCISION IN SEXUAL INTERCOURSE	19

Chapter 4: THE FEMALE SEX ORGANS — 19

49. GENERAL FUNCTION OF THE FEMALE SEX ORGANS	19
50. THE FEMALE SEX GLANDS, THE OVARIES	19
51. DESCENT OF THE OVARIES	19
52. THE OVARY FOLLICLES	20
53. OVULATION	20
54. THE FALLOPIAN TUBES	21
55. THE FALLOPIAN TUBES MAY SUBSTITUTE FOR ONE ANOTHER	21

		PAGE
56.	PASSAGE OF THE EGG THROUGH THE FALLOPIAN TUBE	21
57.	THE WOMB OR UTERUS	21
58.	UTERINE NECK, CERVIX	22
59.	ANTEVERSION, OR FORWARD DISPLACEMENT OF UTERUS	24
60.	RETROVERSION OR BACKWARD DISPLACEMENT OF UTERUS	24
61.	DESCENT OF THE UTERUS	25
62.	PROLAPSUS OF THE UTERUS	25
63.	THE VAGINA	25
64.	THE VULVA	26
65.	THE PERINEUM	27
66.	THE OUTER LIPS	27
67.	THE GREATER VESTIBULAR MUCOUS GLANDS	27
68.	THE INNER LIPS	27
69.	THE FEMALE URETHRA	27
70.	THE VAGINAL ENTRANCE (INTROITUS)	28
71.	THE HYMEN, OR MAIDENHEAD	28
72.	BREAKING OF HYMEN (DEFLORATION)	29
73.	DOES THE HYMEN SERVE ANY USEFUL PURPOSE?	29
74.	THE BOAT-SHAPED DEPRESSION	30
75.	THE CLITORIS	30
76.	THE BREASTS	30

3 Hormones and the Sexual Functions

Chapter 5: THE HORMONES — 32

77.	WHAT IS A HORMONE?	32
78.	THE THYROID GLAND AND THYROXIN	33
79.	THE PITUITARY GLAND AND ITS HORMONES	33
80.	ANTIHORMONES	34
81.	TO UNDERSTAND SEX FUNCTIONS IT IS NECESSARY TO KNOW ABOUT HORMONES	35

Chapter 6: PUBERTY — 35

82.	WHAT IS ADOLESCENCE?	35
83.	PUBESCENCE AND PUBERTY	35
84.	THE PITUITARY SEX HORMONES IN CONTROL: THE GONADOTROPIC HORMONES	36
85.	SEX GLANDS AS DUCT GLANDS	36

		PAGE
86.	THE SEX GLANDS AS ENDOCRINE GLANDS AND SEX HORMONES PROPER	36
87.	CLASSIFICATION OF SEX CHARACTERISTICS	37

Chapter 7: MALE SEX CHARACTERISTICS — 37

- 88. MALE SEX CHARACTERISTICS — 37
- 89. THE FIRST EJACULATION — 37
- 90. THE HORMONAL SEX CHARACTERISTICS OF THE MALE — 38
- 91. OTHER MALE PHYSICAL SEX CHARACTERISTICS — 38
- 92. MALE MENTAL SEX CHARACTERISTICS — 39
- 93. VARIATIONS IN THE MAN'S SEXUAL DEVELOPMENT AND BEHAVIOR — 39

Chapter 8: FEMALE SEX CHARACTERISTICS — 40

- 94. FEMALE SEX CHARACTERISTICS — 40
- 95. THE FIRST MENSTRUAL FLOW, THE MENARCHE — 40
- 96. FEMALE HORMONAL SEX CHARACTERISTICS — 40
- 97. OTHER PHYSICAL FEMALE SEX CHARACTERISTICS — 41
- 98. FEMALE MENTAL SEX CHARACTERISTICS — 41
- 99. VARIATIONS IN THE WOMAN'S SEXUAL DEVELOPMENT AND BEHAVIOR — 41

Chapter 9: MENSTRUATION — 42

- 100. THE EGG'S DEPARTURE FROM THE OVARY — 42
- 101. THE YELLOW BODY (CORPUS LUTEUM) — 42
- 102. THE UTERUS PREPARES FOR PREGNANCY — 42
- 103. THE EGG ARRIVES UNFERTILIZED IN THE UTERUS — 43
- 104. APPEARANCE OF THE MENSTRUAL FLOW — 43
- 105. PERSONAL HYGIENE DURING MENSTRUATION — 44
- 106. SANITARY NAPKINS — 44
- 107. OTHER METHODS OF ABSORBING THE MENSTROUS BLOOD — 45
- 108. INTERCOURSE DURING MENSTRUATION — 45
- 109. DOUCHING AFTER MENSTRUATION — 45
- 110. NORMAL QUANTITY AND DURATION OF MENSTRUAL FLOW — 46
- 111. MENSTRUAL IRREGULARITIES, DYSMENORRHEA — 46
- 112. MENSTRUAL PAINS — 46
- 113. TREATMENT OF MENSTRUAL PAINS — 46
- 114. MORPHINE SHOULD NOT BE USED — 47

		PAGE
115.	MEDICAL TREATMENT OF UNUSUALLY SEVERE MENSTRUAL PAINS	47
116.	SURGICAL TREATMENT OF ACUTE MENSTRUAL PAINS	47
117.	IRREGULAR BLEEDINGS	47
118.	MENSTRUATION IN NEWBORN BABY GIRLS	48
119.	WHEN THE FIRST MENSTRUATION IS SLOW IN COMING	48
120.	TOO FREQUENT AND INFREQUENT MENSTRUAL BLEEDINGS (POLYMENORRHEA AND OLIGOMENORRHEA)	49
121.	VIOLENT OR PROTRACTED MENSTRUAL FLOW	49
122.	TOO LIMITED MENSTRUAL FLOW (HYPOMENORRHEA)	50
123.	WHEN MENSTRUATION DOES NOT APPEAR AT ALL (AMENORRHEA)	50
124.	SUDDEN INTERRUPTION OF MENSTRUATION (SUPPRESSIO MENSIUM)	50
125.	VICARIOUS BLEEDING (MENSTRUATIO VICARIA)	51
126.	BE CHIVALROUS, GENTLEMEN!	51

Chapter 10: THE MENOPAUSE 52

127.	WOMAN'S SECOND CHANGE OF LIFE (THE MENOPAUSE)	52
128.	THE MENOPAUSE IS NOT A "DANGEROUS" AGE	52
129.	A NEW REVOLUTION—IN THE WORLD OF HORMONES	53
130.	WHEN DOES THE MENOPAUSE BEGIN AND HOW LONG DOES IT LAST?	53
131.	CLASSIFICATION OF SYMPTOMS OF THE MENOPAUSE	54
132.	ONSET OF CHANGE OF LIFE, THE CLIMACTERIC PERIOD	54
133.	*Torschlusspanik*	54
134.	THE PRODUCTION OF FEMALE SEX HORMONES DIMINISHES	55
135.	CESSATIÓN OF MENSTRUATION	55
136.	CHANGES IN THE GENITAL ORGANS	55
137.	TENDENCY TO OBESITY	55
138.	CHANGES IN THE ORGANISM HAVE A MASCULINE TREND	56
139.	HOT FLUSHES, PERSPIRING, ETC.	56
140.	CHARACTER CHANGES	56
141.	TREATMENT OF THE MENOPAUSE TROUBLES	56
142.	HORMONE TREATMENT WITH ESTROGENS	57
143.	SHE MAY NOT FEEL ANYTHING AT ALL	57
144.	THE POSTCLIMACTERIC PERIOD	58

		PAGE
145.	SEX NEEDS AFTER THE CHANGE OF LIFE	58
146.	BLEEDING IN THE POSTCLIMACTERIC PERIOD	58
147.	MEN HAVE NO REGULAR CHANGE OF LIFE—STILL	59

4 Sexual Need or Sex Urge

Chapter 11: THE NEED OF THE ORGANISM — 60

148.	ON BALANCE AND LACK OF BALANCE	60
149.	WHAT IS A NEED?	60
150.	THE NERVOUS SYSTEMS OF THE ORGANISM	61
151.	THE VEGETATIVE NERVOUS SYSTEM	63

Chapter 12: DIFFERENT CONCEPTIONS OF SEX NEED — 64

152.	WHAT IS SEX NEED?	64
153.	THE THEORY OF THE NEED OF REPRODUCTION	64
154.	THE THEORY OF EVACUATION	66
155.	PASSIVE AND ACTIVE SEX NEED	67

Chapter 13: PASSIVE SEX NEED — 67

156.	A FUNDAMENTAL DIFFERENCE BETWEEN THE MALE AND THE FEMALE SEX CELLS	67
157.	SEX HORMONES AND SEX NEED	68
158.	WHAT ARE EMOTIONS?	70
159.	ORIGIN OF LIKES AND DISLIKES	71
160.	DEVELOPMENT OF THE FEELING OF PREFERENCES OR LIKES IN CHILDHOOD	71
161.	LIKES AS SENTIMENTS DEVELOPED DURING PUBERTY	72
162.	BEING IN LOVE	73
163.	FROM PASSIVE TO ACTIVE SEX NEED	74

Chapter 14: ACTIVE SEX NEED — 74

164.	DEVELOPMENT OF THE CONTACT NEED	74
165.	WHAT TAKES PLACE DURING SEXUAL EXCITATION?	75
166.	THE NEED OF RELAXATION (DETUMESCENCE)	76
167.	THE SEX CENTER	76
168.	HOW IS THE SEX CENTER INFLUENCED?	77
169.	SYMPTOMS OF SEXUAL EXCITATION	78
170.	HOW MAY THE SEX NEED THEN BE DEFINED?	78

Chapter 15: **SEX NEED IN WOMAN** — 79

- 171. WOMAN'S EARLY MALE IDEAL — 79
- 172. THE IDEAL IMAGE AS BASIS FOR THE CHOICE — 80
- 173. HOW THE WOMAN'S FULL SEXUAL NEED IS AROUSED — 80
- 174. "THE ONE AND ONLY" — 81
- 175. SHE IS HIS—IRREVOCABLY AND FOREVER — 81
- 176. WOMEN AND SEXUAL INTERCOURSE — 81

5 *Living Together*

Chapter 16: **SEXUAL NEED AND SEXUAL INTERCOURSE** — 83

- 177. AN INTRODUCTORY REMARK — 83
- 178. WHAT ARE THE CHARACTERISTICS OF SEXUAL INTERCOURSE? — 83
- 179. WHAT ARE THE CHARACTERISTICS OF LIVING TOGETHER? — 83
- 180. THE THREE STAGES OF LIVING TOGETHER SEXUALLY — 84
- 181. CONDITIONS OF THE ALLUREMENT STAGE — 84
- 182. CONDITIONS OF THE SEXUAL EXCITEMENT STAGE — 85
- 183. THE CONDITIONS OF THE RELAXATION STAGE — 86

Chapter 17: **THE ALLUREMENT** — 86

- 184. THE URGE TO SHOW OFF — 86
- 185. BEING IN LOVE, AND THE DECISION TO DO SOMETHING ABOUT IT — 86
- 186. THE THREE SENSES IN THE ALLUREMENT STAGE — 87
- 187. ODORS (SCENTS) AS LURE — 87
- 188. HUMAN ODORS — 87
- 189. ARTIFICIAL SCENTS, PERFUMES — 87
- 190. LURE AFFECTING THE SENSE OF HEARING — 88
- 191. THE HUMAN LOVE SONG — 88
- 192. LURE THROUGH SIGHT — 88
- 193. SIGNIFICANCE OF THE SENSE OF FORM — 89
- 194. APPRECIATION OF FORM AND FIGURE IS SUBJECT TO CHANGING FASHION — 89
- 195. FAT BUTTOCKS — 89
- 196. THE IMPORTANCE OF COLOR APPRECIATION — 89

CONTENTS

Chapter 18: LOVE PLAY — 90

197. THE THREE SENSES AT PLAY IN THE SEXUAL EXCITATION STAGE — 90
198. TOUCH IN THE SERVICE OF THE SEX NEED — 90
199. THE FIRST INTENTIONAL TOUCH — 90
200. THE DIFFERENCES BETWEEN EXCITATION AND REACTION TO EXCITATION — 91
201. FIELDS OF EXCITATION OR EROGENOUS ZONES — 91
202. EROGENOUS ZONES IN WOMEN — 92
203. EROGENOUS ZONES IN MEN — 92

Chapter 19: SEXUAL INTERCOURSE, COITUS — 92

204. THE SEXUAL ACT — 92
205. LOVE MUST BE MUTUAL — 92
206. THE PRACTICAL CONDITIONS FOR SEXUAL INTERCOURSE — 93
207. THE PRELUDE — 94
208. INSERTION OF PENIS — 94
209. POSITIONS FOR SEXUAL INTERCOURSE — 94
210. ORGASM — 94
211. THE AFTER-PLAY — 96

6 Hygiene of the Couple's Sex Life

Chapter 20: BODY CARE IN SEX RELATIONS — 97

212. CARE OF THE MALE SEX ORGANS — 97
213. CARE OF THE FEMALE SEX ORGANS — 97
214. CLEANSING THE VULVA — 97
215. KEEPING THE VAGINA CLEAN — 98
216. DOUCHING OF THE VAGINA — 98
217. THE HAND-BULB SYRINGE — 98
218. THE DOUCHE BAG — 99
219. WHAT QUANTITY OF FLUID AND WHAT TEMPERATURE IS SUITABLE FOR A DOUCHE? — 99
220. COMPOSITION OF THE DOUCHE LIQUID — 100
221. DOUCHING WITH PURE WATER — 100
222. DOUCHE WITH PHYSIOLOGICAL SALT WATER — 100
223. ADDING A TOUCH OF ACID — 100
224. ADDING A BREW OF CAMOMILE — 100
225. DOUCHE MIXED WITH SPECIAL DISINFECTANTS — 101

Chapter 21: HYGIENE OF SEXUAL LIVING TOGETHER — 101

226. HOW OFTEN IS IT CONSIDERED NATURAL TO HAVE SEXUAL INTERCOURSE? — 101
227. MAN'S DESIRE FOR SEXUAL INTERCOURSE — 101
228. WOMAN'S DESIRE FOR SEXUAL INTERCOURSE — 102
229. WHAT THE ANCIENTS SUGGESTED — 102
230. THE PRESENT-DAY NORM — 102
231. IS IT HARMFUL TO REPEAT SEXUAL INTERCOURSE AFTER A SHORT INTERVAL? — 103
232. DIMINISHED SEX NEED — 104
233. HEIGHTENED SEX URGE — 104
234. EXAGGERATED SEXUAL INTERCOURSE — 105
235. ILLNESS AND OTHER CIRCUMSTANCES INFLUENCING HABITS OF INTERCOURSE — 105

7 Disturbances in a Couple's Sex Life

Chapter 22: WHAT ARE THE CAUSES OF DISTURBANCE IN A COUPLE'S SEX LIFE? — 106

236. INTRODUCTORY REMARKS ON APPARENT AND REAL CAUSES — 106
237. WHAT ARE INHIBITIONS? — 108
238. THE EGO AND ITS ATTITUDE TYPE — 109
239. TOLERANCE AND INTOLERANCE — 110
240. WHAT IS UNDERSTOOD BY MENTAL MATURITY? — 111
241. EGOTISM — 111
242. THE IMPORTANCE OF CHARACTER — 111
243. WHAT IS A COMPLEX? — 112
244. CONFLICTS AND REPRESSED COMPLEXES — 112
245. ALCOHOL AND SEX LIFE — 114
246. PURELY PHYSICAL CAUSES OF DISTURBANCES IN SEX LIFE — 115

Chapter 23: IMPOTENCE — 116

247. WHAT IS UNDERSTOOD BY POTENCE AND IMPOTENCE? — 116
248. NATURAL OR PHYSIOLOGICAL IMPOTENCE — 117
249. IMPOTENCE DUE TO DISEASE OR TO VIOLENT INJURY — 117
250. IMPOTENCE DUE TO INSUFFICIENT SEXUAL EXCITATION — 118
251. THE WOMAN'S PART IN THE DUAL RESPONSIBILITY — 118

		PAGE
252.	ALCOHOL AND IMPOTENCE	119
253.	INHIBITED IMPOTENCE, ALSO CALLED EMOTIONAL IMPOTENCE	119
254.	IMPOTENCE DUE TO IMPOTENCE!	120
255.	TREATMENT OF IMPOTENCE	121

Chapter 24: TOO EARLY EJACULATION — 121

256.	WHAT IS UNDERSTOOD BY TOO EARLY EJACULATION?	121
257.	WHAT CAUSES TOO EARLY EJACULATION?	122
258.	TREATMENT OF THE TOO EARLY EJACULATION	122

Chapter 25: ABOUT THE SATISFACTION OF WOMAN — 123

259.	SIMULTANEOUS ORGASM	123
260.	THE UNAWAKENED WOMAN	123
261.	THE UNSATISFIED WOMAN	123
262.	A SERIOUS OBSTACLE TO HAPPY MARRIAGES	123
263.	SEXUAL NEUROSES	124
264.	THE HIGHLY SEXED OR EROTIC WOMAN	125
265.	THE EASILY SATISFIED WOMAN	125

Chapter 26: FRIGIDITY — 125

266.	WHAT IS FRIGIDITY?	125
267.	SEXUAL COOLNESS	125
268.	WHAT CAUSES SEXUAL COOLNESS?	126
269.	TREATMENT OF FRIGIDITY	127

Chapter 27: GENITAL SPASMS—VAGINISM — 127

270.	WHAT ARE GENITAL SPASMS?	127
271.	WHAT CAUSES GENITAL SPASMS?	127
272.	TREATMENT OF GENITAL SPASMS	128

Chapter 28: DISPLEASURE AT INTERCOURSE (DYSPAREUNIA) — 128

273.	WHAT IS DYSPAREUNIA?	128
274.	DYSPAREUNIA IN MEN	129
275.	DYSPAREUNIA IN WOMEN	129
276.	TEN REASONS WHY WOMEN MAY REFUSE SEXUAL INTERCOURSE	130

	PAGE
Chapter 29: HATRED AND JEALOUSY	130
277. HATRED AND ITS CAUSES	130
278. HATE HINGING ON LOVE	132
279. JEALOUSY	132

8 Marriage

Chapter 30: CHOICE OF A MARRIAGE PARTNER	134
280. IMPORTANCE OF CHOICE	134
281. ABOUT THE AGE FOR MARRIAGE	134
282. GETTING ACQUAINTED	134
283. ABOUT INTERCOURSE BETWEEN ENGAGED COUPLES	135
284. PRENUPTIAL MEDICAL EXAMINATION	136
285. HEREDITARY TAINT	136
286. ENDOGAMY	137
287. EXOGAMY	138
288. TO WHOM IS MARRIAGE FORBIDDEN?	138
289. CHOICE OF A PARENT FOR ONE'S CHILDREN	139
Chapter 31: MARRIAGE AND SEX LIFE	139
290. LIKE "LAW AND RIGHT"	139
291. MARRIAGE AND SEX LIFE ARE CLOSELY LINKED	140
292. MATRIMONY AS A SOCIAL INSTITUTION	141
293. THE MEDICO-HYGIENIC SIGNIFICANCE OF MATRIMONY	141
Chapter 32: DIFFERENT FORMS OF MARRIAGE	141
294. WHAT IS MONOGAMY, AND WHAT IS POLYGAMY?	141
295. NOT POLYGAMOUS, BUT POLYEROTIC	142
296. PRACTICE OF POLYEROTICISM	142
297. CAUSES OF POLYGAMY AND POLYEROTICISM	143
298. HISTORICAL BASIS OF MONOGAMY	144
299. ETHICAL BASIS OF MONOGAMY	145
300. THE MONOGAMOUS "FEELING"	145
301. AN AUSTRALIAN GROUP MARRIAGE	146
302. SCHOPENHAUER'S TETRAGAMY	146
303. THE DISTRICT MANOR IN OELSEBY-MAGLE	147
Chapter 33: ORIGIN OF MARRIAGE	147
304. STEALING THE BRIDE (RAPE)	147
305. PURCHASING THE BRIDE	148

CONTENTS

		PAGE
306.	EXCHANGE OF GIFTS	148
307.	THE DOWRY	149
308.	SECRET MARRIAGES	149
309.	THE WEDDING AS A CONDITION FOR SEXUAL INTERCOURSE	150
310.	THE WEDDING CEREMONY	150

Chapter 34: EARLY MARRIED LIFE 151

311.	THE WEDDING NIGHT	151
312.	BREAKING OF THE HYMEN (DEFLORATION)	151
313.	THE INITIATION	151
314.	THE HUSBAND'S RESPONSIBILITY ON THE WEDDING NIGHT	152

Chapter 35: MARRIAGE IN PRACTICE 153

315.	THE GREAT EXPECTATIONS	153
316.	THE HAPPY MARRIAGE	154
317.	HOW TO KEEP A MARRIAGE HAPPY	154
318.	THE UNHAPPY MARRIAGE	155

9 Sex Life of the Unmarried

Chapter 36: YOUNG PEOPLE BEFORE MARRIAGE 157

319.	EARLY YOUTH	157
320.	SEXUAL ABSTINENCE BEFORE MARRIAGE	157
321.	CHANCES FOR EARLY MARRIAGE	158

Chapter 37: THE UNMARRIED YOUNG MAN 158

322.	THE FRANK YOUNG MAN	158
323.	THE SHY YOUNG MAN	158
324.	THE OVER-AGGRESSIVE YOUNG MAN	159

Chapter 38: THE UNMARRIED YOUNG WOMAN 159

325.	THE FRANK YOUNG WOMAN	159
326.	THE MODEST YOUNG WOMAN	159
327.	THE FRIVOLOUS YOUNG WOMAN	160

Chapter 39: THOSE WHO NEVER MARRY 160

328.	UNMARRIED PEOPLE IN THE OLDER AGE GROUPS	160
329.	NATURAL CELIBACY	161
330.	UNNATURAL CELIBACY	161

	PAGE
331. SUBLIMATION	162
332. SPINSTERS	162

Chapter 40: NONMARITAL SEX RELATIONS — 163

333. FACTS TO BE FACED	163
334. IF SHE GETS PREGNANT	163
335. SEXUAL PROMISCUITY	164
336. PROSTITUTION	164

10 Fertilization, Pregnancy, Childbirth

Chapter 41: PROCREATION — 166

337. TWOFOLD PURPOSE OF SEXUAL INTERCOURSE	166
338. ON THE ORIGIN OF LIFE	167
339. ORIGIN OF THE STORK FABLE	167
340. PATERNITY AND DETERMINATION OF BLOOD TYPE	169

Chapter 42: HEREDITY — 170

341. HEREDITARY ELEMENTS, GENES	170
342. THE CHROMOSOMES MERGE WHEN THE EGG IS FERTILIZED	170
343. NUMBER OF CHROMOSOME PAIRS	171
344. INDIRECT, MITOTIC DIVISION OF CHROMOSOMES, KARYOKINESIS BEFORE FERTILIZATION	171
345. SISTERS AND BROTHERS DO NOT DEVELOP ALIKE	171
346. SEX CHROMOSOMES	172
347. SEX-DETERMINING CHROMOSOMES IN THE EGG CELL	173
348. SEX-DETERMINING CHROMOSOMES IN THE SPERM CELL	173
349. WHAT DETERMINES THE BABY'S SEX?	173
350. THE SPERM CELL ALONE DETERMINES THE SEX	174
351. EQUAL NUMBER OF BOYS AND GIRLS	174
352. WHEN IS THE BABY'S SEX DETERMINED?	175
353. INFLUENCE OF THE PARENTS ON THE BABY'S SEX	175
354. A WOMAN WHO CAN BEAR GIRLS CAN ALSO HAVE BOYS	176
355. CHROMOSOME DIVISION AND CELL DIVISION AFTER FERTILIZATION	176
356. WHAT IS EUGENICS?	176
357. POSITIVE EUGENICS	177
358. NEGATIVE OR PREVENTIVE EUGENICS	177

CONTENTS

	PAGE
Chapter 43: FERTILIZATION	177
359. THE UNFERTILIZED EGG	177
360. SEXUAL INTERCOURSE IS THE NORMAL METHOD OF FERTILIZATION	178
361. IF SEXUAL INTERCOURSE CANNOT TAKE PLACE	178
362. FERTILIZATION IN SPITE OF THE HUSBAND'S IMPOTENCE	178
363. FERTILIZATION IN SPITE OF THE WIFE'S IMPOTENCE AT SEXUAL INTERCOURSE	178
364. THE STEEPLECHASE OF THE SPERMATOZOA	178
365. THE LAST SPURT	179
366. THE SPERM CELL PENETRATES INTO THE EGG	179
367. ACTUAL FERTILIZATION, FUSION OF THE PRONUCLEI	179
368. A MIRACLE HAS HAPPENED	180
Chapter 44: PREGNANCY	180
369. CLEAVAGE OF THE ZYGOTE	180
370. TWINS FROM A SINGLE EGG	180
371. OTHER TWINS, TRIPLETS, ETC	180
372. THE TRANSPORTATION OF THE ZYGOTE (FERTILIZED OVUM OR EGG) THROUGH THE TUBE	181
373. TUBAL PREGNANCY, EXTRAUTERINE PREGNANCY (ECTOPIC PREGNANCY)	181
374. TUBAL ABORTION AND TUBAL RUPTURE	181
375. FORMATION OF THE GERMINAL DISK	182
376. THE WHOLE NEW HUMAN BEING IS DEVELOPED FROM THE GERMINAL DISK	182
377. THE CELLS OF THE GERMINAL DISK MAY SUBSTITUTE FOR EACH OTHER	183
378. WHEN RESERVE CELLS START OUT ON THEIR OWN; TERATOMA FORMATION	183
379. FURTHER DEVELOPMENT OF THE EMBRYO	184
380. HOW THE EMBRYO FEEDS	184
381. THE UMBILICAL CORD	185
382. THE PLACENTA	185
Chapter 45: SYMPTOMS OF PREGNANCY	186
383. THE FIRST MISS	186
384. MORNING SICKNESS	186

385. DURATION OF PREGNANCY VOMITING	187
386. TREATMENT OF PREGNANCY VOMITING	188
387. CHANGES IN THE BREASTS	188
388. CHANGES IN THE ABDOMEN	189
389. CHANGES IN THE GENITAL ORGANS	189
390. MOVEMENTS OF THE FETUS	190
391. SOUND OF THE FETUS	190
392. STRUCTURE AND POSITION OF THE FETUS	190
393. X-RAY EXAMINATION OF THE PREGNANT WOMAN	190
394. SPECIAL PREGNANCY TEST	191
395. THE PRINCIPLES OF THE RABBIT TEST	191
396. THE FROG TEST (OR XENOPUS) AND THE TOAD TEST	192
397. OTHER PREGNANCY TESTS	193
398. HOW SOON AFTER IMPREGNATION MAY CONCEPTION BE DETERMINED?	193
399. DURATION OF PREGNANCY	193

Chapter 46: HYGIENE DURING PREGNANCY — 194

400. PREGNANCY IS A NORMAL CONDITION	194
401. GENERAL HYGIENE DURING PREGNANCY	194
402. EATING DURING PREGNANCY	194
403. KEEPING REGULAR DURING PREGNANCY	195
404. NEED OF CALCIUM DURING PREGNANCY	195
405. NEED OF IRON DURING PREGNANCY	195
406. HOW TO DRESS DURING PREGNANCY	196
407. EXERCISE DURING PREGNANCY	196
408. BATHING, SPONGING, AND DOUCHING DURING PREGNANCY	196
409. CARE OF NIPPLES AND BREASTS DURING PREGNANCY	197
410. SEXUAL INTERCOURSE DURING PREGNANCY	197
411. TUBERCULOSIS AND PREGNANCY	198
412. SYPHILIS AND PREGNANCY	198
413. DIABETES AND PREGNANCY	198
414. GERMAN MEASLES AND PREGNANCY	199
415. VARICOSE VEINS AND HEMORRHOIDS DURING PREGNANCY	199
416. ALBUMEN IN THE URINE	199
417. RISK OF PUERPERAL CONVULSIONS OR PRE-ECLAMPSIA	199
418. PUERPERAL CONVULSIONS (ECLAMPSIA)	200
419. IF SYMPTOMS OF A DISEASE OCCUR DURING PREGNANCY	201

		PAGE
420.	ARRANGEMENTS WITH A HOSPITAL OR A PRIVATE NURSING HOME SHOULD BE MADE IN AMPLE TIME	201
421.	THE LAST DAYS OF PREGNANCY	201

Chapter 47: CHILDBIRTH — 202

422.	POSITION OF FETUS AT DELIVERY	202
423.	SIZE OF BABY'S HEAD IN RELATION TO BIRTH TRACT	202
424.	THE BIRTH FORCE	202
425.	ONSET OF LABOR	203
426.	LABOR IS INDEPENDENT OF THE CHILDBEARING MOTHER'S WILL	203
427.	FREQUENCY OF LABOR PAINS	203
428.	DURATION OF LABOR	203
429.	PAINS AT REGULAR INTERVALS	204
430.	ANESTHETICS IN CHILDBIRTH	204
431.	PERIOD OF DILATATION	205
432.	BREAKING OF THE BAG OF WATERS	205
433.	THE PERIOD OF EXPULSION	205
434.	CARE OF THE NAVEL	206
435.	APPARENTLY STILLBORN	206
436.	THE AFTERBIRTH—CLOSING PHASE OF CHILDBIRTH	206
437.	TREATMENT OF THE BABY'S EYES	207
438.	THE NEWBORN BABY	207
439.	MAL POSITION OF THE FETUS	208
440.	DIFFICULT BIRTH (DYSTOCHIA)	208

Chapter 48: THE LYING-IN PERIOD — 210

441.	IMPORTANCE OF LYING-IN PERIOD	210
442.	WHAT HAPPENS TO THE ABDOMINAL ORGANS AFTER CHILDBIRTH?	210
443.	RISK OF PROLAPSUS OF THE UTERUS	210
444.	RISK OF PUERPERAL FEVER	210
445.	RISK OF BLOOD CLOT (EMBOLISM)	211
446.	DURATION OF THE LYING-IN PERIOD	211
447.	EXERCISES FOR WOMEN AFTER CHILDBIRTH	212
448.	THE AFTER-PAINS	212
449.	NURSING THE BABY	213
450.	DISTURBANCES IN NURSING	213
451.	COMPOSITION OF MOTHER'S MILK	215

		PAGE
452.	RETURN OF MENSTRUATION AFTER CHILDBIRTH	215
453.	SEXUAL INTERCOURSE AFTER CHILDBIRTH	216
454.	HOW LONG AN INTERVAL SHOULD ELAPSE BETWEEN TWO PREGNANCIES?	216
455.	THE CYCLE IS COMPLETED	216

11 Interruption of Pregnancy

Chapter 49: ABORTIONS AND MISCARRIAGES — 218

456.	WHAT IS MEANT BY INTERRUPTION OF PREGNANCY?	218
457.	WHAT ARE MISCARRIAGES AND ABORTIONS?	218
458.	HOW FREQUENTLY DO ABORTIONS OR MISCARRIAGES OCCUR?	218
459.	WHAT ARE THE FORMS OF INTERRUPTIONS OF PREGNANCY?	219

Chapter 50: MISCARRIAGES — 219

460.	THE TWO FORMS OF MISCARRIAGE OR SPONTANEOUS INTERRUPTION	219
461.	ACCIDENTAL MISCARRIAGE	219
462.	POSSIBLE INFLUENCE OF EXTERNAL FACTORS	219
463.	HABITUAL MISCARRIAGE	220
464.	THE IMPORTANCE OF THE RH-FACTOR	220
465.	BLEEDING AT MISCARRIAGE	221
466.	PAINS ACCOMPANYING MISCARRIAGE	221
467.	WHAT IS DELIVERED IN A MISCARRIAGE?	221
468.	TREATMENT OF MISCARRIAGE	222
469.	THE FETUS AND THE AFTERBIRTH MUST BE COMPLETELY REMOVED	222
470.	CONFINEMENT IN BED AFTER A MISCARRIAGE	222
471.	CONSEQUENCES OF A MISCARRIAGE	222

Chapter 51: INDUCED ABORTIONS — 223

472.	TWO FORMS OF INDUCED ABORTIONS	223
473.	DISEASES ENDANGERING THE PREGNANT WOMAN'S LIFE OR HEALTH	223

12 Regulation of Fertilization

Chapter 52: PROBLEMS OF FERTILITY — 225

474.	WHAT IS THE CRUX OF THE PROBLEM?	225
475.	THE GREAT POPULATION SURPLUS OF THE PAST	225

	PAGE
476. BUT STERILITY IS ON THE INCREASE	226
477. THE LAW OF GRADUAL STERILITY	226
478. THE PRACTICAL APPROACH OF INDIVIDUAL PROBLEMS	226

Chapter 53: PSEUDO STERILITY — 227

479. WHAT IS PSEUDO STERILITY?	227
480. GUIDANCE IN INTERCOURSE	227
481. FERTILIZATION TERMS	228
482. DETERMINING THE TIME OF FERTILIZATION	229
483. KNAUS' TABLES	229
484. IMPORTANT INFORMATION FOR CHILDLESS MARRIAGES	230

Chapter 54: STERILITY — 230

485. WHAT IS STERILITY?	230
486. WHOSE "FAULT" IS IT?	231
487. EXAMINATION AND TREATMENT OF THE HUSBAND	231
488. AN EVALUATION OF STERILITY TESTS FOR THE HUSBAND	232
489. INVESTIGATION OF THE PENETRATION OF SPERM CELLS INTO THE MUCOUS CLOT	233
490. EXAMINATION OF THE WOMAN	233
491. INFANTILISM AS A CAUSE OF FEMALE STERILITY	234
492. CHANGES IN THE VAGINIA AS CAUSES OF STERILITY	234
493. LONG AND NARROW CERVICAL CANAL AS CAUSE OF STERILITY	234
494. STERILITY CAUSED BY RETROVERSION OF THE WOMB	235
495. CHANGES IN THE UTERINE MUCOUS MEMBRANES AS A CAUSE OF STERILITY	235
496. BLOCKING OF PASSAGE BY UTERINE TUMORS	236
497. INFLAMMATION OF THE FALLOPIAN TUBES AS A DIRECT CAUSE OF STERILITY	236
498. EXAMINATION OF FALLOPIAN TUBES BY BLOWING AIR THROUGH THEM	236
499. TESTING BY INJECTION OF A TRACER INTO THE TUBES	237
500. TREATMENT OF CHANGES IN THE FALLOPIAN TUBES	237
501. ADHESIONS AS CAUSES OF STERILITY	237
502. DEFICIENCY OF OVARIAN FUNCTION	238
503. STERILITY WITHOUT ANY DISCOVERABLE CAUSE	238
504. ARTIFICIAL FERTILIZATION (INSEMINATION)	239

	PAGE
Chapter 55: CONTRACEPTION	239
505. CONTRACEPTION OR NOT	239
506. PRACTICAL REMARKS ABOUT SEXUAL ABSTINENCE	240
507. TWO POSITIVE METHODS FOR THE PREVENTION OF PREGNANCY	241
508. STERILIZATION OF THE FEMALE	241
509. STERILIZATION OF THE MALE	241
510. CASTRATION OF THE FEMALE	241
511. CASTRATION OF THE MALE	241
512. EVALUATION OF THE FIVE COMPLETELY EFFECTIVE METHODS FOR THE AVOIDANCE OF PREGNANCY	242
513. UNCERTAIN METHODS OF PREVENTING PREGNANCY	242
514. STERILIZATION BY HORMONE TREATMENT	243
515. COITUS ANTE PORTAS	243
516. CAREZZA (COITUS RESERVATUS)	243
517. COITUS INTERRUPTUS	244
518. DOUCHING	244
519. SPERM-BLOCKING MEANS	245
520. VAGITORIA CONTRACEPT	245

13 Masturbation

Chapter 56: MASTURBATION, SELF-GRATIFICATION	246
521. WHAT IS MASTURBATION?	246
522. PRACTICE OF MASTURBATION	246
523. HOW THE PRACTICE OF MASTURBATION WAS FORMERLY REGARDED	246
524. FEAR OF THE CONSEQUENCES OF MASTURBATION	247
525. ABOUT MASTURBATION AFFECTING THE BRAIN	247
526. THE INFLUENCE OF MASTURBATION ON BEGETTING AND CONCEIVING	248
527. ABOUT THE LOSS OF MATTER AT MASTURBATION	248
528. MASTURBATION AND SEX HORMONES	248
529. THE SOLITARY PERSON	249
530. MASTURBATION IN ADOLESCENCE	249
531. IT IS THE CHARACTER THAT IS THREATENED BY MASTURBATION	250
532. TREATMENT OF MASTURBATION	251

14 Sexual Abnormalities

Chapter 57: HORMONE-CONDITIONED ABNORMALITIES — 252

533. INFLUENCE OF HORMONES — 252
534. ADIPOSOGENITAL DYSTROPHY — 252
535. EARLY AND PRECOCIOUS SEXUAL MATURITY — 253
536. CASTRATION OF MEN AND BOYS — 253
537. INFLUENCE OF CASTRATION ON SEX NEEDS — 254
538. ARTIFICIAL MENOPAUSE — 255
539. TRUE AND FALSE HERMAPHRODITISM — 256
540. INTERSEXUALISM AND GYNANDROMORPHISM — 257
541. GYNECOMASTIA AND HIRSUTISM — 257

Chapter 58: ABNORMAL SEX LIFE — 258

542. HOMOSEXUALITY AND ANALOGOUS CONDITIONS — 258
543. PEDERASTY — 259
544. AUTOEROTICISM — 260
545. EROTOMANIA — 260
546. NYMPHOMANIA (ABNORMALLY STRONG SEX URGE IN WOMEN) — 260
547. SATYRIASIS (ABNORMALLY STRONG SEX URGE IN MEN) — 260
548. ALGOLAGNOSIS (SENSUOUS PLEASURE THROUGH PAIN) — 261
549. FETICHISM — 261
550. EXHIBITIONISM — 262
551. SCOPTOPHILISM — 262
552. SODOMY, BESTIALITY — 262
553. NECROPHILISM — 262
554. UROLAGNOSIS AND COPROLAGNOSIS — 262
555. CLEPTOLAGNOSIS AND PYROLAGNOSIS — 263
556. WHERE IS THE BORDERLINE BETWEEN NORMAL AND ABNORMAL SEX LIFE? — 263

15 Diseases of Sex Life

Chapter 59: VENEREAL DISEASES — 265

557. WHAT IS UNDERSTOOD BY VENEREAL DISEASES? — 265
558. HOW ARE VENEREAL DISEASES TRANSMITTED? — 265

	PAGE
559. CONTAGION THROUGH OBJECTS	266
560. PREVENTION OF VENEREAL DISEASE	267
561. NEW METHODS OF TREATMENT OF VENEREAL DISEASES	268

Chapter 60: GONORRHEA — 269

562. WHAT CAUSES GONORRHEA?	269
563. HOW CAN GONORRHEA BE TRACED?	269
564. DISSEMINATION OF GONORRHEA	270
565. GENITAL GONORRHEA IN THE MALE	270
566. URETHRAL GONORRHEA (URETHRITIS GONORRHOICA) IN THE MALE	270
567. URETHRITIS ANTERIOR	271
568. URETHRITIS POSTERIOR	271
569. GONORRHEA OF THE PARA-URETHRAL DUCTS	271
570. GONORRHEA OF THE URETHRAL MUCOUS GLAND DUCTS (PERI-URETHRAL INFILTRATIONS)	271
571. GONORRHEA OF THE LYMPHATIC VESSELS AND THE LYMPHATIC GLANDS (LYMPHADENITIS GONORRHOICA)	272
572. GONORRHEA IN THE PROSTATE GLAND (PROSTATITIS GONORRHOICA)	272
573. GONORRHEA IN THE VESICAL GLANDS (SPERMATOCYSTITIS GONORRHOICA)	273
574. GONORRHEA OF THE EPIDIDYMIS (EPIDIDYMITIS GONORRHOICA)	273
575. EXTRAGENITAL GONORRHEA IN MEN	273
576. GONORRHEA OF THE ANUS (PROCTITIS GONORRHOICA) IN MEN	273
577. OPHTHALMO-BLENNORRHEA	274
578. THE QUARTERMASTER ON SS IGNOTA	274
579. GONORRHEA IN THE JOINTS	274
580. OTHER LOCALIZATIONS OF GONORRHEA	275
581. GENITAL GONORRHEA IN WOMEN	275
582. GONORRHEA IN THE URETHRA (URETHRITIS GONORRHOICA) IN WOMEN	275
583. GONORRHEA IN THE GREATER VESTIBULAR GLANDS (BARTHOLONITIS GONORRHOICA)	276
584. GONORRHEA IN THE CERVICAL CANAL (CERVITITIS GONORRHOICA)	276

		PAGE
585.	GONORRHEA OF THE FALLOPIAN TUBES (SALPINGITIS GONORRHOICA)	276
586.	EXTRAGENITAL GONORRHEA IN WOMEN	277
587.	GONORRHEA OF THE RECTUM AND THE ANUS (PROCTITIS GONORRHOICA) IN WOMEN	277
588.	GENITAL GONORRHEA IN LITTLE GIRLS	277
589.	TREATMENT OF GONORRHEA	277
590.	SYRINGE AND VACCINE TREATMENT	277
591.	SULFA DRUG TREATMENT	277
592.	ARTIFICIAL FEVER COMBINED WITH TREATMENT BY SULFA DRUGS	278
593.	PENICILLIN TREATMENT	278
594.	WHEN MAY A GONORRHEA PATIENT BE SAID TO BE CURED?	279

Chapter 61: SYPHILIS — 279

595.	WHAT CAUSES SYPHILIS?	279
596.	HOW IS SYPHILIS TESTED?	279
597.	WHAT IS A WASSERMANN REACTION OR TEST?	280
598.	ACQUIRED SYPHILIS	280
599.	PRIMARY SYPHILIS	281
600.	THE HARD CHANCRE	281
601.	ADJACENT LYMPHATIC GLANDS SWELL	281
602.	SECONDARY SYPHILIS	281
603.	CHANGES IN THE SKIN	282
604.	CHANGES IN THE MUCOUS MEMBRANES	282
605.	TERTIARY SYPHILIS	283
606.	WHEN THE SKIN AND THE INTERNAL ORGANS ARE AFFECTED	283
607.	CHANGES IN THE ORGANS OF CIRCULATION	283
608.	THE EFFECT ON THE BONES	284
609.	CHANGES IN THE SPINAL CORD	284
610.	EFFECT ON THE NERVOUS SYSTEM	286
611.	THE PATELLAR REFLEX	286
612.	TEST OF THE SPINAL FLUID ("SPINAL CORD TEST") IN SYPHILIS	286
613.	CHANGES IN THE BRAIN	287
614.	SYPHILIS DURING PREGNANCY	287
615.	CONGENITAL SYPHILIS	288
616.	SYSTEMATIC WASSERMANN TESTS	288

	PAGE
617. THERAPY OF SYPHILIS	288
618. WHEN MAY A SYPHILITIC BE CONSIDERED CURED?	290
619. HOW LONG SHOULD A SYPHILITIC BE KEPT UNDER OBSERVATION?	290

Chapter 62: VENEREAL ULCERS 291

620. VENEREAL ULCERS	291
621. WHAT ARE BUBOES?	291
622. TREATMENT OF BUBOES	291

Chapter 63: THE FOURTH VENEREAL DISEASE 291

623. THE FOURTH VENEREAL DISEASE—LYMPHOGRANULOMA INGUINALE	291
624. THE FREI TEST	292
625. TREATMENT OF THE FOURTH VENEREAL DISEASE	293

Chapter 64: NONVENEREAL DISEASES OF THE SEXUAL ORGANS 292

626. NONVENEREAL DISEASES OF THE SEXUAL ORGANS	292
627. THE ITCH (SCABIES)	293
628. CRAB LICE OR MORPIONS	293
629. VENEREAL WARTS (CONDYLOMAS)	294
630. BLADDER RASH (HERPES)	294
631. SIMPLE URETHRAL INFLAMMATION (URETHRITIS SIMPLEX)	294
632. INTERTRIGO	294
633. PRURIGO VULVAE	295
634. PRURIGO GRAVIDARUM	295
635. THE WELANDER SORE	295
636. BARTHOLINITIS	296
637. VAGINITIS (COLPITIS, ELYTRITIS)	296
638. INFLAMMATION OF THE INTERNAL FEMALE GENITALS (ENDOMETRITIS AND ANNEXITIS)	296
639. CONSTRICTION OF THE FORESKIN (PHIMOSIS)	297
640. PARAPHIMOSIS (SPANISH COLLAR)	297
641. INFLAMMATION OF THE FORESKIN (BALANITIS)	297
642. GANGRENE OF THE PENIS—GANGRENOUS CHANCRE	297
643. ENLARGEMENT OF THE PROSTATE	298
644. CATHETER TREATMENT OF ENLARGED PROSTATE	298

		PAGE
645.	SURGICAL TREATMENT OF ENLARGED PROSTATE	299
646.	HORMONE TREATMENT OF ENLARGED PROSTATE	299
647.	INFLAMMATION OF THE EPIDIDYMIS (EPIDIDYMITIS) AND INFLAMMATION OF THE TESTES (ORCHITIS)	299
648.	TUBERCULOSIS OF THE MALE SEX ORGANS	300
649.	TUBERCULOSIS OF THE FEMALE SEX ORGANS	300
650.	TUMORS IN THE SEX ORGANS	301
651.	CANCER OF THE MALE SEX ORGANS	301
652.	CANCER OF THE FEMALE SEX ORGANS	301

16 Sexual Education

Chapter 65: TEACHING CHILDREN ABOUT SEX — 303

653.	THE SEX LIFE OF CHILDREN	303
654.	WHAT DOES A CHILD KNOW ABOUT SEX?	304
655.	NO TEACHING OF SEX DURING PUBERTY!	304
656.	WHY IS IT CONSIDERED DIFFICULT TO TEACH CHILDREN ABOUT SEX?	305
657.	THE TWO REAL DIFFICULTIES TO BE OVERCOME	306
658.	WHAT PARENTS DARE NOT TELL THEIR OWN CHILDREN	306
659.	AT WHAT AGE SHOULD CHILDREN LEARN ABOUT INTERCOURSE?	307
660.	SUGGESTIONS FOR TEACHING CHILDREN ABOUT SEX	307
661.	SEX EDUCATION AT SCHOOL	308

Chapter 66: SEX EDUCATION OF ADULTS — 308

662.	ADOLESCENTS	308
663.	PARENTS	309
664.	TRAINING OF TEACHERS AND PHYSICIANS	309

Chapter 67: SIGNIFICANCE OF SEXUAL EDUCATION — 309

665.	ONE MUST BE MATTER-OF-FACT	309
666.	THE VALUE OF SEXUAL EDUCATION SHOULD NOT BE UNDERESTIMATED	310
667.	BUT SEXUAL EDUCATION ALONE IS NOT ENOUGH	310

I
THE HUMAN ORGANISM

Chapter 1: THE LIVING BEING

1. *The Human Organism*   Nothing in the world has been the object of wider scientific research and greater philosophical speculation than the human organism. Egyptian sages and, before them, the philosophers of India and China observed the myriad functions and activities of human life and pondered on the mystery of death. Their thinking resulted in the conception that the "life spirit"—what we call "the soul" and which even today remains as much of a scientific mystery as ever—was the essence of a human being's life, the organism being the mortal frame into which life had been breathed and, as such, subservient to the "life spirit."

The ancient Greeks were the first to introduce the theory of body fluids. Temperaments could be *choleric* or quick to flare up; *phlegmatic* or placid; *melancholy* or pessimistic; *sanguine* or optimistic, according to the special mixture of the body fluids. The microscope, first constructed in 1590, made it possible to observe minute parts of the body on a much enlarged scale. In that way scientists obtained such detailed knowledge of the *nervous system* that, in the past century, it came to be considered the core of the human organism, the link between physical and psychical man, between body and soul. Finally, in the present century the increasing knowledge of hormones has afforded a greatly extending scope for understanding the interdependence and interplay between the human organism and the urges, longings, desires, thoughts, and actions of human beings.

2. *Structure and Functions of the Human Organism* In order to comprehend anything as complicated as how sexual life manifests itself in the individual and in sexual intercourse, a basic knowledge of the structure of the human body is essential. In some respects the knowledge we have is of comparatively recent origin. The human organism has sometimes been compared to a machine, a not very apt comparison, inasmuch as a machine can neither reason nor reproduce itself. This purely materialistic conception is as far from the truth as was the idea of the ancient sages who regarded the body as a mere shell in which the "life spirit" or soul lived its own independent life.

A more apt comparison would seem to be to liken the human organism to a nation consisting of many members, more or less independent, paying taxes and working like the rest of us and thus contributing their individual share to the maintenance, growth, development, well-being, and normal teamwork of the whole. At the same time, like the rest of us, they may cheat the tax collector, lose the urge to work, or directly counteract the good of the community. This may not only have a bearing on the general state of affairs, but may bring about such disturbance that the disorders react on those members that provoked them.

The *psyche* was formerly called the *soul* or *spirit,* and even today the words *spiritual* or *soul-like* are used in the sense of *psychological* or *mental.* The words psychical, spiritual, "of the soul" may be used interchangeably, because, in reality, they have exactly the same meaning. The word *mental* belongs in the same category; it is the Latin equivalent of psychical.

Here I want only to say that the *psyche,* or mental life of an individual, means the total consciousness of an individual and the forms in which it shows up, or, as *psychology* has it: the theory of the psyche—its *manifestations* or *symptoms.* It is necessary, then, that we learn as much as possible about the human body and its functions, and this will help us to understand the psychological phenomena which are overwhelmingly important in the matter of human sex life.

3. *The Organs* Each of the parts of the body adapted to a specific function is called an *organ:* the tongue for speaking and tasting; the ears for hearing; the eyes for seeing, etc. Some organs have several functions. The skin, for example, has the task of holding together the underlying tissue and several other important functions in addition. The sense of temperature, feeling, and touch is determined by the skin, and through its pores a number of waste products are excreted. The glands are organs; the stomach is a very complicated organ; the liver, the kidney, the lungs, the heart, and the brain are organs. The muscles and the blood are also types of organs.

4. *The Cell* Each organ is composed of tissues and these tissues are made up of microscopic elements called cells, which vary in shape and function. The skin consists of two layers of tough, flat cells, cemented together like bricks in a wall and forming "the wall" or protective covering of the organism. The red blood corpuscles are tiny, coin-shaped cells which lend their red color to the almost colorless blood plasma. The muscles are made up of long, flexible muscle cells. Each organ, and consequently, the entire body, is a mosaic of myriads of tiny cells. Each organ has its very special form, its definite appearance, and its own special function.

5. *The Single-celled Organism* In the organic world there are living organisms which consist of just one single cell. They are called *protozoa*. The *amoeba* is such an organism. It usually lives in ordinary ditch water and is the most primitive form of an independent organism. Bacteria, also, are unicellular organisms, such as the bacteria of venereal diseases which will be described in greater detail later. The amoeba consists of a *cell membrane,* enclosing the *protoplasm.*

In the protoplasm there is a *nucleus* (as in almost all of the cells of the human body); one or more minute *nucleoli;* and *vacuoles,* containing nutritional elements. That, in the main, is all the single-celled organism consists of. And yet the amoeba (so tiny that one drop of water contains millions and millions of them) is an independent *living* being. It can move, absorb nourishment, digest, and excrete waste. Like every other living organism it absorbs oxygen from the air and exhales carbon dioxide, which means that a process of combustion takes place in it. Moreover, it is capable of reproduction.

6. *Division of the Cell* The reproductive process of an amoeba is the most primitive form of reproduction we know. First the cell, and then the nucleus, stretches lengthwise. Then the nucleus and nucleoli divide. The protoplasm shrinks completely at the middle or near the middle, and divides. Thus we have two new amoebas of the identical composition as the original cell. The cells in the human organism follow in all essentials the same principles when they split—the so-called mitotic division, or cleavage by *mitosis*. It is described in greater detail in section 344 where the behavior of the *chromosomes* during the cell division is also outlined.

Chapter 2: GLANDS AND SEX LIFE

7. *Glandular Cells and Glands* In various areas in the human organism are cells endowed with the capacity of producing a substance or of absorbing some substance from the blood and secreting it again into the blood, more often in a changed composition. These cells are *glandular cells*. They are frequently found in groups sometimes linked by *connective tissue*, and that is how a *gland* originates. A gland, then, is an organ consisting entirely, or mainly, of glandular cells and capable of producing some dynamic substance and secreting it to the surrounding area.

8. *Open Glands* An *open gland* is one from which the glandular product passes through a duct or canal to the place where it is needed, or from where it is to be expelled from the body. If the glandular product is destined for use in the organism itself, or in the body of another person, it is called a *secretion*. For instance, the *salivary glands* contain cells capable of secreting saliva; and the male sex glands produce seminal fluid with spermatozoa. On the other hand, if the product is a *waste prod-*

uct which the organism must only rid itself of, it is called an *excretion*. The *sweat glands*, for instance, contain sweat gland cells which exude sweat, and the kidneys contain glandular cells which excrete urine.

9. *Ductless Glands* Many glands, however, have no outlet. These are called *ductless* or *endocrine glands*. Their glandular products are emptied directly into the blood stream which circulates through them, and are carried through the whole body. The product of a ductless gland is called a *hormone*. The word hormone is derived from the Greek *hormao* which means "I activate," or, more colloquially, "I start." The idea is that the hormone brings a message by way of the blood stream to the organs. Or, as it was formerly expressed less correctly, the hormone "arouses" the organs to *increased* activity, or sometimes "depresses" their activity.

10. *Sex Glands and Sex Cells* The *sex glands* include open as well as ductless glands. They secrete hormones which are absorbed by the blood, and also produce the fertilizing cells proper, or sex cells which in man are called the *sperm cells* and in woman the *egg cells*. These find an outlet through special ducts. When a male sex cell unites with a female sex cell it fertilizes the female sex cell. Whereupon the egg acquires the capacity to grow and multiply so that, in the course of nine months, it develops into an entirely new being, the baby.

11. *Functions of the Sex Organs* The sex or genital or reproductive organs are in the closest, most intimate communication with the entire body by means of hormones. As we shall see, certain of these organs also have the task of producing male or female sex cells and bringing them into contact with each other. The internal female sex organs, moreover, must shield and nourish the fetus during its development, and bear the child. The woman's sex functions, in a wider sense, also comprise the breasts from which the baby secures nourishment.

2

THE SEX ORGANS

Chapter 3: THE MALE SEX ORGANS

12. *General Function of the Male Sex Organs* The male sex glands (the testes) produce the *male sex cells*, which pass out of the body into the female genital organs at the time of intercourse by way of a special duct. On their way out the sex cells are mixed with other glandular secretions from the male genitals, and the final product is called the seminal fluid, which contains the fertilizing *spermatozoa*.

13. *The Male Sex Glands: the Testes* The male sex glands are the two testes. As early as six weeks after an egg has been fertilized and an embryo begins to take shape, the beginnings of sex glands may already be traced, high up in the abdomen of the tiny being.

14. *Sex Glands Initially Bisexual* It is a peculiar fact that at this early stage we find initial male and female sex glands in the same embryo. Only gradually, as the growth of the fetus progresses, will it be revealed whether these early beginnings develop into male or female, whether the infant will be a boy or a girl.

15. *Descent of the Testes* Simultaneously with the growth of the testes in the embryonic stage (in which case, of course, the initial female sex glands are not developed) they descend so that at the birth of the baby boy they have normally passed down into the *scrotum*.

16. *The Scrotum* As a rule the left testis is slightly larger than the right, and often hangs down further. The testicles are divided from each other by a rather strong partition. This partition has great practical importance: if one testicle is diseased, the other may not be directly infected. Examples of diseases affecting the testes are inflammation attending *mumps, tuberculosis,* and *gonorrhea.*

Nature seeks to maintain them at a rather uniform temperature by letting the muscles of the scrotum wall contract in cold, making the surface full of wrinkles and furrows, and thus diminishing the area that gives out heat. When it is hot the scrotum expands, and through its very large sweat glands the surface is moistened, and cooled by evaporation. During sexual excitement the scrotum may contract.

17. *Imperfect Descent of the Testes* It sometimes happens that a testicle has not descended completely at the time the baby is born, but is located in the abdominal cavity or in the inguinal canal. This condition is often accompanied by hernia in some form, and it may be unilateral as well as bilateral. In some cases the gradual descent of the testes may continue through boyhood, either spontaneously or helped along by proper medical treatment. If the testicles have not been eased to their place in the scrotum before the boy reaches his fifteenth or sixteenth year, an operation may become necessary. Such cases, however, are not frequent.

18. *Sensitivity of the Testes* Questions have been raised as to the possible purpose of the permanent location of the very sensitive testes in what is really a rather exposed place, such as the scrotum. The sensitivity of the testicles is evidenced in that sudden pressure on them causes a very definite sensation of pain and nausea. A blow on them may cause fainting and vomiting. It has long been a matter of common knowledge that un-

descended testes prove to have little or no sperm-producing ability.

Recent research clearly indicates that the capacity of the testes to produce sperm is lost when the temperature rises above a certain limit, one which the temperature in the abdominal cavity evidently exceeds. It is also stated that men who are professionally exposed to high temperatures (stokers and others) not infrequently become *sterile*. Temporary sterility follows prolonged fever.

19. Structure of the Testes The testes resemble horsechestnuts in shape and size. A testicle is divided into tiny lobules each containing several greatly convoluted, mutually connected, fine tubules from $\frac{1}{5}$ to $\frac{1}{3}$ millimeter thick. These are glandular tubules. The two testes together contain tubules to a length of nearly half a mile. The hormone-producing cells are located among these hairlike tubules.

20. Seminal Cells The seminal cells are constructed on almost the same principle as an old-fashioned round brick chimney. The bricks are the gland cells which develop in three stages from the outer wall toward the middle of the tube. In growing they mature and divide and are provided with a tail-like appendage. They are then *sperms* or *spermatozoa*.

21. The Spermatozoa A sperm consists of a *head*, a *middlepiece*, a *tail*, and a barely discernible *tail thread*. The appearance is rather like that of a tadpole, which caused Leeuwenhoek when he demonstrated the spermatozoa in 1677 to give it the slightly incorrect name of *spermatozoon* (literally "small semen animal"). The spermatozoa are very small. From the top of the head to the tip of the tail thread they measure only $\frac{1}{25,000}$ of an inch which means that one thousand sperms placed behind one another would form a procession about as long as a match.

22. Number of Sperms In about half a thimbleful there are more than 100 million sperms. A single ejaculation (which as a rule amounts to about 3 to 5 milliliters) contains an average of 345 million spermatozoa.

This number is particularly impressive when we remember that on our globe there are at all times no more than about 200 million women capable of having children. Since one sperm suffices to fertilize an ovum it would mean that in theory one single ejaculation contains more than enough *male sex cells* to fertilize all sexually mature women on earth.

23. *Life Expectancy of the Sperms* It has been firmly established that sperm cells, when kept in a proper place, may remain alive up to 205 hours, i.e. about nine days and nights, after the ejaculation. And sperm cells have, autoptically, proved to be alive in female sex organs—thus at a relatively low temperature—for three and one-half weeks after sexual intercourse. However, it is of greater interest to know how long semen cells may live in the sex organs of a living female.

24. *The Chromosomes* The head of the spermatozoon is no more than about $1/5000$ of an inch long, and about $1/12000$ of an inch broad. The front part consists of a substance capable of a certain resistance, called the cap. As does practically every cell in the organism, it has a nucleus containing 48 minute colorable elements called *chromosomes*. Inherent in them are all the hereditary dispositions or *genes* capable of transmission from the father to the child. If we consider that the semen cell, the spermatozoon, is really the father's sole contribution to the new human being, it is, indeed, a very impressive thought. Every quality the child inherits from its father comes from the head of a tiny "tadpole" not more than $1/5000$ of an inch or so long, and, to narrow it down still further, from a few minute grains in that head.

It is not only physical qualities like a Roman or a pug nose, delicate or coarse hands, arched or flat nails, height, girth, a certain way of walking or of getting up, a special timbre of the voice; also inherited are such qualities as a gift for mathematics, alertness or sluggishness, superficiality or thoroughness, a hot temper or a calm good nature. All of them are qualities characteristic of the father which may later, by heredity, prove to be characteristic of the child.

25. *The Epididymis* The epididymis is the small banana-shaped body located on top of and behind each testicle. The epididymis does not contain sex gland cells, but serves as a kind of temporary storeroom. It consists of rather thick winding tubes measuring about five and a half to six and a half yards, in which sperms received from the testicle are stored. According to recent

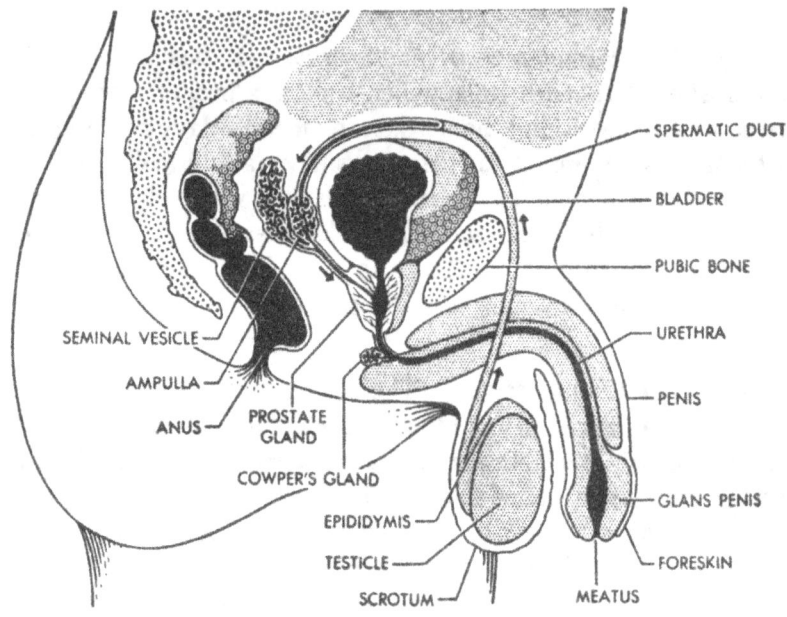

MALE ORGANS (side view)

research (Walker) the epididymis also has another function: it secretes independently a substance which contributes to the maturing of the sperms.

26. *Vas Deferens* From the epididymis the sperms pass through the *vas deferens,* a tube which is about twenty inches long, up into the abdomen where the *vas deferens* runs along both sides of the bladder and passes behind it.

27. *Pseudo-cryptorchism and Hernia* As mentioned earlier, the testes are, to start with, located high in the abdominal cavity, and descend into the scrotum during the embryonic stage, leaving the abdominal cavity by way of the so-called *in-*

guinal canal through which the *vas deferens* later enters that cavity. The passage of a testicle may have left an opening wider than the *vas deferens* and its surrounding blood vessels can fill. In such cases the testicle—particularly if something presses on the scrotum—may sometimes slip back up into the abdomen.

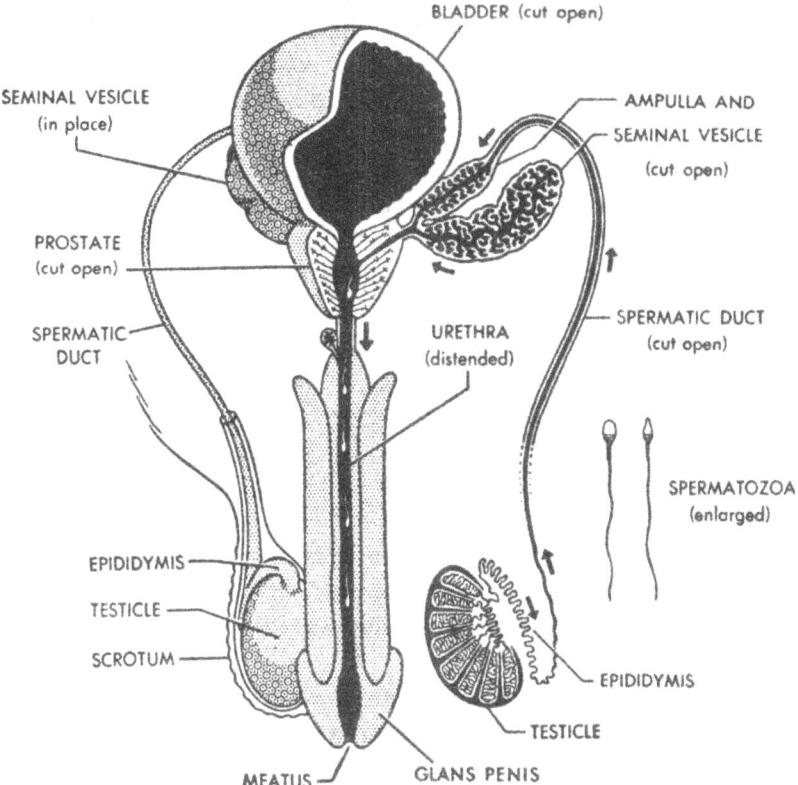

MALE ORGANS (front view)

Furthermore, through the aperture and canal by which the organs in the abdominal cavity have a certain connection with the upper part of the scrotum, part of the intestines or some other abdominal contents may sometimes try to make their way into the scrotum. If it shows only as a bump in the groin it is called an *inguinal hernia;* if, however, it extends right down into the scrotum the name is *scrotal hernia.* In most boys the aperture closes shortly after birth. But it is evident that every boy and man, purely because of the descent of his testes, may suffer a hernia via this so-called hernia gate.

28. *Vesical Glands*   Near the end, the *vas deferens* widens somewhat on both sides and forms the *ampulla*. Almost where the enlargement takes place the *vas deferens* receives the outlets from two big glands located behind the bladder, the so-called *vesical glands*. Formerly they were called the seminal vesicles because they were believed to serve only as a temporary storage place for *semen*, as is the case in certain animals.

It is now known that they are glands in their own right, secreting a special substance which seems to be concerned with the strength and degree of the sex urge. It has also been suggested (Steinach) that the secretion from the vesical glands heightens the vitality of the sperms, since well-developed vesical glands seem to go together with great fecundity. The secretion from these glands is sticky and, as a component of the seminal fluid, contributes to its final character.

29. *Urethral Crest*   The last part of the way, the *ampullae* pass through the big ring gland which is called the *prostate*, then end side by side in the ejaculatory ducts on the urethral crest, a tiny elevation on the posterior wall of that part of the urethra which is on a level with the prostate gland.

30. *The Prostate*   The prostate grows around the junction of the ureter with the bladder. It weighs about 0.7 oz. In shape and size it rather resembles a large chestnut with a hole through it.

From an evolutionary point of view the prostate corresponds to the female uterus. And corresponding to the uterine cavity in woman there is in man an opening or canal from the urethra leading into a small "pocket" in the prostate about midway between the outlets of the *ampullae*. This tiny "pocket" is of no physiological importance to the male, but must be mentioned because certain venereal germs, namely the gonococci, which cause gonorrhea are apt to lodge there in the later stages of the disease.

The prostate is composed of numerous small glands producing a fluid with a peculiar smell. This fluid is endowed with the amazing and very important quality that when mixed with the spermatozoa it makes them come "alive" and able to move along. The mixing process does not take place till the moment the seminal fluid is about to be ejaculated. Then the prostate fluid is secreted into the urethra through at least twenty small holes located around the *urethral crest* and rains down upon the spermatozoa. The sperms immediately attain their full capacity for motion, and by lashing their whiplike tails are able to move forward at a speed of a fifth of an inch a minute.

31. *The Urethra in the Male* As we know, the urethra serves in both sexes to excrete urine from the bladder. In the male it also has the function of expelling the seminal fluid. It runs in the form of an S lying down, from the bottom of the bladder to the tip of the male genital organ, the penis. The part of the urethra located in the penis is about six to eight inches in length and at least five millimeters in diameter.

32. *Closing of the Bladder During Ejaculation* During the ejaculation *colliculus seminalis* and adjacent parts are capable of swelling in such a way that they close off that part of the urethra which is connected with the bladder. Thus there is no risk that any urine, which might destroy the sperms, gains contact with them. Another common effect of this blocking-off process is that a man generally finds it impossible to urinate immediately after ejaculation.

33. *Bulbo-urethral Glands* The two big bulbo-urethral mucous glands are located at the curve of the urethra and produce a transparent secretion-like glycerine. Through specific ducts this secretion reaches the urethra. Its purpose is a double one: first, it serves as a lubricant easing the introduction of the penis into the female genital tract. Its second function is to cleanse the urethra of any remnant of urine which might injure the sperms, and finally, to form a sticky sheath around the sperms making them more liable to adhere to the interior of the female genitals. In addition to these big bulbo-urethral mucous glands numerous tiny glands have their outlets in the urethra

in various spots along the duct. The bulbo-urethral (mucous) glands are automatically emptied before sexual intercourse or coitus.

34. *What Is a Reflex?* If a fly alights on your hand while you are occupied by something else, you will shoo it off without stopping to think about it. An unconscious gesture like that is called a *reflex movement*. The sensation of the legs of the fly on the hand, the so-called "irritant," is "telephoned" from the sensory nerves of the hand through nerve centers to the spinal cord.

The message, however, does not reach the cortex of the brain, the supposed seat of consciousness. It is conducted through nerve cells in the spinal cord, the *reflex center* of this reflex, to other nerve filaments, namely those which activate the muscles of the arm, and for that reason the action need not reach one's consciousness at all. By reflexes in general we mean certain manifestations of life which come about through exterior or interior activation but without the will or conscious decision having anything to do with it. A good example of a reflex movement in the human organism is the so-called patellar (knee-cap) reflex.

35. *Various Types of Reflexes* Reflex actions occur incessantly all through the body. There are the reflexes which seemingly need not be learned by practice, and might best be called *nonacquired reflexes*, as for instance, secretion of saliva when we eat. Then there is the reflex of winking the eyelids, and the reflex we are dealing with here: the secretion of the mucous glands when sexually excited. The second category of reflexes comprises practiced or *acquired reflexes*, such as walking, or playing a musical instrument.

A special type of acquired reflex is the so-called *conditioned reflex*, first demonstrated by the ingenious Russian physiologist Pavlov the nature of which is evident from his classical experiment. He discovered that when a dog is given a piece of meat its salivary glands begin to secrete saliva. If, at the same time, one of its hind legs is dipped in cold water, or if a certain note is sounded, the secretion of saliva will occur after some time of practice. It is sufficient for the hind leg to be immersed in cold water, or for a certain note to be sounded, to activate the secretion of saliva. It is *not* necessary any more to offer the dog meat at the same time.

Finally, if a reflex occurs exclusively via a secondary nerve center it is called an *isolated reflex*. If primary nerve centers are involved too (for instance the brain centers), the reflex which then becomes more complicated, is called a *coordinated reflex*.

36. *The Male Organ, the Penis* The physician's term for the male member the copulatory or uniting organ is *penis*. In the present time the majority of adults are familiar with this term. As a rule the penis hangs down flaccidly and is about one and a half times the size of its owner's thumb, somewhat bigger in hot weather and smaller in cold weather. The brownish skin covering the penis is very thin and elastic, and provided with numerous sweat and sebaceous glands.

Other species in the animal world offer great contrast. For example, male birds generally have no penis. To hold the hen and ensure contact with its copulatory organ the cock has to seize the hen by the neck with its beak and keep it down. Originally the penis was a wartlike thorn in the spermatic cord. In dogs, rodents, carnivora, bats, and monkeys, for instance, quite a solid bone remains in the penis. This bone is not present in the human male, whose penis therefore is entirely flexible.

37. *Pubic Hair, Pubes* The hairy growth on and around the genital organs in both man and woman is called *pubic hair*. On the male this hairy covering extends from about the root of the penis and scrotum more or less high up on the abdomen. There it often grows into a peak ending somewhat below the navel. Pubic hair is rather coarse as a rule, and differs from hair in other parts of the body by its triangular structure. For that reason pubic hair is quite curly.

38. *Erection of the Penis* It is amazing that the penis which in its flaccid state measures only about three to four inches, can become hard, thick, stiff, and long, *erected*, as it is called, in which case its ordinary size may be almost doubled.

The erected penis, then about six inches long, is sometimes called by the Greek term, *phallos* (phallus).

39. *The Erectile System*   The penis consists almost exclusively of *spongy* or erectile tissue made up of a great number of crisscrossing muscular filaments comparable to the fibers in a sponge. The spaces between these muscle threads are filled with blood constantly pumped by the heart through the arteries into the penis. The blood leaves it through veins which carry it back to the heart. The muscle filaments are controlled by ganglia similar to those that direct the activity of the mucous glands. These ganglia or nerves, in other words, are nerves not subject to the person's will, but activated by influences of which he is not necessarily conscious.

Normally the muscle filaments in the spongy elements of the penis are contracted and the interstices between them leave space for only a relatively small quantity of blood. However, they relax under the influence brought to bear through the ganglia, with the result that the interstices expand and permit the influx of more blood. The heart, which constantly pumps blood into the penis at a certain pressure immediately fills the bigger space with blood. And that causes the erection of the penis. At the same time the veins leading back to the heart *from* the penis are partly blocked.

40. *Purpose of Erection*   The purpose of penis erection is to attain the essential shape for introduction into the female genital tract. This is necessary if the penis is to function as a copulatory or mating organ.

41. *Erection without Any Sexual Purpose*   If the exit of blood from the penis is obstructed, accumulation of blood in the penis may result; it is blocked, and this may bring about erection. It may happen, for instance, if the bladder is very much distended as is often the case in the morning. However, this so-called *early morning erection* disappears as soon as the bladder is emptied. Accumulation of feces, or too much air pressure in the rectum, may also cause erection.

42. *The Penis Head*   This part of the penis is formed by the tip of the tumescent or erectile tissue which encases the urethra and forms what looks like a thick hood around the ends of the two bigger spongy elements. The penis head is covered by a delicate, slightly moist membrane. This membrane is very delicate thin skin, amply equipped with sensory nerves and the *spongelike elements.* The penis head is therefore very sensitive to the touch.

In many men a slight touching of the penis head arouses more than anything else a feeling of sexual voluptuousness or pleasure, where a stronger touch is felt as pain.

43. *The Foreskin, Prepuce*   In a male infant the penis head is covered by a fold of skin which is a prolongation of the penis skin. Out in front it forms a double fold, and is anchored in the furrow behind the penis head. On the lower side of the penis head the foreskin is attached more firmly by the thin foreskin band. In a newborn baby boy the foreskin most frequently looks like a tiny pouting mouth with a very small hole, just barely large enough to permit the passage of the urine. In rare cases the aperture is so narrow that it has to be dilated artificially to prevent urination from being blocked completely. On the inside of the foreskin, or prepuce, there are varying numbers of sebaceous glands which are also on a part of the penis head. These sebaceous glands exude a secretion which together with the waste cell tissue from the surface, form a pasty substance called *smegma.* If this is not removed regularly it may sometimes cause inflammation of the prepuce.

44. *Stricture of the Prepuce (Phimosis)*   If the foreskin is so tight that it makes urinating difficult, or if the foreskin in the adult cannot be pushed back over the *glans* the term *stricture of the prepuce* is used. This sometimes occurs in newborn babies and in big children and adults, as a result of certain inflammations. It is generally possible to manipulate the prepuce, expanding it so as to permit the urine to pass. Only in rare cases is it found necessary to perform a special operation on the foreskin.

45. *Normal Enlargement of the Prepuce*   However, as the boy grows older the prepuce or foreskin generally distends, gets more commodious. When he reaches his fourteenth or fifteenth year this foreskin is usually so loose and easy that it may be pushed or pulled back over the penis head which is then exposed and protrudes uncovered. For many persons, however, this is only feasible many years later. It is considered normal if the foreskin can be pulled back before a man has completed his twenty-fifth year.

46. *Circumcision*   The surgical removal of the foreskin, so that the glans penis protrudes uncovered, is called circumcision. It is estimated that about one sixth of the male population of our globe, corresponding to about 175 million, have been circumcised. Circumcision is often practiced at puberty and in many primitive peoples it is considered an initiation into manhood. The Jewish religion prescribes that male infants when they are one week old must have part of the foreskin removed in such a manner that what remains may be pulled back over the penis head. This operation was originally performed by nonprofessionals, but today it is done by medical men.

47. *Circumcision as a Shield against Venereal Disease.* Quite apart from its ritual significance, circumcision must now be considered as a practical hygienic measure. After circumcision the penis head is no longer covered and thus easily risks abrasions or irritation by contact with diapers and other clothing. However, the delicate skin of the penis head naturally grows coarser and in time acquires the appearance of ordinary skin. It is true that being uncovered it is more exposed to the onslaughts of bacteria, yet the operation usually occurs at a time when those germs which are really dangerous in this connection, the bacteria of venereal diseases, are least likely to gain access to the penis head and do harm. Gradually then, the excellent result is so achieved that as the boy is growing up, his penis head becomes capable of considerable resistance to germ infections. And it is a fact that syphilis—the great offender in this connection—is almost unknown in persons who are circumcised.

48. *Significance of Circumcision in Sexual Intercourse*
While the skin of the penis head grows coarser as a result of circumcision, it also becomes less sensitive. Thus the male partner will reach his climax and ejaculation more slowly than an uncircumcised person. This can only be regarded as an advantage in intercourse, since it is not a rare occurrence for a woman to experience difficulty in attaining her orgasm simultaneously with the man.

Chapter 4: THE FEMALE SEX ORGANS

49. *General Function of the Female Sex Organs* The most important parts of the female genitals are the sex glands, *the ovaries*. They produce the female sex cell: the *ovum* or *egg*. From one of the ovaries (both of which are located in the cavity of the pelvis) the egg passes through the connecting *Fallopian tube* into the *uterus*. From there it is either expelled through the vagina as an unfertilized egg, or after nine months of protection and growth inside the uterus, born as a new human being. Finally, in connection with the female sex organs we must mention the mammary glands charged with the nutrition of the newborn infant.

50. *The Female Sex Glands, the Ovaries* The two ovaries lie well hidden and protected within the pelvis, one ovary on each side. The right ovary is located so near the appendix that if one organ is affected the other easily follows suit. In shape and size the ovaries look like thin-shelled almonds. Their total weight varies from less than one quarter of an ounce to about one half ounce, and they contain follicles for 70,000 to 400,000 eggs. Of this enormous quantity a maximum of only 500 reach full development during a woman's lifetime. Only a very limited number are fertilized, sometimes none at all.

51. *Descent of the Ovaries* As mentioned before, the male and female sex glands—testes and ovaries—at their initial, embryonic stage are located high up in the abdomen. While normally the testes descend the whole way down into the scrotum of the male child before birth, the ovaries of the female child only move into the small, true pelvis where they remain, well protected, for the rest of their existence.

52. The Ovary Follicles If we examine a cross section of an ovary in the microscope we notice near the rim, in the cortex, a lot of tiny beginnings of ova, or vesical follicles, which do not develop further. Among these follicles are a smaller number surrounded by a special layer of cells (as a rule about 30,000). When a girl approaches puberty these begin to grow: they are then called ovary follicles, formerly termed the Graafian or primary follicles. A well-developed ovary follicle consists of an outer cortex of cells arranged like palisades encircling a moat.

Inside the "moat" is the follicle fluid, and protruding like a tiny peninsula we see the "egg-hill." There the egg sits well protected, surrounded by yet another circle of cells. When around the end of the seventeenth century, scientists thought they were gazing at human eggs in an ovary, what they really saw were the follicles.

53. Ovulation Every month one, or possibly two, Graafian follicles that have ripened into eggs, emerge from the ovary. This takes place in the following manner: Because of the constantly growing pressure of the fluid within, the follicle bursts and the egg is forced into the abdominal cavity where almost invariably it is caught in one of the Fallopian tubes. At the time this getting rid of the egg (called ovulation) takes place, the woman may experience painful contractions of the uterus, at times a little like birth pangs. These pains, because the ovulation generally takes place about midway between two menstruations, are called *in-between pains* and sometimes indisposition.

The great majority of women experience no unpleasantness at ovulation. However, at the same time the *body temperature* rises abruptly by 0.5 to 1 degree and remains at this higher temperature until the occurrence of a menstruation. This fact may be used to calculate the time of ovulation. Finally, sometimes a woman's sexual tone and feeling may be influenced by ovulation, as a rule in the way that she is more strongly drawn toward the other sex.

54. *The Fallopian Tubes* The shape of the Fallopian tube or tuba recalls an ancient herald's trumpet. The Greek word for trumpet, *salpinx*, is traced in the term *salpingitis* (inflammation of the tubes). The two Fallopian tubes externally coated by the peritoneum, extend from the uterus on both sides of the true pelvis. They end in a small appendage like a tiny chestnut leaf that can cover the ovary like a hand with spread fingers and catch the egg when it is about to be ejected from the follicle.

55. *The Fallopian Tubes May Substitute for One Another* In the normal course of events the tube on the right receives the egg from the right ovary, and the tube on the left, that from the left ovary. But it is quite possible that an egg from the right ovary may be caught in the left tube. This is an important factor where one of the tubes has deteriorated through disease or has been removed by surgery. It is still possible for a woman to conceive and become a mother with only one ovary in one side and one tube in the opposite side.

56. *Passage of the Egg through the Fallopian Tube* In contrast to the male spermatozoon the egg has no spontaneous movement. It is passively carried through the tube, wafted on by *cilia*, tiny hairs inside the tube which in brief jerks manage to push the egg toward the uterus. This is a slow process; the passage through the Fallopian tube which is about five inches long takes about fourteen days.

57. *The Womb or Uterus* A woman has two ovaries, two Fallopian tubes, but only one womb or uterus. In a virgin the uterus is shaped like a medium-sized pear, the narrow end pointing downwards. It is slightly more than three inches long and weighs about one and one-half oz. The upper, larger part is called the uterine body, the lower part, the neck or cervix. The *uterine body* is hollow and consists mostly of nonstriated muscles, i.e. muscles not controlled by the will, in contrast to mus-

cles in the arms and legs. The interior is entirely lined with a thick coat of glandular tissue so that only a small triangular cavity, the *uterine cavity,* is left. At the two upper corners of the triangle the two Fallopian tubes enter the womb below, the uterine body narrows into the uterine neck or cervix.

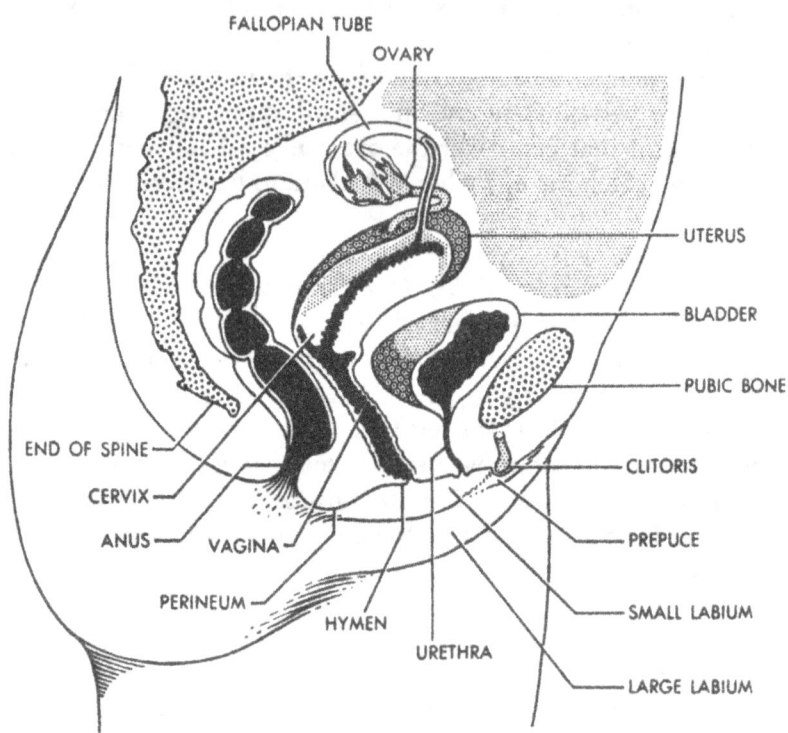

FEMALE ORGANS (side view)

58. *Uterine Neck, Cervix* Like the womb the cervix is hollow, a fibro-muscular tube, but with not nearly as many glands as the womb. The cervical cavity is more like a duct, the cervical *canal,* which is blocked by a *mucous plug,* formed by the gland secretions of the cervix into the vagina is called the *external uterine os* or just the *os.* The point where it connects with the interior of the uterine body, is called *the internal os.* In a woman who has never had a child the external uterine *os* in size and shape looks like a shoestring hole. In women who have borne, it has changed into a slit or a star-shaped aperture. This

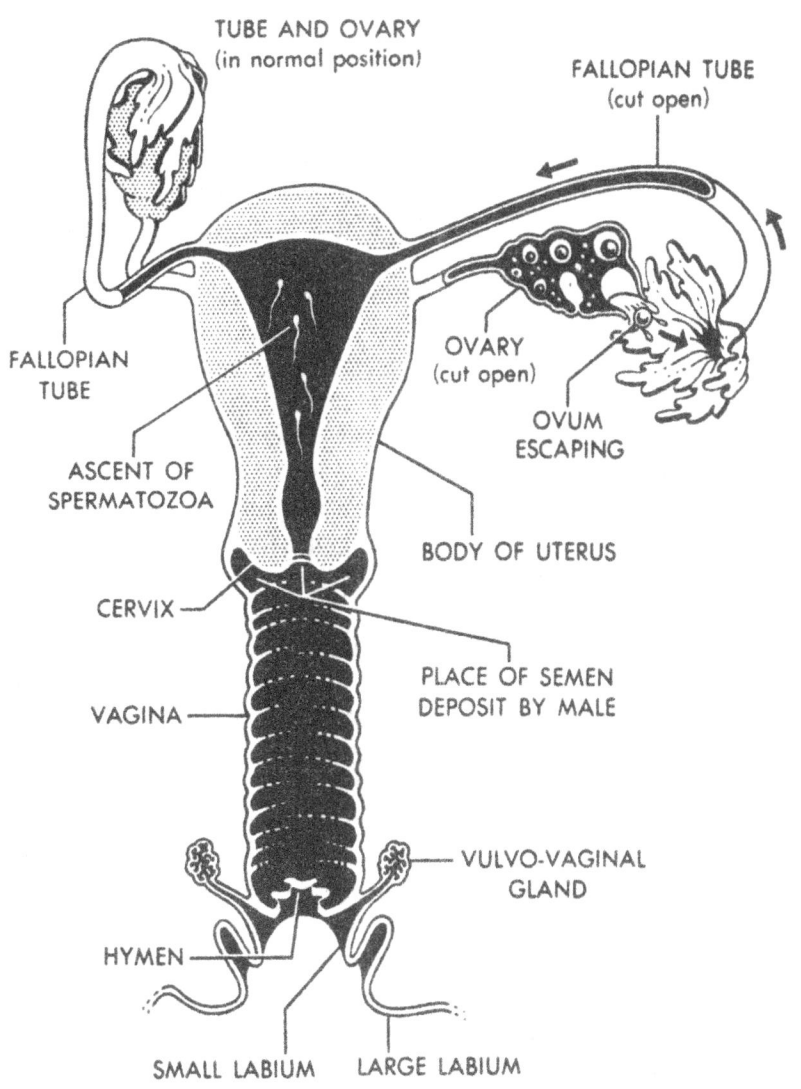

FEMALE ORGANS (front view)

change in the external *os* is the most definite distinguishing mark by which to establish whether or not a woman has had a child (or a miscarriage). The lower part of the uterine neck protrudes into the vagina and is coated with an extremely delicate and vulnerable membrane equipped with numerous nerve elements making it at least as sensitive as the glans penis in the male.

59. *Anteversion, or Forward Displacement of Uterus* The long axis of the uterus is not in direct prolongation of the lengthwise axis of the vagina for the uterus is slightly forward-bent whereby the uterine *os* is turned a little backwards and downwards. Moreover, the cervix and the uterine body meet at almost right angles causing the *fundus uteri* to stick out straight while the anterior surface of the *corpus uteri* rests on the bladder.

60. *Retroversion or Backward Displacement of Uterus* The uterus is kept in place in its normal position of moderate anteversion or forward displacement by a complicated system of strong ligaments. If these ligaments stretch and lose their resiliency—as may be the case after childbirth—the uterus may rise to an upright position or may be bent backwards. In other cases retroversion of the womb is congenital. It is a condition which may very well be present in a woman without her being aware of it, and in our day and age the tendency is to consider retroversion of the womb as something not particularly out of the ordinary.

Frequently, however, certain troublesome symptoms accompany the condition. The woman may have a sensation as if the uterus were actually sinking into the vagina, though there is no indication that such is actually the case. Pain in the small of the back occurs frequently, and sometimes the woman will mention that she has difficulty in urinating and that coitus is accompanied by pain. She may also complain of pains when emptying her bowels, though this is an infrequent occurrence. Further symptoms of a more than ordinary nature indicated as accompanying backward displacement of the uterus are: headaches, pressure in the diaphragm, indigestion, a feeling of faintness and general fatigue. Sometimes the condition may also bring on coughing and hoarseness.

61. Descent of the Uterus If the ligaments have become so slack as to permit a rather considerable change in the position of the womb, it may slip clear down into the vagina. This state which we call *descent of the uterus* is accompanied by a distinct sensation of heaviness in the abdomen. Should that feeling of heaviness become too pronounced, the complaint usually has to be treated by insertion of a uterus ring, also called a pessary, to keep the uterus in place.

62. Prolapsus of the Uterus If the uterus comes down so far that the cervix becomes visible at the vulva, that condition is described as a *prolapsus of the uterus*. It should be treated by a doctor without delay. For in this abnormal position the mucous membrane covering the cervix, an extraordinarily delicate and vulnerable membrane, risks injury by rubbing against clothing, sanitary napkins, etc. Bacteria may make their way through the injured mucous membrane at this point, situated so near the urethra and the anus, thus causing severe inflammation. If a prolapsus of the uterus cannot be contained by means of a uterus ring, it may become necessary to have recourse to surgery.

63. The Vagina The vagina is a fibro-muscular tube about three inches long and one inch broad so built that the front and back walls touch. Only deep in, at the very back, the vagina is more commodious. Around the uterine neck or cervix it forms a smaller anterior vaginal vault and further back a larger posterior vaginal vault in which the seminal fluid may be deposited. There are any number of individual variations in the size of the vagina that need not have any relation to the size of the woman. The walls of the vagina are very solid and consist of numerous strong, elastic muscle fibres that become active during intercourse and in labor. The interior is lined with a moist membrane corrugated almost like a washboard. Such moist membranes in the body are called *mucous membranes*.

In women who have borne more than one child, the mucous membrane is frequently smoother and the vagina generally more gaping, a condition which tends considerably to diminish the erotic sensations at coitus. A great number of micro-organisms live in the vagina, keeping it a trifle moist and, as a rule, also helping to keep it clean.

64. The Vulva The *vulva* or *cunnus* is bordered in front by a fatty cushion covered with pubic hair, called *mons veneris,*

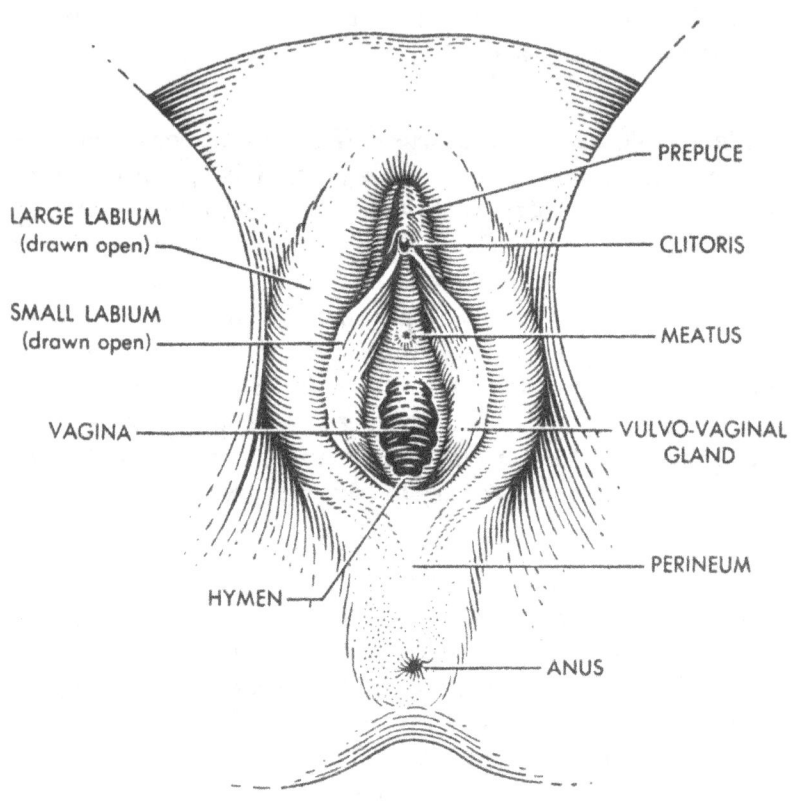

VIEW OF THE VULVA

the mount of Venus, and behind by the so-called *perineum* connecting the vulva and the anus. Along the vulva on both sides lie the outer and inner labia (or lips). In the vulva there are four organs which we shall mention specifically: the *clitoris,* the *urethra,* the *vaginal orifice* or *entrance,* and the *boat-shaped depression* behind it.

THE SEX ORGANS

65. *The Perineum*   The perineum as mentioned before is located between the vulva and the anus. During labor this has to stand very considerable stretching, made possible by numerous tensile elements in it. None the less the perineum has a tendency to tear—it happens in one-third of all births. The damage, however, is rarely very great.

66. *The Outer Lips*   The outer labia or lips average more or less three inches in length, from below one inch to more than an inch in height, and they are more or less three-fourths of an inch large. Normally they touch each other, thus closing off vulva.

In front they are two-thirds covered with *pubic hair* (*pubes*) which continues into the pubic hair on the *mons veneris*. Here the hairiness stops in an almost straight, horizontal line—in contrast to the pubic growth in man which often grows in a peak up the abdomen. The structure of the outer labia is somewhat similar to the interior of the penis. It is the same principle of erectile tissue that may swell with an influx of blood to such an extent that the labia become firm or even hard.

67. *The Greater Vestibular Mucous Glands*   In the outer labia we find the *greater vestibular mucous glands*. They produce a lubricating liquid comparable to that produced by the large mucous glands of the male urethra. This lubricating fluid is secreted into the vulva. If the large female mucous glands suffer inflammation they may swell considerably. Such inflammations are very painful as a rule and are often, though not always, due to gonorrhea.

68. *The Inner Lips*   The inner lips are two small skinlike folds as a rule a little moist, wherefore they tend to stick together. In some cases one of the inner labia is much higher than the other and protrudes like a big flap outside the outer labia.

69. *The Female Urethra*   The female's urethra, in contrast to the urethra of the male, has no direct connection with normal sex life. It is only from two and a half to a little more than three inches long, and leading from the lower part of the bladder, has its outlet in the vulva between the clitoris and the vaginal orifice. It is equipped with a closing or occluding muscle which, with the passage of the years, tends to grow lax so that old women often have trouble retaining their urine, a cause of great embarrassment to neat old ladies. Old men, on the other hand, often suffer because they are *not* able to get rid of their urine.

70. The Vaginal Entrance (Introitus) Normally the vaginal opening, introitus, is almost closed because the walls of the vagina lie so close together that the entrance rather resembles a capital H. The outlets of the two large mucous glands are located near the vaginal entrance.

71. The Hymen, or Maidenhead In women who have had no sexual relations, the vaginal orifice is more or less closed by a membrane, most often a thin membrane, the so-called *maidenhead* or *hymen*. As a general rule this membrane is broken at the first coitus or attempt at coitus. However, it is important to know that it may also break from other causes, for instance by strenuous physical exercise, violent riding, or by an unfortunate fall, and, of course, by a direct blow in the sex organs. We particularly wish to emphasize this. Many marriages have failed at the very outset because the young bridegroom was obsessed by a preconceived idea that a hymen must look *just* so. Every young man should know and realize that there are many variations of the normal, unbroken hymen.

I have, for instance, seen hymens that closed the entire vaginal orifice. When a young girl with such a hymen has her first menstruation no blood flows. It is not till the second or third time, when the pressure is too great to bear, that she consults a doctor. Then the tense hymen is lanced; the blood gushes out and her menstruation henceforth follows a normal course. There may be hymens that cover the entire vaginal orifice, but with a tiny aperture in the center; or hymens that are perforated and full of holes like a sieve. Other hymens cover the posterior part of the orifice. That is the form which is generally and, as we have seen, mistakenly described as the only acceptable edition of an intact hymen. There may be hymens that appear as fringes on both sides of the vaginal entrance; another type resembles a broken hymen—a hymen that protrudes like folded scallops or flaps round the entire vaginal orifice, or around a part of it. One would almost have to be a professor in legal medicine and to have seen hundreds of broken and intact hymens to be able to declare with definite authority whether a certain hymen *is* or *is not* intact.

So we must understand how ridiculous it is when a newly-married bridegroom pronounces judgment in this matter and risks ruining his marriage at the start for the simple reason that he was not properly informed.

72. *Breaking of Hymen (Defloration)* As we said before, the hymen generally breaks at the first coitus or attempt at coitus. This is called *defloration*. Young women often have very exaggerated ideas of how painful that is. One of the reasons for this is that formerly a favorite way of describing defloration was: *the bursting of the hymen.* When the hymen gives way there may be a brief lancing pain, a little blood, but rarely any copious bleeding. But this is far from the general rule. If the coitus is prepared and preceded by love play and the female genitals have been moistened by the secretions of the mucous glands, the breaking of the hymen may even pass unnoticed. Young women, therefore, need not harbor any fears or anxieties about their first coitus on *that* account. In about 15 per cent of all cases the hymen does not break at all at coitus, but remains intact. However, it does break at parturition, when a woman has her first child.

73. *Does the Hymen Serve Any Useful Purpose?* The opinion has been advanced that at the primitive stages of human life sexual intercourse began at a very early age when the boy's penis was not yet fully developed. Thus the presence of the hymen at that time not only was no hindrance to coitus, but, on the contrary, a necessity, because it made the vaginal opening sufficiently narrow to make it fit the otherwise too small penis. In that ancient period the hymen was not broken, but it was gradually dilated. That this hypothesis might be correct is borne out not only by the fact that in many primitive peoples to this

day early childhood marriages are often customary. It gains support also by the fact mentioned above that the hymen among civilized peoples in many cases does not break at all at intercourse, but in about fifteen per cent of all cases remains intact.

74. The Boat-shaped Depression In women with unbroken hymens, that part of the vulva which lies between the introitus and the perineum is shaped like a more or less definite, rather oblong depression called the boat-shaped depression. We know of several cases where the ignorance of young husbands was such that they did not realize that to carry on intercourse the penis must be introduced into the vagina. When finally they consult a doctor because it has at last dawned upon them that something is not quite as it should be, it is revealed that they made the mistake of taking the boat-shaped depression for the vagina.

75. The Clitoris The clitoris is an organ of great importance to woman's sex life. As will be seen, it rather resembles a small penis, and, in an evolutionary sense, that is what it really corresponds to. It is a vestige from that phase in the embryonic stage when nature had not yet given a definitely male or female direction to the genital organ of the embryo. Apart from the fact that the urethra does not pass through the clitoris, it is really like a penis *in miniature;* it has a *clitoris head* (*glans clitoridis*) richly equipped with voluptuous-sensory nerve ends, and surrounded by a fold of skin, a hood, corresponding to the foreskin in the male. Like the penis, it consists largely of spongy, erectile tissue capable of *erection*. In its flaccid, neutral state the clitoris is a little more than half an inch long, but may become twice that in its erected state.

As we shall see later, the clitoris is the female organ the touching of which more than anything else causes keen sexual enjoyment in a woman.

76. The Breasts In a more general sense the mammary glands or the breasts also can be considered as a female sex organ. The breast consists of fifteen to twenty-five groups of small grape-shaped glands buried in soft, fatty tissue. Each of the glandular groups have outlets, the so-called lacteal ducts, leading to the nipple (*papilla*) where they end in a bunch close together. During the last part of their passage below the zone of pigmentation (*areola*) that surrounds the nipple, the lacteal ducts extend and become tiny "milk-sacs." The nipple may protrude quite considerably when cold, or when sexually activated, or when the baby is nursing. The color of the nipple may be pink or beige in fair women; in brunettes and dark-haired women it is more brown, sometimes almost black, and often surrounded by a brownish aureole. Apart from its high prestige and function as the organ for nursing babies, the breast plays a certain part in several of the phases of sexual union; thus, it is not an unessential erogenous zone. And we shall see in the following that the breast is very intimately related to the most essential female sex functions. This relation thus exists in regard to development; and in regard to its activity as a milk-producing organ it is constantly influenced by the female sex hormones. However, let us first look more closely at what is meant when we speak of hormones, especially sex hormones.

3
HORMONES AND THE SEXUAL FUNCTIONS

Chapter 5: THE HORMONES

77. *What Is a Hormone?* Hormone is the name given to a substance internally secreted by a ductless gland. There are many different hormones, produced by different glands. From these glands the hormones pass into the blood stream that carries them all over the organism; in that way the hormones get into contact with all organs in the body. A hormone, however, influences or activates only those organs or tissues for which it is designed, for only these are sensitive to that particular kind of hormone. In the same way that a cell in the nervous system sends out an impulse via a nerve thread to a group of cells in an organ, so a ductless gland, by way of the blood stream, sends out an impulse to an organ in the shape of a hormone. This hormone then exercises either a constructive or an obstructive influence. It helps either to stimulate or depress the activity of the organ in question. Some hormones—the so-called essential or controlling hormones—play a special part. Their function is regulation of the hormone production of certain other endocrine glands. In that way you might say that the hormone-producing endocrine glands practice a kind of teamwork, a fact of great significance to the normal development and functioning of the body. If, therefore, the hormone production of a gland is deficient or fails entirely it may result in a vital disturbance of the normal balance of the organism. However, from animal glands that secrete the

same hormones as the human being, it is now possible to manufacture certain artificial preparations having the same effects as the natural hormones. Should the hormone production of a certain gland be faulty, the lacking quantity may be substituted by giving the person injections of that hormone or of the hormone-like substance, or in tablet form provided these do not deteriorate or lose their effect by passing through the alimentary canal.

78. *The Thyroid Gland and Thyroxin*   The thyroid gland, imbedded in the front of the throat, offers an example of hormonal action. It is an integral endocrine gland, that is, it has no outlet to the exterior. The hormone it produces is called thyroxin. If, for some reason, the thyroid gland produces *too much* of this hormone the blood will contain greater quantities than normally. Should the gland manufacture a nonbeneficial variety of the hormone the patient may change in a number of ways. His heart will beat more quickly, he will lose weight, and the nervous system become more sensitive than usual. Imagine a skinny, perspiring person with palpitations of the heart, with trembling hands, a complete nervous wreck not able to keep still for a moment, chasing from one place to another. That is the picture of a person *poisoned by thyroxin*, and not a rare case at all. The opposite happens if the thyroid gland produces *too little* thyroxin. Then the person may become fat, lazy, and phlegmatic, with a too slow heartbeat. Such a person may derive much benefit from extra doses of thyroxin. The important thing, however, is to find the correct dose on the advice of a physician.

79. *The Pituitary Gland and Its Hormones*   In the head, behind the eyes and above the nose, located in a small saddle-shaped bone pit below the surface of the cranium like a small spur from the brain and better protected than anything else in the human body, we find a small gland, the size of the kernel of a hazel nut. Its name is the hypophysis or the pituitary gland. It consists of an anterior, intermediate and a posterior lobe. It is an endocrine gland the importance of which has only been investigated during rather recent years. However, despite its rather insignificant weight it has proved to be an organ of such importance that some people have found cause to believe it was

the seat of the soul. In fact, the hypophysis is a sort of *grand central* for a lot of vital manifestations, among others those connected with growth and reproduction.

For here many hormones are secreted. Up to the present it has been estimated that the number of apparently different hormones produced by the pituitary gland is about twenty. The anterior lobe, for instance, produces the hormone regulating growth. If there is an excess of it, one may become a giant; if there is too little, one may become a dwarf. This hormone has been isolated in a pure state, and is used in various preparations, such as Antuitrin G, Phyol, and Crescormon for treatment of dwarfism.

Another pituary hormone regulates the growth of those parts of the body which protrude. If an oversupply of this hormone is produced in the body, an individual develops a big nose, a thick tongue, large hands and feet, long legs, long arms, etc. If too little is secreted, the opposite development may take place. In the anterior lobe, moreover, those hormones are produced which exercise influence on the sex organs, the milk secretion, the suprarenal glands, and basal metabolism.

80. *Antihormones* In many animals, as well as human beings who have been treated with certain hormones of unknown species (among them the sex hormones mentioned from the anterior lobe of the pituitary gland) over a considerable period, the blood has been found to contain certain substances—*antihormones*—which counteract the effect of the hormones used in treatment. So far, we do not know where the production centers of these antihormones are located, neither do we know exactly how they function nor anything definite about their nature. But it must be realized that if an organism does not of itself produce a sufficient quantity of a certain hormone, and one consequently wants to add hormone of an unknown species, there is the definite risk that if the hormone preparation is taken over a comparatively long period, the condition may become worse instead of better, because antihormones may be formed which further diminish the effect of the hormone of which the organism already produced too little. People should be aware that in some cases hormone treatments are beneficial only to a

certain extent. If carried beyond that they may have the opposite effect. On the other hand, the possibility is not excluded that some time in the future antihormones may be used to remedy complaints due to too plentiful hormone production.

81. *To Understand Sex Functions It Is Necessary to Know about Hormones* The above explanations present some idea of what a hormone really is, and of the very essential role which the pituitary gland in particular plays among the body's hormone-producing glands. In the following sections we shall show how the hormones really run like a red thread through human sex life. As a result we no longer need regard the elemental sexual drives or urges as something mysterious and arbitrary, but may understand them and conceive of them in their truly powerful and harmonious correlation.

Chapter 6: PUBERTY

82. *What Is Adolescence?* When we talk of adolescence we mean the traditional time of youth in its widest sense. It covers the period from shortly after the tenth year until attainment of complete physical and psychic maturity, as a rule between twenty and thirty. This period is of great psychic importance since its course, to a great extent, determines the entire physical, emotional, and psychic condition of the individual in later years.

83. *Pubescence and Puberty* Pubescence approximately corresponds to the first half of adolescence. Pubescence in the average normal girl begins soon after the eighth or ninth year. For about that time the figure, until then angular and boyish, begins to develop into more rounded and softer forms, further accentuated about the eleventh or twelfth year, when the female pelvis grows larger. Moreover, a considerable increase of fatty tissue is noticeable, particularly on the shoulders, breasts, throat, hips, buttocks, and mons veneris. About halfway through pubescence, those sexual characteristics directly connected with the *reproductive capacity* appear. This transition is called *puberty*.

84. The Pituitary Sex Hormones in Control: the Gonadotropic Hormones   It is believed all of the hormones produced by the pituitary gland have contributed to bringing about the changes that have taken place in both sexes. But they seem to be *exclusively and solely* responsible for the revolution in the *sex* functions which puberty brings and which, in temperate zones, takes place generally when the boy is about thirteen to fifteen years old and the girl twelve to fourteen. For about this time the pituitary gland starts to produce a significant amount of hormones, identical in boys and girls, which circulate through the entire body. These only leave their mark in one particular spot in the boy and in the girl, namely on their sex glands: the boy's testes, and the girl's ovaries developing in size. A general term for sex glands is *gonads,* and the hormones that affect and stimulate them are called *gonadotropic hormones,* or *gonadtropins.*

85. Sex Glands as Duct Glands   The gonadotropic hormones from the pituitary gland then, affect the gonads or sex glands. They "start" the boy's testes, which now—and not until now—begin producing spermatozoa, and they "start" the girl's ovaries, the ripening of follicles and the ovulation. When that is accomplished boy and girl are nubile, ripe for sexual union. The youth is capable of begetting children, and the girl is capable of becoming pregnant.

86. The Sex Glands as Endocrine Glands and Sex Hormones Proper   Further sexual maturity is reached, in addition to the gonadotropic hormones of the pituitary gland taking a message to the testes and the ovaries telling them to start functioning as *open glands,* to produce seminal fluid and let eggs ripen and emerge. These hormones also alert the sex glands (testes and ovaries), telling that they must begin to function as *endocrine glands,* and as endocrine glands they must also produce special hormones on their own.

The hormones produced directly by the testes and the ovaries, are called the essential sex hormones. In contrast to the gonadotropic hormones they differ in the two sexes. And it is they that more than anything else make puberty a revolutionary period in the life of the human being. Their action causes the sexually dormant children to grow into sex-conscious men and women.

87. Classification of Sex Characteristics Fifty years ago the sex characteristics of the two sexes were divided into so-called "*primary* and *secondary* (or *dependent*) sex characteristics," and later, into the *essential* and the *accidental* sex characteristics. A clear definition of the exact meaning of one or the other was never arrived at, however.

Nowadays a more modern manner of classifying the sex characteristics is the purely descriptive device of distinguishing between *genital* and *extragenital* (genitals being the sex organs, as we have mentioned before). Among the *genital* sex characteristics we find the sex glands, their products and outlets and the further apparatus of sex, while the *extragenital* sex characteristics comprise the other physical and psychic sex differences that are more or less, or perhaps entirely, independent of the activity of the internal secretions of the sex glands.

At the present phase of our knowledge this classification already seems somewhat dated. Therefore it is my suggestion that the sex characteristics of each sex be henceforth divided into *genital, hormonal,* and *other physical distinctions*, and finally, psychologically distinguishing marks.

Chapter 7: MALE SEX CHARACTERISTICS

88. Male Sex Characteristics These are: a. the special structure of the male sex organs; b. the activity of the testes as open glands, i.e. production of spermatozoa; c. the activity of the testes as endocrine glands, i.e. production of male sex hormones.

89. The First Ejaculation When the production of sperm has started, this, as a rule, soon manifests itself in the growing boy as *ejaculations* in connection with his sexual activity. The so-called nocturnal emissions, frequently accompanied by erotically tinged dreams, may also occur at this time.

90. The Hormonal Sex Characteristics of the Male In the testes among the *tubuli contorti* are the so-called interstitial cells. Under the stimulating effect of a pituitary gonadtropin these testicular testes cells begin manufacturing a hormone. This is the male sex hormone proper. Its action causes the boy's larynx to grow and it also develops his vocal cords, making his voice deeper. It is the influence of this hormone that makes the male beard sprout, develops the muscles and chisels the grown man's finished form out of that of the undeveloped boy: the man's broad shoulders, narrow hips, strong limbs, thickened neck, and powerful chest. In the armpit the axillary growth of hair appears. The penis develops, as well as the testes, the pubic growth around the penis starts, and spreads without definite limits; hairy growth often appears on the abdomen and the chest as well. And last, but not least: the adolescent suddenly discovers that he looks at the members of the opposite sex with different eyes. He notices the female form and contours, feels a protective urge well up within him, sees those creatures he formerly regarded with scorn as "just girls" become unapproachable, and, at the same time, fear- and awe-inspiring mysterious beings.

It is all so new! A revolution is taking place within him. His own body is the stage for this great event. It is altogether most confusing. The male sex hormone has not yet been totally isolated. Since 1931, however, about thirty *androgenes*—i.e. substances which have an effect similar to that of the male hormone—have been prepared from male urine testis-tissue or manufactured synthetically. They are now used in treating various complaints both in men and in women, either as injections or by grafting, or by rubbing the product into the skin; also in some cases, as tablets. The best-known of them is *testosterone*.

91. Other Male Physical Sex Characteristics On a number of other physical points, whose connection with the sex glands cannot always be established directly, great differences exist between man and woman. For instance, in general body structure, dental structure, bone structure, hairiness, the chemical composition of the blood, etc. On pp. 15–31 you will find a survey of a series of physical differences between man and woman.

92. *Male Mental Sex Characteristics* A great many scientific attempts have been made to establish the particular male and female psychic sex characteristics. However, the investigations and research cannot be said to have brought any definitely valid results. One great difficulty tending to thwart such research is inherent in the fact that every individual from birth through childhood and adolescence is definitely influenced by innumerable social and sexual traditions.

In reality, modern psychology is inclined to take the view that most of the qualities formerly ascribed to psychic sex differences were simply due to the widely differing conditions in which the two sexes grow up, both in regard to general education and training, and especially in regard to sex morals. To this must be added the further source of error that no normal man or woman is capable of judging sex differences from a purely sexless standpoint.

93. *Variations in the Man's Sexual Development and Behavior* Finally, it should be emphasized initially here that within each sex there are enormously great variations in the sexual development and behavior. This has been documented by various authorities, as by the extensive research undertaken by Dr. Kinsey, the American professor of zoology. A relatively good conception of the sexual development is gained by examining the so-called *total outlet* of the individuals. The term total outlet means all forms of sexual activity resulting in an orgasm, that is to say, without ejaculation before puberty, and with ejaculation after puberty. It appears that about fourteen years is the average age for the first orgasm with ejaculation, and that 95 per cent of all men of this group have been sexually active at the age of fifteen. Those entering puberty early experience all through the life almost twice as high an average of total outlet as in the case of those with a slower development. As a rule, it is those with the higher intelligence who reach earliest the age of puberty. On an average, adult men have outlets total two or three times a week, but great variations exist in this area. For instance Kinsey reports the case of a physically healthy and normal man who for thirty years had only one ejaculation, while others had ten to

twenty ejaculations or more per week over a long period of years. The great width of variation thus indicated is essentially due to hereditary, psychological and social factors which will gradually be dealt with in detail in the following pages. Here it should only be mentioned that *infantilism* means that the individual, after the time when puberty normally occurs, remains at a partly childish, *infantile* stage which, amongst other things, is characterized by a more or less deficient development of the sex organs and the sex functions.

Chapter 8: FEMALE SEX CHARACTERISTICS

94. *Female Sex Characteristics*   These comprise: a. the special structure of the female sex organs; b. the activity of the ovaries as open glands, i.e. the ripening of the eggs, ovulation and its consequences; c. the activity of the ovaries as ductless glands, i.e. hormone-producing glands.

95. *The First Menstrual Flow, the Menarche*   The most definite sign that a girl has reached puberty is the onset of menstruation. This is a direct consequence of ovulation and the effects of the female sex hormone. Menstruation is such an important part of the female sex functions that it will be dealt with in a special chapter. The first menstrual flow is called the *menarche*.

96. *Female Hormonal Sex Characteristics*   It is the female sex hormone produced by the ovaries that transforms a girl into a woman. The budding awareness that the opposite sex arouses in her is an entirely new and bewildering interest which threatens to upset and completely revolutionize her former attitude. The change generally results in a certain *shyness*, which in this connection is usually called *modesty*, and only rarely does it result in the opposite sex. As in the case of the boy, the sex hormone also stimulates the development of the girl's sex organs. The outer labia generally grow fuller, more filled with blood, and pubic growth appears. It is characteristic that the pubes do not go further than just above the *mons veneris* where a rather sharp borderline is in evidence. The axillary hairs begin to grow in the armpits, the girl's figure becomes more rounded, soft lines and curves gradually predominating. This is actually caused—quite prosaically—by deposit of fatty tissue, but the forms show up as pleasing curves, firm, full hips, small softly-cupped breasts, round, narrow shoulders. No croaking voice, nor prickly mustache here. No, the girl is all soft and yielding; and all of this is due to the female sex hormone. This hormone originates in the follicles, and the term for it most often used currently is *estrin*.

In section 142 we shall consider a number of *estrogens,* meaning substances that produce the same effect as estrin. Those estrogens, which may be prepared synthetically, are hardly identical with the pure female sex hormones, but they are greatly employed for combating those ailments that are supposed to be caused by a deficiency of estrin. The ovaries produce yet another sex hormone, *progesterone* which, together with estrin, is a determining element in the normal development of a number of female sex characteristics. This will be described in greater detail in the next chapter. It is significant to note here, however, that supplementing the estrogens in the body with a supply from the outside seems to stimulate its secretion of progesterone.

97. *Other Physical Female Sex Characteristics* The female is generally smaller than the male. Her skin is softer, she has a clearer complexion, and altogether presents more extragenital physical characteristics.

98. *Female Mental Sex Characteristics* What was said about the male psychic sex characteristics as described in section 92, is true of the female too.

99. *Variations in the Woman's Sexual Development and Behavior* Just as in the male, the interplay of the many factors of a hereditary, psychological, and social nature, etc., in the woman is of such a complex and complicated nature that there necessarily must be great variations in the woman's sexual development and behavior. Also this will be gradually dealt with on the following pages. However, the research of the next years

will probably bring forward new views in this respect. In respect to female infantilism the facts stated about men under section 93 apply also to women.

Chapter 9: MENSTRUATION

100. *The Egg's Departure from the Ovary* Stimulated by the gonadotropins an egg ripens and emerges (one about every twenty-eight days) from one of the ovaries about midway between the menstrual periods. It is caught in one of the Fallopian tubes, and its transportation toward the uterus, helped along by the cilia in the interior of the tube, starts immediately. The passage through the tube takes about fourteen days. However, before the egg gets as far as that, several other things have taken place in various locations in the female organism.

101. *The Yellow Body (corpus luteum)* When the egg has left the follicle in the ovary, the follicle, stimulated by another gonadotropic hormone from the pituitary gland, the so-called *luteinizing hormone*, is transformed into what is called the *yellow body* or *corpus luteum*. This consists of cells, endocrine glandular cells containing a yellow pigment which starts secreting a hormone by the name of *progesterone* as soon as the egg has left the ovary. This hormone circulates in the blood stream and causes a number of changes.

For example, the hormone conveys a message to the mammary glands that an egg has emerged; that pregnancy may eventually occur; that the mammary glands, therefore, may have to deliver milk to a newborn baby in nine months, and so had better start right now making the necessary preparations. In this activation, which really causes certain tissue in the breasts to grow, estrin takes part. It is possible that the hypophyse also has some influence in this relation, but so far that point has not been fully clarified.

102. *The Uterus Prepares for Pregnancy* Both the ovarian hormones—estrin and progesterone—make their effect felt by the uterus. Its mucous membrane begins to develop; its muscular walls become thicker. More veins appear, and also more uterine glands. During this whole period the uterus is under the influence of a hormone from the intermediate and the posterior lobes of the pituitary gland. The function of this hormone is to make the uterus contract. This cannot be brought about, however, as long as the uterus is also under the influence of the progesterone; in other words, as long as the corpus luteum is at work. The uterus distends as it develops, and the many veins crisscrossing its surface form a regular system of canals. The underlying purpose of all this is to prepare the womb to receive the egg now on its way from the ovary toward the uterus, and which may be fertilized during its passage through the Fallopian tube.

Thus the womb prepares to shelter the embryo for eight to nine months, and to provide it with all the many different substances it needs for thriving and developing. And such a tiny egg, which in the course of only some months will become a small human being, makes very immoderate demands. The uterine cells literally go about building a little nest for the egg. The blood stream carries nourishment to the womb, sugar, protein, fat, salts, water, and vitamins. The uterine wall is used as a storeroom, and it cannot be too well stocked. There is a dearth of blood vessels to carry all these supplies; that is why it is necessary to build extra rails and sidetracks. There is a hammering and knocking, beating and thumping in the busy workshop day and night.

103. *The Egg Arrives Unfertilized in the Uterus*   All this activity goes on for about fourteen days. Then, suddenly, the progesterone fails to arrive. Corpus luteum has been waiting for a message—a hormone—from the egg that it has been fertilized. If this message is not delivered within fourteen or fifteen days, corpus luteum perishes, production of progesterone stops, and the unfertilized egg is left to shift for itself.

104. *Appearance of the Menstrual Flow*   The oxytocin, which during this time has directed its constant efforts at making the uterus contract, but was prevented by the progesterone from achieving this, now has a free rein. The uterine muscles, which in the past fortnight had grown considerably bigger and stronger,

therefore, suddenly contract. The veins burst, the accumulated cell tissue, all the material for the nest, a coating of uterine mucous membrane, blood, mucus, and the egg itself—the cause of the whole chain of creative events—are forced out of the womb through the vagina. It is this process that is called the menstruation, menses or monthly bleeding.

105. *Personal Hygiene During Menstruation* Of course, strict cleanliness is very important during menstruation. Only one generation back it was generally believed that a woman should not bathe her genitals during bleeding, because of the danger of abdominal inflammation. Nothing could be further from the truth. On the contrary, if partly dried blood particles are allowed to remain in the same place for several days they provide an excellent soil for the thriving of bacteria of various sorts which thereupon penetrate into the vagina and can cause abdominal inflammations. So it is important to know how to practice proper general hygiene during menstruation. Cold must be avoided, and sponging with cold water, therefore, is not recommended. But cleansing the genitals with tepid water is not only harmless, but directly helpful. During a menstrual period one may change one's underclothes as often as desired without any risk, provided they are sufficiently warm, dry, and, above all, *clean*. Warm underwear is recommended because regular pleasant warmth will often relieve the discomfort of menstruation. One should eat and drink as usual during menses. Since a woman menstruating is generally more tired than usual she needs extra sleep and rest at this time. In some cases sponging the skin around the genital organs with boiled water or a solution of borax, and powdering or rubbing the skin with a little oil or vaseline, is practical.

106. *Sanitary Napkins* These are generally used for the absorption of the menstruous blood. They must be changed frequently, *how* frequently is hard to say. It is certainly not possible to state any hard and fast rule, because the quantity of blood women lose differs in each individual, and it also depends upon how absorbent the sanitary napkins are. As a general rule, of course, as soon as the sanitary napkin begins to chafe, smell, or cause discomfort in some other way, it is time to change.

107. Other Methods of Absorbing the Menstruous Blood During the last days of menstruation when there is less bleeding, it is possible for a woman to be "safe" with just a small wad of cotton placed between the outer labia to absorb the small amount of blood still seeping out. But it is definitely objectionable to use this method from the outset. Cotton, inserted into the vagina or in the introitus between the inner labia will, if the bleeding is relatively plentiful, quickly absorb so much blood that it becomes like a firm, tight object blocking the regular flow of menstrual blood. Any drugstore can supply safe sanitary napkins as well as descriptive literature as to their use.

108. Intercourse During Menstruation While they menstruate some women feel a great sex urge and have a decided need for sexual intercourse at this time. In this connection it must be remembered that introducing the penis into the vagina really means introducing a foreign body with the attendant risk of bringing bacteria right up into the vagina and perhaps further on into the womb. However, these considerations that are often advanced in regard to intercourse during menstruation, seem to be of a rather theoretical nature.

At any rate, it is a fact that many women do have intercourse during their menstrual period, and apparently without any harmful consequences. The problem of sexual intercourse during menstruation will, therefore, if the desire is present, above all be a question of whether the partners themselves find it desirable or not, and that is a matter they must decide for themselves.

109. Douching After Menstruation When the menstrual flow has stopped completely, it is usual to take a cleansing douche with boiled water adding a weak borax or physiological salt-water solution. It may also be expedient to put a little lactic acid into the douche water. Two tablespoonfuls of ordinary granulated sugar and a teaspoonful of powdered borax dissolved in about two pints of boiled water may also be used.

110. *Normal Quantity and Duration of Menstrual Flow*
The quantity of menstrual bleedings vary widely in each individual woman. Some women only bleed for two or three days, and only very little; others may bleed for a week or more, often very copiously, particularly at the outset. It is not infrequent for a woman to have to change sanitary napkins six or eight times on the first day. On an average, the bleeding may be said to last for three to six days, most severe at the start, and gradually decreasing during the remaining days.

111. *Menstrual Irregularities: Dysmenorrhea* Dysmenorrhea actually means menstrual irregularity in general. Menstrual pains therefore only constitute one of the forms of dysmenorrhea. As every form of dysmenorrhea may be accompanied by some mental disturbance, though as a rule rather slight, it might be a good thing to supplement the treatment of the various individual forms of dysmenorrhea that we shall now look into with some measure of mental hygiene.

112. *Menstrual Pains* The violent uterine contractions on the first day of bleeding may cause menstrual pains. Many women may experience pains so severe that they must remain in bed. The appearance of the pains vary greatly in different women and at different times. They may set in before the bleeding occurs, or not start until bleeding commences. In some cases the pains come only every second or third time, or they may stay away if a change in living conditions has occurred in the meantime. In the case of office workers, for instance, they may stay away during vacations, and start again when the girls resume their regular work. In this respect mental factors play a certain part. We know, of course, that good tidings or temporary happy conditions may cause menstrual pains to disappear completely, whereas bad news or a crushing sorrow may make them more violent.

113. *Treatment of Menstrual Pains* In most cases the menstrual pains will disappear if a woolen article, a heating pad or something hot is put on the abdomen. The effect of most old household remedies is undoubtedly due to the feeling of warmth and comfort they bring.

114. Morphine Should Not Be Used   Some commercial tablets contain morphine. The use of them may be habit forming, wherefore they should be taken only under doctor's orders, and closely checked, the more so since there are other remedies for overcoming menstrual pains.

115. Medical Treatment of Unusually Severe Menstrual Pains   During the first few days of menstruation many women have to take some anetic (pain-allaying) or sedative tablets, to dull the pains sufficiently to be endured. In recent years, however, it has been found that hormone treatments with progesterone or with *estrogen* a few days prior to the expected menstrual period will often diminish the pains considerably.

116. Surgical Treatment of Acute Menstrual Pains   In many women who have not given birth the cervical canal of the uterus is so narrow that the passage of menstrual blood is accompanied by acute pains, particularly if there is excessive bleeding and if, at the same time, the cervical muscles contract convulsively. In such cases it is often possible to alleviate or avoid the pain by dilation of the cervical canal. That is done by means of the dilatators, smooth cylindrical instruments in a variety of sizes. To begin with, the smallest dilatator is placed for some minutes in the cervical canal; then follow the others, increasing in size, until the cervix has been sufficiently distended to permit the passage of the menstrual blood without difficulty. Many women get along with a dilatation like that two or three times a year. It can be done by any physician with surgical training, and it is virtually painless.

117. Irregular Bleedings   The term "irregular bleedings" may mean many different things. If the bleedings appear at the *normal time*, but are abnormally large or last an excessively long time, the condition is called *menorrhagia*. Bleedings at other times than at the normal menstrual period, and without connection with it, are called *metrorrhagia*, particularly if they have the character of a hemorrhage.

In more popular terminology "irregular bleedings" practically always refer to metrorrhagia. Such a condition always requires close attention. It is frequently the symptom of a beginning miscarriage, and, in a woman whose menstruations have ceased completely, a metrorrhagia may herald some serious abdominal illness. All this will be described later.

Sometimes the term "functional uterine bleeding" is used to describe a uterine bleeding that appears when no organic illness is present. But since it must be taken for granted that such a bleeding too is caused by a disturbance in some organ somewhere—perhaps far removed from the uterus—the term is unfortunate. We therefore suggest that until the cause of the bleeding has been established in each case, the term *cryptogenous* or *cryptogenetic uterine bleeding* (from the Greek *kryptos* (hidden) and *genesis* (origin) be used, thereby indicating that the real cause has not yet been discovered. As to treatment of irregular bleeding there is one general rule: Consult a doctor as soon as possible.

118. *Menstruation in Newborn Baby Girls* In rare cases bleeding through the vagina has been observed in newborn girls during the first couple of days after birth. This strange phenomenon frightens young mothers. Their fear, however, is entirely groundless. This is in reality an ordinary menstruation caused by hormones accumulated in the blood of the fetus immediately prior to birth; it lasts a few days and then stops spontaneously. The baby girl suffers no harm from it, and menstruation will not as a rule be observed in her until the time for its normal appearance comes.

119. *When the First Menstruation Is Slow in Coming* The first menstruation, the *menarche*, generally, in temperate zones, appears when the girl is about twelve to fourteen years of age, as mentioned above. In warmer climates it is apt to come earlier; in colder climates, somewhat later. However, even in temperate climates the appearance of the first menstruation is subject to rather wide variations. Many girls menstruate as early as eleven years of age, while on the other hand it is not rare to see a first menstruation delayed until the girl is sixteen or seventeen. Therefore, one may say that there is no cause for anxiety even if the girl gets to be near twenty before the first menstruation appears. Only if she has trouble or discomfort at regular monthly intervals without any bleeding is there any real reason to investigate the matter and see if an abnormal condition has developed.

120. *Too Frequent and Infrequent Menstrual Bleedings (Polymenorrhea and Oligomenorrhea)* As formerly indicated the general rule is for the menstrual flow to appear every twenty-eight days. This *menstrual cycle*, however, varies widely in different individuals. In some women menstruation comes punctually every three weeks, or at even shorter intervals. This frequent menstruation, as a rule, is called *polymenorrhea*. Other women menstruate every four or five weeks in which case the term is *oligomenorrhea*. Fundamentally, it is not possible to say that one cycle is more normal than the other. It may therefore be set down as a principle, that *if the menstrual flow appears at regular intervals it is normal*. If greater irregularities occur (such as delayed, or too early, appearance) of more than a few days this may be symptomatic of some pelvic disturbance, and a doctor should be consulted. It has often been observed that after childbirth the menstrual cycle changes permanently or temporarily. If, for instance, the cycle was four weeks before the woman gave birth, it may change to three weeks or so.

121. *Violent or Protracted Menstrual Flow* The quantity of blood as well as the duration of the menstrual flow may also be subject to wide individual variations, as also the quantity of blood discharged need not be the same in two consecutive months. A condition of unusually violent or unusually prolonged menstrual flow is called *hypermenorrhea*. A single occasion of violent or protracted bleeding is called a *menorrhagia*. A general guiding line for determining whether a menstrual flow is too large or too protracted is this: Does the woman feel tired after the blood has ceased to flow, and, especially, does it take some time for her to regain her strength? If she feels fit and has a sensation of her body being lighter than before the bleeding, all is well. But if she remains tired after an unusually copious menstrual flow this may be a warning that she suffers from some pelvic complaint which should be seen to by her physician.

122. *Too Limited Menstrual Flow (Hypomenorrhea)* If, at the time a normal menstruation is due, only a very small quantity of pale, hardly blood-colored discharge is secreted, that, generally, is a symptom that the woman is anemic or that her general health is debilitated. However, it may also indicate the presence of some atrophy, that the uterus or the ovaries are wasting away. It is, as a rule, combined with oligomenorrhea; and the treatment will depend upon the cause of the ailment.

123. *When Menstruation Does Not Appear at All (Amenorrhea)* Amenorrhea, or absence of menstruation, is a symptom that may be due to: a. hormone disturbances; b. mental causes; c. a change in manner of living, for instance, when a girl is studying hard for graduation, or during a vacation, or change of work or residence; d. anemia and other states of ill health; and of course, e. pregnancy. It is a peculiar fact that a woman's fear of an unwanted pregnancy and her idea that it may have come about, may be the cause for her missed menstruation. This would seem to document her erroneous supposition that she is pregnant. If the first menstruation, the menarche, has not appeared at all, the term *primary amenorrhea* is used; if menstruation ceases after having appeared normally for some time, it is called *secondary amenorrhea*. Formerly, amenorrhea was treated for a fortnight with an estrogenic preparation, and after that for seven days with progesterone. Better results are now being obtained by treating the condition with a compound of gonadotropins. It goes without saying, of course, that eventual anemia and other states of weak health must be treated separately. It is also of the greatest importance that possible deficiencies or errors in nutrition be corrected.

124. *Sudden Interruption of Menstruation (Suppressio Mensium)* A special form of amenorrhea is the so-called *suppressio mensium*, a sudden interruption of menstruation already started, or an absence of an expected menstrual flow which had given warning of its coming by premenstrual symptoms. This, as a rule, is caused by an acute inflammation of the genital organs, particularly of the womb, or by a sudden contraction of blood vessels brought about, for instance, by a too sudden and severe cooling off of the abdomen. More rarely, the cause will be of a more general nature, as for example, the effect of a violent emotional shock.

125. *Vicarious Bleeding (Menstruatio Vicaria)* Menstruatio vicaria means discharge of blood from other spots than the uterus, but correlated to the menstrual cycle. Such bleeding may either coincide with the normal menstruation or—more frequently—be a substitute for it. It may appear, for instance, as a nose bleed, which is the most common form, or by vomiting or spitting blood, bleeding from the gums or from the eye's conjunctiva; or, if the person has hemorrhoids, the blood may come from them. In some women it appears constantly, with the regularity of normal menstruation, in others only once, or a couple of times. Slight cases receive no treatment; more complicated cases should always be referred to a doctor, since the causes may be many and varied, and the cure must depend upon the origin of the ill.

126. *Be Chivalrous, Gentlemen!* I am most anxious to have my masculine readers understand what a real burden it is for a woman to endure the discomfort of menstruation every month from about her thirteenth to, approximately, her forty-fifth year. The only interruptions in this schedule are pregnancies and following periods of nursing her babies. It means that out of this whole period of about thirty years, she spends altogether five to six years in this way. She must wear a sanitary napkin in a most awkward place. The sanitary napkin may chafe and cause the greatest discomfort, and must be changed frequently in order to remain hygienic. No matter where she is she must manage this change, she must have clean sanitary napkins ready and must be able to get rid of the soiled ones. Moreover, she must develop the ability of standing the pain without showing it in any way. That is difficult since her ordinary powers of resistance are diminished as long as the menstrual flow lasts.

Physically she is more easily exhausted and much more susceptible to hardship, and probably also more receptive to infections than otherwise. Mentally and emotionally she is hypersensitive. She loses courage if she is rebuked, feels so very, very tired, yet generally carries on her work as usual. All this occurs almost one whole week out of every single month the year round. If she works behind a counter she must present the same smiling appearance for the customer. If she remains at home and looks after house and children she must receive her husband with the same graciousness and cheerfulness as ever when he comes home after his day's work. The man is spared all this, and it is up to him to show chivalry in this matter, and to remember that this process in the woman is very closely bound up with his own desire to become a father some day, or with his happiness at already being a father. Should a man ask a girl for a date and she declines, or she makes him feel that she would rather not go out, he ought to think that in one out of five cases she is menstruating and, still more frequently, about the fact that she is expecting "the curse" and therefore feels uneasy about going swimming or dancing, to the movies, or to some other place, or risk conditions in which she would find herself at an unpleasant disadvantage, if the menstrual flow should suddenly start. Do be chivalrous, gentlemen!

Chapter 10: THE MENOPAUSE

127. *Woman's Second Change of Life (the Menopause)* The menopause is a temporary state in a woman's life and reveals itself in a variety of ways, of which the definite cessation of menses is the most important, for it terminates the woman's function as a reproductive being. The so-called *artificial menopause* (which will be described later) brings about exactly the same result.

128. *The Menopause Is Not a "Dangerous" Age* Many young women feel some anxiety at the idea of the menopause because they have been told by the older generation what a very "dangerous" age it is. This expression "dangerous age" has no basis in fact, generally speaking. The menopause is a *normal* condition and, in its normal course, presents no feature more "dangerous" than the first change in female life, which was puberty. If, nevertheless, the menopause formerly to many women did become a "critical" period it was largely due to the fact that women's and—not least—men's knowledge of these things was quite limited. And it is now our task to aid in lifting this cover of ignorance and misunderstanding so those women facing menopause may be prepared for it and, if need be, take their precautions.

129. *A New Revolution—in the World of Hormones* First of all, the ovaries stop producing hormones; because of the close teamwork between the hormone-producing glands in the entire body, the hormone production of the pituitary gland, the thyroid, and the suprarenal glands as well, undergo certain changes. Every symptom connected in any way with the menopause may, in reality, be ascribed to modifications in the hormone production and the upsetting of the body's balance. In many ways this is similar to the state of puberty.

130. *When Does the Menopause Begin and How Long Does It Last?* No hard and fast rule can be given about the beginning of the menopause. As a general rule it may be said that the change of life begins when the woman is somewhere between forty-five and fifty. But a great many variations occur. In some women the menopause begins—or rather faint symptoms of it, without any actual menopause—already in their thirties. In others, the change does not start until they are in their fifties. Well-known gynecologists firmly maintain that the earlier menstruation began in the young girl the longer it will continue, and *vice versa,* the later it started, the earlier it ceases. However, there are many exceptions to this rule.

As to how long the change of life lasts, there is also no definite answer. Some women (however, they are in the minority) only experience a few hot flushes in connection with the rather sudden cessation of their menstruation, and that constitutes *their* change of life. However, in most women menstruation ceases gradually, over a period of one to three years, possibly characterized by more or less pronounced "change-of-life" symptoms. Some women, however, have to stand these discomforts for a protracted number of years.

131. *Classification of Symptoms of the Menopause* The symptoms that, along with the gradual cessation of menstruation, are present during those years of change of life should properly be listed as symptoms of hormone disturbances and are of a physical as well as of a psychological nature.

132. *Onset of Change of Life, the Climacteric Period* In many cases the ovaries increase their function as *endocrine glands* which means that they will produce more hormones than normally. This occurs simultaneously with curtailment of their activity as *open glands,* i.e. as dischargers of eggs. The previously mentioned effects of female sex hormones may then sometimes become very pronounced. At this stage of the climacteric period the woman may feel more of a *woman* than ever before. Often she feels much more violently attracted to the opposite sex than she ever imagined possible even in her most abandoned dreams. This attraction *may* show up as a restless chasing after sexually exciting interludes, to such an extent that it sometimes takes on the character of a panic. The German expression *Torschlusspanik* (panic at the closing of the gates) aptly describes this condition which to a great extent is responsible for the change of life being called "the dangerous age."

133. *Torschlusspanik* This refers to the panic that seizes some people when they want to get in or out a door and suddenly find it closed. The term is a very striking one. The woman realizes that her days as a female in the most closely defined sense of the word, are on the wane. While they lasted she was aware of the power a younger or a mature woman wields over men—as the *masculine* sex. She has enjoyed her own victories and perhaps used her influence. She now fears being dethroned, and the jealousy with which she watches every least step of her husband often makes a wife's change of life a real burden to him too. She accuses him of eying women in the street, of having clandestine affairs, and so on.

134. *The Production of Female Sex Hormones Diminishes*
The aforementioned state of accelerated production of sex hormones in a woman's climacteric period is rarely of long duration. It is only temporary, and is followed by the opposite: greatly diminished hormone production. And then appear a number of symptoms pointing to the disappearance of the hormone in question, and with them the disappearance of some of the typically female characteristics.

135. *Cessation of Menstruation* Menstruation occurs at longer intervals. From five to eight weeks or more may now elapse between two menses, eventually interspersed with periods in which the menstrual flow appears at shorter intervals. But gradually the woman stops menstruating altogether. Simultaneously with the menses becoming more and more rare, they also, as a rule, decrease in amount. If, formerly, a woman bled for four or five days, soon she will bleed for only two or three days, then only for one day, less and less, until complete cessation.

136. *Changes in the Genital Organs* That the bleeding stops is due to changes in the ovarian functions. By and by the walls of the uterus grow thinner; its lining of mucous membrane shrinks, and the uterine neck grows smaller, hardly protruding into the vagina any more. The vaginal walls generally shrink a little too, and become more smooth. Sometimes, at the onset of the change of life a discharge may appear, accompanied by a most unpleasant itching. The external genitals, as a rule also shrink somewhat, as the fatty tissue of the *labia majora* has a tendency to break down. Very troublesome itching in the vulva is often a sign of the approach of the menopause.

137. *Tendency to Obesity* The attractive distribution of those plump charms, formerly so pleasing, changes. These charms develop a tendency to spread. The lady gets a "tummy" or "spare tires" when she is unable to keep her weight down. But her full cheeks are getting peaked, and often vanish. To counteract this tendency, a woman must be careful not to eat too much and see to it that she gets plenty of exercise. In recent years these measures are often being supplemented by treatments with thyroxin preparations. *But beware;* such treatments should be used only under a doctor's care and supervision.

138. *Changes in the Organism Have a Masculine Trend* During the change of life a woman's whole appearance may get a masculine touch. The hair, woman's crowning glory, may show a tendency to fall out. But, simultaneously, a tiny mustache may sprout and shade the upper lip—particularly in dark women. The voice often gets deeper and somewhat husky.

139. *Hot Flushes, Perspiring, etc.* The familiar classical symptoms—in addition to the menopause proper—are: sudden hot flushes, excessive perspiring, unexpected blushing, palpitations of the heart, restlessness, feelings of "pins and needles" in fingers and toes, and spells of dizziness. All these may come on suddenly and disappear just as suddenly. The symptoms signify a lack of balance in the nervous system. After the favorable results of hormone treatments registered in recent years in combating these symptoms one is entitled to draw the conclusion that this upset in the nervous equilibrium is hormonal in origin.

140. *Character Changes* Emotional changes in woman at the change of life are not nearly as widespread as people generally imagine. Real mental illnesses (insanity) seldom occur. It is mostly a question of more or less temporary changes in character. During her change of life a woman often becomes irritable, and may take trifles far more seriously to heart than one would expect in view of her age and judgment. Her enthusiasm may also be quickly aroused, and may vanish just as promptly. She may laugh easily and her tears, in particular, come at the slightest provocation. The main character symptom of her condition is a lack of former balance. In that respect, the climacteric period recalls the state of puberty, so there would seem to be some justification for making a direct comparison between these two great changes in a woman's life, also in regard to their psychological aspects.

141. *Treatment of the Menopause Troubles* Sometimes the changes in character take root before the physician is consulted. They have come to stay. In those cases there may be some basis for some type of psychotherapy. Another, often supplementary, treatment consists in giving the organism a proper dose of *estrogen* to make up for a deficiency in *estrin*.

142. *Hormone Treatment with Estrogens* We shall here mention the most important of the estrogens that may be used in such hormone treatment. The first estrogen that was prepared in a state of purity was estrin. This substance is present in great quantity in the urine of pregnant women from which it was first isolated. Great quantities of it are also present, but in modified form, in the urine of mares with foals. The manufacture of estrin, known since 1929, is now based on such urine. Another estrogen, *estradiol*, extracted in various forms from the ovaries of pigs, from human placenta, from the testes of stallions and the urine of pregnant women and mares with foals, produce a much stronger estrogen effect than estrin, and may possibly be a purer form of it. On the other hand, we have a weaker edition of estrin in the closely related *estriol*, that may be extracted from human placenta and from the urine of pregnant women.

As a matter of fact, estrogens appear rather prolifically in nature. Estrin in its pure state is produced from palm kernels. A most important development has been the synthetic production, since 1939, of estrogens. Collectively such synthetic estrogens are called *estrols*, and are widely employed. Estrogens are administered as injections, as suppositories, in drops or tablets, or as an ointment to be rubbed into the skin. The effect of these preparations is often remarkably successful, but in other cases only poor results are obtained, and in this connection it should be emphasized that they are dangerous if used indiscriminately over long periods for which reason the treatment must be under a doctor's careful supervision.

143. *She May Not Feel Anything at All* I should like very much to point out that there are many women to whom the foregoing carries no message, because they had practically no trouble with their change of life. In those cases menses diminish very gradually, both in quantity and frequency, "hot flushes," perspiration, itching, mustache, obesity, and irritability are happily

absent. And these women tranquilly make the transition into the period which, with a term derived from the Latin word *post* ("after"), we call the postclimacteric period.

144. *The Postclimacteric Period*   When once she has the change of life well behind her, many a woman feels better than she ever did when she was capable of menstruating. She has now reached a more relaxed period of her life. It is true that this period requires some resignation in many women, but in others it proves to offer many chances for personal development they had never before thought of taking up.

145. *Sex Needs After the Change of Life*   Even among sensible, grown-up persons there is a very widespread, but quite mistaken, belief that sexual desire or the needs of a sex life disappear after the menopause. As for women who have loved their husbands body and soul during a long marriage, the sexual need will hardly be affected at all. The two of them, husband and wife, will be able to enjoy many fine years of happy sex life together. And they need no longer have any anxiety that the wife may conceive, an anxiety which in the years preceding the menopause could interfere a good deal with their sexual union. There have been examples cited by authorities of how the sex urge may last up to a woman's old age. In one case a widow seventy years old who married again twenty years after her menopause found her need as well as her capacity for enjoyment as great as before.

146. *Bleeding in the Postclimacteric Period*   Menstrual irregularities during the period that the change of life is in progress need not cause any anxiety, if these irregularities are limited to menstruations growing less frequent and plentiful. However, one must be most vigilant about bleeding that takes place after the definite cessation of menstruation. If the woman takes some hormone preparations which many women do to prolong their youth to some extent, by taking too big doses she may risk the continuation of her bleedings. Thus such bleedings may be due to the preparation but this is by no means always the case. In many instances bleedings in the postclimacteric period will be a symptom of some abdominal ailment and may be the first and only sign of cancer. It is, therefore, extremely important that a woman who bleeds after her regular menstruation has stopped immediately consult her doctor and submit to a *gynecological examination*. This type of an examination is an investigation of the external and internal genitals (the latter to be observed through the vagina) to find out whether their appearance is normal and whether they feel normal to the touch.

147. *Men Have No Regular Change of Life—Still . . .*
In the male there is no definite period corresponding to the change of life in woman when hormone production affecting the reproductive capacity ceases or diminishes. A man may, in fact, continue to beget children until far up in his old age. However, a number of characteristic symptoms common to most men often make their appearance, pointing to a *pseudo-change of life* which in frequent instances may be favorably affected by a hormone treatment, and for this very reason proves to be something in the direction of a change of life. The woman who is undergoing her own change of life ought to pay attention to these male symptoms because her understanding is so badly needed. Just at the time the woman's change of life sets in, when she is approaching her fifties, many men begin to fall off a bit, they are no longer up to par. It dawns on them that they haven't at all realized those dreams they cherished in their youth. And, still worse, perhaps it may become clear to them that they will never realize them. Rheumatism, a feeling of fatigue, lack of pep, too high blood pressure may irk them. A man also finds that he can not stand as much as formerly. He may no longer be in the forefront where his work is concerned, he sees how younger men are being preferred. All this, and a lot more, make him feel lonely and depressed and he suddenly realizes that what he needs is nothing less than *a friend*. His lack of psychological balance that at least to a certain extent must be regarded as due to certain modifications in the nervous system may require some sort of real psychotherapy. But the very best cure for him often proves to be the friendship of an understanding wife.

4

SEXUAL NEED OR SEX URGE

Chapter 11: THE NEED OF THE ORGANISM

148. *On Balance and Lack of Balance*   It has been clearly demonstrated in a variety of ways that a general striving to gain and maintain balance is a basic law of nature. Its manifestations can be found in everyday life, as well as what is encountered in the complicated work of atomic scientists. Stated in the more involved scientific manner: Every phenomenon in the universe is subject to what is called the law of equilibration or the law of tending toward a balance. According to this law, every need is the expression of a momentary lack of balance, and every process or activity is a striving to re-establish balance. Thus a need consists of latent or potential energy. And a process or activity exists in different forms of motor or kinetic energy. Stated most simply then, potential energy manifests itself as a need and kinetic energy manifests itself as a process or activity. Therefore, in the human body such interactive functions act to regulate the heartbeat, respiration, secretion of glands, the activity of the nerves, and all other functions in the organism including the mental or psychological ones. The balance in that case is called the *biological equilibrium* or *homeostasis*.

149. *What Is a Need?*   It has just been explained that a "need" means tied-up, potential energy in a system that corresponds to a lack of balance in that system, as in the organism of the human body, for instance. Over the years this potential energy when referred to in relation to a living organism has been given many different names, such as impulse, drive, urge, instinct, tendency, or inclination, etc. The term most frequently employed at the present time is *need*. We talk of a need of emptying our bowels, a need of having children instead of mother instinct, need of survival instead of urge for survival, sex need in preference to sex urge, etc.

Some needs are *complex needs* composed of several *separate needs*. For instance, the need of survival consists partly of a number of physical needs or so-called visceral needs, deriving their name from being related to various internal organs (the Latin word for entrails being *viscera*). Thus, there is the need of food, and of liquids, the need of air. On the other hand, the need of survival consists of *psychological* or *mental needs*, such as the need of knowledge, of judgment, of justification, and the need of possessing something, of self-assertion, of security, etc.

Some of these needs may be further subdivided: the need of food, for instance, may be specified as need of carbohydrates, salt, vitamins, etc.; and the need of salt, may be specified still further as ordinary salt (sodium chloride), copper salt, iron salt, etc.; and the need of vitamins, in A, B_1 and B_2.

The means by which needs are satisfied are called *satisfactors*. For instance, the need, *hunger*, will excite processes such as seeking food, eating and digesting it until the hunger with the food as "satisfactor" has been stilled. Persons, objects, events, and ideas may be "satisfactors"; the person, object, etc., that does *not* satisfy a need might be called a *dis-satisfactor* of the need in question.

Moreover, some needs which cannot be satisfied in the world of reality may obtain a measure of gratification in the realm of imagination. The gratification which such *inhibited needs* obtain is one of the basic reasons for the success of most romantic novels, motion pictures, and plays. In the field of sex they influence the so-called erotic daydreaming and, also, to a certain extent, masturbation.

150. *The Nervous Systems of the Organism* The various needs that jointly make up the sexual need are intimately linked to processes in the nervous systems of the human body—this need, our particular subject, will be dealt with in the following chapters. In order better to understand the next few chapters a certain knowledge of the nervous system is requisite.

It is a generally known fact that the cerebrum, which is the seat of consciousness, receives by way of the ordinary nerves —the so-called *sensory* nerves—sensory impressions resulting from seeing, hearing, smelling, tasting, and impressions of touch, pain, heat, cold, etc., by means of the eyes and ears, the nose, tongue, skin, etc. It is not, however, a matter of general knowledge that the cerebrum is also connected via subsidiary brain centers with two special nervous systems (basic divisions of the entire nervous system) that regulate a great many of the so-called *vegetative functions*, i.e. functions, particularly in the internal organs, necessary for the normal thriving and growth of the organism. These two nervous systems, the joint name of which is the *vegetative nervous system*, are the *sympathetic nervous system* and the *autonomic nervous system*, and both of them influence (*innervate*, as it is called) to a great extent the *same* internal organs, but in absolutely opposite ways.

Their effect on the organs corresponds closely to the effect of certain hormones in the body, and for that reason it must be concluded that the hormones in question work through the instrumentality of either the sympathetic or the para-sympathetic nervous system. Actually, both of these systems are *autonomous* or self-governing. They are able to activate vegetative functions such as, secretion of saliva, peristaltic movements, chemical transformation of foods, and they are also capable of influencing the heartbeat and the respiration, *without the aid* of the consciousness or the will. However, they are widely connected with the so-called *somatic nervous system* under which the *sensory nerves* mentioned above belong as they are also connected with the *motor nerves*, which are designed to excite the motor muscles in the trunk and the extremities. Through certain subsidiary brain centers the vegetative nervous system is also in direct connection with the cerebrum. This means, that the cerebrum, which represents our consciousness, receives information about a number of vegetative processes. Consequently, it is able to influence them through influencing the vegetative nervous system.

For instance, it is possible to exercise will power to keep urinating under control; the same applies to evacuating of feces. One also may consciously stop breathing at least for a while. Moreover, it is a well-known phenomenon that the heartbeat may be accelerated by concentrating on it.

Since the interplay of the sympathetic and para-sympathetic nervous systems definitely influences the feelings of an individual, in regard to exciting them in the first place, and influencing their further course (a matter which will be described in greater detail), it is best to pause a moment to look into the separate functions of these two nervous systems in particular.

151. *The Vegetative Nervous System*   The autonomic nervous system capable of being influenced by the hypophysis-hormone *pituitrin* has charge of a mainly constructive activity in the organism, the activity of *assimilation*. When a person is resting, or asleep, it is principally this nervous system that functions. In this condition the pupils contract, the heartbeats slow down, the delicate blood vessels relax, the activity of the digestive tract increases, the secretion of sweat decreases, sugar is stocked in the sugar storeroom of the liver, and there is a mounting activity of the saliva glands and other glands busy with the digestive function. A point, especially pertinent to our subject here, is this that a number of delicate muscles in and around the genital organs relax, among others in the erectile tissues; this may bring about erection as described in sections 39 and 75.

In contrast to this autonomic nervous system, the sympathetic nervous system acts mainly as a destructive or *dissimilating* agent in the organism. When this nervous system enters into action a great variety of things take place. The pupils dilate; perspiration increases; the heart beats quicker; the bronchies whose task it is to supply air, with its contents of oxygen, to the lungs, dilate; the delicate blood vessels contract; the tiny muscles which cause the hair to stand on end on one's head and elsewhere, also contract; the activity of the digestive tube diminishes. More *adrenalin* is secreted from the suprarenal glands and sugar is released from the sugar stock in the liver so as to be available for the increased combustion processes in the muscular tissue, etc. In brief, the organism is getting out of balance.

The function of the *sympathetic system* seems to be to prepare the organism for battle. This system puts it in fighting condition by cutting the flow of blood to the digestive organs to some extent. In compensation, the activity of the heart, lungs, and brain increases and the muscles receive an added supply of sugar to facilitate increased muscle activity. If greater pressure or activation is brought to bear on the organism through the sympathetic nervous system, the result may be copious perspiring, staring, glazed eyes, goose pimples, or hair "standing on end."

Chapter 12: DIFFERENT CONCEPTIONS OF SEX NEED

152. What Is Sex Need? The normal sex need or urge has been defined partly as the urge of an individual of one sex to achieve sexual union with an individual of the opposite sex, and partly as the drive or need for survival of the species. It is, therefore, together with the individual need of survival, the strongest urge in nature. However, neither of these definitions reveals anything about the deeper quality and contents of this strong need. As a result, through the years, a great many scientists have investigated the matter with a view toward exploring and elucidating these provisional definitions further.

153. The Theory of the Need of Reproduction It would seem rather natural to regard the sex need as purely a need for reproduction, the urge of an individual to live on in another being beyond the span of his natural life. And in former days this old theory was strongly held by well-known scientists.

One of the arguments *in favor of the theory* is this: The reproductive need, like the need for survival in all living beings, is a necessary condition for the continuation of life. In other words, it is a primitive, deeply-rooted quality inherent in life, like eating, drinking, breathing, moving about, and registering impressions. The reproductive need, as defined above, is present in all living beings. It is found even in the protozoa, one-cell organisms which would seem to be a direct indication that the reproductive need is a quality inherent in the very nature of the cells and in their mysterious structure as yet insufficiently investigated.

The main point *against the theory* is this: Although most men want to procreate, the need for reproduction is regarded as more specifically a female characteristic. It is a fact that a woman may yearn for a child of her own without feeling any desire for a sexual partner. That would seem to indicate that the female reproductive urge, or need of children, is not tied to the sexual need if, by that term, we mean the urge or need to achieve sexual union with a person of the opposite sex. The mother instinct is roused, but the sexual instinct may still be dormant. Another sign that might indicate the divorce of the mother instinct from sexual desire is this: In women with a strong maternal instinct, it is a fact that while their sexual passion is at its height, thoughts of a possible child generally are relegated to the background. Furthermore, it is a fact, that many persons state openly they do not desire children. Finally, it appears, that parents who have adopted children often consider they have paid a fully valid tribute to the need for survival of the species in raising children born by others.

A modern evaluation of the need for reproduction should run somewhat like this: From a purely biological point of view the very fact that the male organism secretes special sex cells, the spermatozoa, destined for the reproduction of the species, and the female organism, on its part, produces the egg cells, must be considered as *one* manifestation that the human species has a need of reproducing itself. *Another* manifestation pointing in the same direction, is the sexual need, defined as the urge or need of an individual of one sex to achieve sexual union with an individual of the opposite sex. Consequently, the sexual need and the reproductive need are not *identical*. From the point of view of the species the sexual need is a *link* in the chain of the reproductive need. From the point of view of the individual, the reproductive need in *some* persons may be a part of the individual sexual need. But in *other* persons it is not necessarily so. This must be taken into consideration when looking at the final definition of what sexual need is.

154. *The Theory of Evacuation* Another theory advanced is that sexual need was a need of evacuation. The genitals become engorged with sex fluids, the evacuation or discharging of which generated those pleasurable sensations that were the essential purpose of the sex urge.

This theory is an ancient one. According to Havelock Ellis, medieval ascetics called woman "a temple built over a sewer." In France, a brothel is sometimes referred to as *La Cloaque* (the sewer), and Michel de Montaigne wrote: "When all is said and done, I find that Venus is nothing more than the pleasurable excitement obtained by evacuating our vessels, just as Nature makes evacuation of other parts a pleasure." Martin Luther often compared sexual desire to the need for urinating and said that to marry was as necessary as to urinate.

As it gradually became clear that woman does not give off (evacuate) any essential substance during intercourse, this theory, to be valid, had to limit its application principally to the male. However, in order not to exclude the female completely from this theory, attention has been called to the fact that a mother often experiences a pleasant feeling of relaxation when she nurses her baby. In advancing this thesis, however, the theoretical men entirely overlooked the fact that mother's milk would then have to be considered as one of the sex fluids. And that would definitely conflict with the general concept of what a sex fluid consists of.

Experience proves, however, that in many men the sexual desire *after* evacuation of their seminal fluid may be just as strong as *before*. Furthermore, though woman does not, as we just mentioned, give off any special substance during intercourse she is capable of feeling an extremely strong sex need. From study of fishes we know that in spite of the fact that male and female fish discharge their sperm and eggs directly into the water, the two partners endeavor to get as close to each other as possible during the period in which they evacuate their sex substance. In frogs there is a very lengthy and quite definite attempt at contact between the male and the female during the sexual act, to such degree that this act is called "the clasping process."

The concept that sex need is purely a need of evacuation does not tally with the facts currently being revealed. On the other hand, the latest results of research on the whole matter of sex need provide evidence for the conclusion that the evacuation need represents an essential part of the total sexual need in the male, as we shall see later. Consequently, the evacuation need must be taken into consideration when we come to the final definition of the human sexual need.

155. *Passive and Active Sex Need*   What makes it so difficult to give an over-all valid presentation of the various needs that jointly constitute the sex need is that the whole thing is variable. It is not an absolute quantity. Apparently, the sexual need of a young man not in love with any one in particular, differs greatly from that of the lover immediately before, during, and after sexual intercourse. And at almost every phase of sex need there is a definite difference between the male and the female sex needs.

Since, however, the sex need shows up so differently depending upon whether it is a latent, rather passive state, directed on a person of the opposite sex, or whether it more demandingly and actively clamors for direct satisfaction through sexual intercourse, I shall choose first in the following sections to describe *the passive (latent) sex need* after a few analogies taken from the manifestations of *the sex need in animals*. Next, I shall describe *the active sex need* and conclude with a more detailed characterization of some special peculiarities about the female sex need, after having presented a final definition of sex need as such.

Chapter 13: PASSIVE SEX NEED

156. *A Fundamental Difference between the Male and the Female Sex Cells*   Before we can make a final attempt at characterizing the sex need as such, there still remain several questions to be considered. First, there is the fact that a peculiar difference exists between the man's spermatozoa capable of fertilizing an egg, and the woman's egg cell ripe for being fertilized, compared with the other cells in the male and female body.

Right up to the very moment of fertilization the female egg cell *in regard to chromosomes* has exactly the same structure as the other cells in the body. That is not the case with the male spermatozoon, for it differs from the other cells as to chromosome composition. It could be concluded, therefore, that the fully developed sperm cells in the male could be regarded as foreign bodies which the organism will strive to get rid of, just as it always endeavors to get rid of any foreign matter. If that is a correct conclusion we have here a fact to explain why the sex need in the male, and exclusively in the male, comprises a genuine need of evacuation conditioned by a real physical lack of balance. This in turn might be considered the reason why men need not be sexually awakened, but have a direct primitive need of evacuating their seminal fluid from early youth. Such a conclusion indicates, therefore, that it is entirely natural for the man to take the initiative in the matter of intercourse.

157. *Sex Hormones and Sex Need* At puberty the sex hormones cause the genital organs in both sexes to develop and the entire organism becomes conditioned toward the opposite sex. It takes place in the following manner: An individual's own sex characteristic develops as a result of the teamwork between many hormones, some of which appear only at the approach of puberty. This transformation is accompanied by the rather fundamental need of comparison and appraisal already present in the child. Thus the individual's interest in the corresponding, though different, development of sex characteristics in the opposite sex. Furthermore, the sex hormones, either by activating the genital organs directly, or via the vegetative nervous system, set off the production of sperm and the ripening of eggs with ensuing ovulation. This creative activity brings about a state of fluctuation, a balance and lack of balance, in the sex organs. The cerebrum is kept informed of this ebb and flow that consequently makes a strong imprint on the individual's consciousness.

In the male, the upsurge of sex activity is evidenced by erection and spontaneous evacuation of seminal fluid and pollutions, both manifestations that are set going directly from the nerve centers in the vegetative nervous system. This shows that in the male there exists a real need of discharge, determined by purely hormonal factors. This need is present from the onset of puberty. Anything analogous to that can hardly be said to exist in the female. Only about 20 per cent of women indicate having noticed any fluctuations in their sex feelings, and scarcely more than half of this group state that their sex urge is greatest immediately before and after menstruation, i.e. at a time when the production of sex hormones would seem to be particularly prolific. However, more recent experiments in hormone research have established that by injecting estrogens in certain female animals, and progesterone in others, it is possible to awaken a desire for mating, that is, a sexual need that shows up in the animals as *heat*. This must be regarded as evidence that sex hormones constitute a definite factor in the basic sex needs of the animals in question. In this connection it should be mentioned that by giving women estrogen injections it is possible to bring about marked changes in the vaginal mucous membrane. However, we possess no certain evidence as to whether or not these changes are accompanied by special fluctuations in the sexual needs of these women.

Altogether, it is hard to gather reliable data about sexual fluctuations in women because such fluctuations are not, as in the case of animals, accompanied by visible, objective symptoms. That means that we have only the women's own, generally vague, descriptions on which to base our opinions in that respect.

Some women—rather few, it must be admitted—nevertheless indicate a rise in their sex urge in connection with menstruating. Several possible explanations have been advanced for this. One authority has concluded that the prominent place menstruation holds in the minds of women might cause them to put a special interpretation on other events of a sexually tinged nature. Another authority believes that the increased sex need could be explained perhaps as a more urgent need for tender care due to the physical and psychic lack of balance characteristic of menstruation. Personally, I believe that the phenomenon—at least in the case of women who have experienced an orgasm—finds its explanation in the swelling of the genital organs during menstruating. The woman interprets this as a tumescence with its attendant urge for detumescence that constitutes an essential component of the sex need. At the same time I am of the opinion that the significance of the above-mentioned psychic elements is basic, precisely because the emotions hold the most prominent place in the yearnings characteristic of the passive sex need, as shall be considered in the following section.

158. *What Are Emotions?* The history of psychology indicates that psychologists throughout the centuries have had to admit their complete ignorance as to the real nature of *emotions*, what they are, how they originate. Scientists have had to be contented with describing them and otherwise explained them as processes in the consciousness more particularly characterized by a number of physical reactions caused, it was believed, by the emotions.

However, in the middle nineteenth century the famous American physiologist, psychologist, and philosopher, William James, and the Dane, Carl Lange, almost simultaneously but independently of one another, advanced the hypothesis that emotions are not the cause of physical phenomena. On the contrary, they considered that *the physical phenomena cause the emotions.* As James wrote: "We feel sad because we weep; angry because we strike blows; fearful because we tremble."

The emotions are linked to fluctuations in those organs that are connected by nerves to the vegetative nervous system. Fluctuations dependent upon the *para-sympathetic system* are accompanied by the so-called pleasurable emotions or *feelings of well-being,* whereas physical changes linked with the *sympathetic nervous system* incite un-pleasurable feelings or *feelings of discomfort.*

When we recall what was said about balance and lack of balance in the organism and the explanations of the connection between the vegetative nervous systems and the cerebrum, the seat of consciousness, we are able to formulate the following summary: *Emotions are the conception by consciousness of the momentary balance or lack of balance in the organism. A state of balance is always accompanied by a feeling of pleasure or well-being. A state of lost balance in the organism represents an un-satisfied need, and is accompanied by a feeling of restlessness and discomfort.* Need of food produces a feeling of hunger—not the opposite cause and effect relation. Need of flight produces fear—not the other way round, and so on. A state of lost balance which is equivalent to a need (the definite nature of which the consciousness does not know and cannot define) brings about a vague feeling of discomfort. Thus one says he "feels uncomfortable" or "out of sorts."

159. *Origin of Likes and Dislikes* I have regarded it quite important to give a detailed description of how individual feelings of well-being or the opposite based on purely biological processes in the body originate. Such consideration is, in my estimation, essential, for these feelings, purely as a matter of habit reaching back to early childhood, have a marked tendency to team up with sensory impressions in the cerebrum, impressions and ideas of external objects and interior imaginings. It is by this means that the feeling of well-being or the opposite, is transferred to the person, object, idea, etc., thus sensed, in the guise of likes, or dislikes. Such a feeling or emotion directed toward an object or a person is called a *sentiment*.

160. *Development of the Feeling of Preferences or Likes in Childhood* From the very earliest days of childhood a number of feelings of likes and dislikes are in the process of formation. The first of them seems to be connected with the feeding and the movements of the infant. The pleasure it feels at the fulfillment of the body's need for nourishment creates sympathy for the mother's milk, and the discomfort of finding an obstacle to the need of kicking and moving, makes the baby feel dislike for the blanket the moment it finds out that it is the blanket that blocks its movements. It is characteristic in this respect that the feelings accompanying the satisfaction of a need, respectively its failing to be satisfied, are not only linked to the "satisfactors," respectively the "dis-satisfactors" proper, but also to the persons, objects, etc., who provide them. Thus, the baby's fondness for the mother's milk is quickly transferred to the mother who might be called a "conditional satisfactor." just as a person who repeatedly gives a dog a stone instead of the bone it expects very soon will come to be regarded as a decided dis-satisfactor as far as the dog's need of a bone is concerned. In that way the person becomes the object of the dog's dislike.

As the great variety of needs arise during childhood, and as they are satisfied or frustrated, the child creates in its own mind a mass of complexes. His needs are satisfied or frustrated almost always through the action of grownups who, in the eyes of the child, possess unlimited means of providing for its needs—which is correct to a great extent—or the grownups themselves are the satisfactors of these needs. In effect, this means that the different feelings of complexes and the opposite in the child become tied to quite distinct ideas and notions so that a certain behavior in its environment arouses the child's likes or dislikes as the case may be. It is with this background the child enters upon puberty.

161. *Likes as Sentiments Developed During Puberty* The greatly increased hormone production in puberty is the cause of many and changing states of unbalance in the vegetative nervous system. These states of disturbed equilibrium bring about a state of unbalance in the brain too, and in the *somatic nervous system* that show up in different ways. We are familiar with very young persons' physical restlessness. They can't keep still, must always be on the move—that may account for some of the popularity of jitterbugging, competitive, different sport forms, and other tiring exercise they love at that period. It could be called a motor-need. So-called mental needs also appear: need of self-assertion, of security, of help, care, entertainment, a religious need, etc. To these belongs also the need of being with others, or the urge young people often feel in the opposite sense, as desiring to avoid company, and show a most peculiar love of contradiction incomprehensible to their surroundings and most of all to the parents "who can't make him out at all any more."

All this is the young person's way of expressing his consciousness of the Ego, refusing to acknowledge the new need, as we shall explain later. Furthermore, as a rule at this period one or more strongly individual needs, the existence of which the person so far has not been aware of himself, begin to become *conscious* needs. One becomes aware that one prefers the company of a certain type. This selection of type is generally based upon impressions from one's childhood of persons whom one was particularly fond of or particularly liked to be together with and is frequently, to an amazing degree, determined by outward things.

A beloved schoolteacher who perhaps wears uniquely shaped, gold-rimmed spectacles may throughout one's life leave an immediately *potential liking* for *all* persons who wear gold-rimmed spectacles of the same or similar shape. And in the same way, the hair or tone of voice of a mother or a nurse, an uncle's familiar figure, the supercilious manners of an admired playmate, etc., etc., may pay a decisive contribution toward molding one's favorite type.

Should a person of one of those types meet another person who proves to be a "satisfactor" of one, or better still, more of these needs, the body's state of defense will relax, and those needs that are as yet unsatisfied become less urgent in the calmer and more pleasurable state of mind now obtaining. The other person, therefore, seems to be a "satisfactor" of even more needs than are involved originally, and the organism gets more and more relaxed. The feeling of well-being thus registered by the consciousness is directly transferred to the other person as a strong current of sympathy.

Later, the mere thought of that person may be enough to produce a pleasant feeling. This reaction, in turn, through the influence of the brain on the vegetative nervous system, may react back on the organism which snaps into balance. That would mean that the very strongly anchored form of attraction that is one of the chief characteristics of being in love, has now originated in the mind.

162. *Being in Love*   Being in love is, generally speaking, a condition having something in common with being seasick. Both conditions can be regarded as quite serious only by the victim and possibly by former victims similarly smitten. In others, who are not directly involved, it seems to call forth a certain spirit of teasing. Being in love, then, is actually a pure manifestation of *feeling*, a feeling expression of liking for another to unlimited and overflowing degree. Therefore, the psychological sign of being in love is the immense intensification of the influence radiating from the beloved. In all this extravagant feeling, essentially the same in men and in women, there is hardly any *active* sexual element.

That violent infatuation or excess of love, although it may also occur at a more mature age, is particularly the privilege of adolescence. Its content is an all-embracing feeling of fondness and we shall now examine more closely how this feeling comes to form the basis of the active sex need.

163. *From Passive to Active Sex Need*   That extravagant fondness based upon a certain person's capability of satisfying the most significant—but not all—needs active at the moment of falling in love determines the desire that drives the lover to want to obtain proof that the beloved is also able to satisfy other needs initially regarded as less essential or not recognized at all.

When it appears to the men and women that there is an opportunity to satisfy these previously unsatisfied needs a contact need arises. This creates the feeling of trust in the possibility of satisfying those mental and physical needs which were before regarded as less important. In both the male and female this contact need forms the passive sexual need. In the man there is also included the need for evacuation. The existence of the contact need in both sexes and the evacuation need in the male is the basis for the totally developed active sexual need. If the need is mutual and circumstances permit, such a development occurs.

Chapter 14: ACTIVE SEX NEED

164. *Development of the Contact Need*   In describing the passive sex need, it was mentioned that the contact need is awakened when the consciousness pleasurably registers that the organism is set at rest and soothed, if the person may touch and obtain contact with another person with promised qualities as a "satisfactor." On such an occasion the sympathetic nervous systems do not disturb the constructive activity of the para-sympathetic nervous system.

The presence of the other person is felt by means of pure sensory agents, such as sight, hearing, perhaps smell. If the contact need is very marked it will not be stilled by these sense agents alone. The organism will demand a still stronger realization of the presence of the "satisfactor." This may be achieved through further sense agents, such as the sensory nerves and taste nerves. It makes no *qualitative*, but only a *quantitative* difference whether the contact need is gratified through sight, hearing, and smell alone or whether it is further gratified by tactile means. The strongest of such tactile impressions (caresses) are conveyed via the so-called *erogenous zones*, areas in the body richly equipped with nerve ends. Among them are the lips, and the tongue (kissing), the latter provided with taste nerves. The *contact need* then is an essential component part of both the passive and the active sex need. This need encompasses the urge to achieve intimate contact, body and soul, with another person, normally a person of the opposite sex. It corresponds to what formerly was termed *the urge of approach* or *the contractile urge*.

165. *What Takes Place During Sexual Excitation?* Those very strong sensory impressions that reach the cerebrum, particularly through the very sensitive nerves of the areas of sexual excitation or erogenous zones, influence the brain so forcibly that new impulses issue from it to the vegetative nervous system. This message is probably sent via the sexual center, which we shall describe a little further on. The vegetative nerve system thus becomes activated. This mounting activation apparently includes the sympathetic and certainly some parts of the parasympathetic nervous system, the latter causing these *erogenic parts* in both sexes to swell. Direct touching of these tumescent elements will have the same effect and often with particular force, because the sensory agents here as in most other parts of the vegetative nervous system may be transferred directly through a very short reflex arch to those parts of it that activate the tiny muscles and blood vessels of the tumescent elements. Simultaneously the mind attempts to close off as far as possible all impressions except those mentioned here. This brings about an intense feeling of unbalance which, however, will be extremely pleasurable because the impressions are so closely bound up with the idea of satisfying the insistent urge of the contact need, as well as the need of obtaining relief from the pressure

created by the swelling of the sex organs. In the male, moreover, the need of evacuation—which is always present in varying degrees—clamors for satisfaction.

This condition is called excitation, or sometimes *tumescence* a very apt expression with which to describe *both* the high level of nervous excitement and the swelling of the genital organs at this most active stage of the active sex need.

166. *The Need of Relaxation (Detumescence)* Sexual excitation as was noted in the previous section, represents a definite state of unbalance in the organism. The factors that cause this condition to terminate and re-establish balance are not known with any degree of certainty. As the tumescence is the result of innumerable activating reflexes, some of them very strong, the most probable supposition would be that the reflex centers of the brain which are particularly sensitive, are the first to tire. This supposition checks with the observation that according as the sexual excitement is reaching its climax the consciousness tends to wane, particularly in the woman, whose sex needs as a rule are highly mental. At the same time the influence of consciousness on the vegetative nervous system is obstructed and, as mentioned before this system is able to function independently of the cerebrum and may, therefore, manifest its activity unhindered and, in the true sense of the word, "automatically." Ejaculation of the semen and the rhythmical contractions of the vaginal muscles belong to the fullest extent in that category.

Thus, during the growing tension of tumescence, a definite need for emotional and physical *de*-tension originates. This need is called *the detumescence need,* and it includes the discharging or evacuation need of the male too.

167. *The Sex Center* Many attempts have been made to explain the mechanics of tumescence, but with scant success. However, it has proved possible to point to a special *sex center* located in the brain. We know now that it is located in that part of the brain which is called *corpora mamillaria* which is in two-way communication, *reversible communication,* with other centers which are partly located in the cortex of the cerebrum.

However, not much detailed knowledge is available about the functions of the sexual center. One theory which has been advanced is that varying degrees of sensitivity in the sex center might determine the intensity of the sexual need. According to that view, lack of sensitivity would entail frigidity, and too high a degree of sensitivity would make a person too highly sexed. The normal would then be an intermediate degree of sensitivity. But I, for one, have not been able to find any convincing proof to support this reasoning.

168. *How Is the Sex Center Influenced?* It *has* been proved, however, that the sex center is influenced from the outside by ordinary sense impressions. Thoughts, ideas, pictures, and memories that crowd into the mind may also be carried by way of the *association center* or perhaps through several association centers to the sex center. Sex impulses may be quite strongly activated by pictures, words, sounds, created by associations originating in a person's own mind and imagination.

It is regarded as certain that the sex center is to some extent subject to hormonal action. However, scientists do not agree as to whether the sex center is directly affected by the sex hormones or whether these affect the sense centers and the association center so that the sex center is indirectly affected in this way.

What we previously called the sexual need of the organism has been represented as resulting from impulses originating in the sex center and reaching the organism via the nervous center. However, a good deal of evidence would seem to act counter to this explanation. It must, for instance, be considered as proved that the male sex hormones have an active, and probably a considerably more direct, influence on those centers in the spinal cord that control penis erection and ejaculation. In my opinion the sex center is but an association center serving as a relay station between the mind and a *previously sexually excited organism*, the latter condition brought about by teamwork between different hormones (of which the sex hormones play a most prominent part) and the autonomous nervous system. However, the question is not yet solved, and I, therefore, feel bound to keep to a description of the most current conception of the function ascribed to the sex center.

169. *Symptoms of Sexual Excitation*   To be exact, we can only describe *the symptoms* of the sexual excitation of the organism: *the brain* is erotically conditioned, i.e. the imagination and thoughts turn to sexual matters. Nerve impulses, working through the *erection center* located at the lower end of the spinal cord in man and through a corresponding center in woman, set the blood coursing through the veins to the sex organs, the penis in man, and the uterus, clitoris and vulva in woman. These organs then become congested, the whole tumescence system in both man and woman swell.

The skin, particularly in the face and chest, becomes hot and flushed due to influences conveyed through other nerve paths in the vegetative nervous system. There are counterpart reactions in other species. For example, in rabbits the inside of the eyelids grows red; in the pig the ear is so congested that it actually droops. In many monkeys the blood courses to their face and nipples, or to the upper thigh and the posterior (*buttocks*), and surrounding parts. Moreover, there is a congestion of the female uterus. In the animal world these symptoms appear immediately prior to the mating season, and in all animal species so far examined, the female does not permit the sexual act to be initiated until the vulva and its adjacent parts have been congested for some time. It will thus be seen that in animals, congestion is a necessary preliminary to the sexual act. In human beings the so-called *nervous element* in sexual desire is sometimes more in evidence than the congestive, or so-called *vasomotor element*. That is the reason why vasomotor changes may pass unnoticed in human beings, although they do exist.

170. *How May the Sex Need Then Be Defined?*   It may be established that the sex need, which represents the need of survival of the species, is a very strong need. The urge is closely linked, on the one hand, to special cells called sex cells. In the male the need is also associated with the structure of sex cells; and, on the other hand, to the nervous systems and the hormones of the body and their interrelation and teamwork, in both sexes.

The sexual need in its passive phase consists of a contact need in both sexes and a discharge need limited to the male. Directly connected with the gratification of the contact need, a detumescence need arises. In the male, this consists of a need of discharge, often of rather visceral nature, whereas in woman it most frequently shows a more psychic trend. Fluctuations in the woman's sexual needs would seem to be mainly fluctuations in her psychogenic or emotional needs. As yet there is no proof of their being linked to hormone conditions; moreover, fluctuations seem to exist in a maximum of only 20 per cent of women. In the male, the sexual fluctuations depend to a certain extent on emotional needs, but probably mainly on the extent of his discharge need, a need that forces him to take the initiative in sexual intercourse, whereas woman usually must first be awakened sexually by artificial methods.

Chapter 15: SEX NEED IN WOMAN

171. *Woman's Early Male Ideal* The foregoing considerations should clarify the fact that the sex needs in human beings are closely linked to purely physical phenomena that to a great extent have been clarified and defined. As a matter of natural logic, sex needs must exist in all *female* individuals as something normal in principle. If in certain women we find a defective or an abnormal sex need, it must be taken for granted that the fault lies with the abnormal reactions of the organism. The reactions of the organism in regard to the unfolding of sex need may have been given a special twist or direction according to the environment in which the woman was raised or finds herself. We must realize what a fundamental influence environment, including adolescent associations and parental instruction, exercises on the development of sex needs in women.

Many women, even those of the present day, look upon men as their superiors. Possibly for that reason, and because such a woman is usually physically less strong in comparison to him, a number of needs are created in her at a very early moment. Man seems to her to be able to satisfy these needs. They are needs such as: the need of security, care, self-respect, harmony, desire for children, etc. In principle, such a woman's attitude in regard to man is, therefore, effectively mapped out at an early age. How true that is may be gathered from the fact that the female of the species, already as a little girl, chooses a hero who becomes her male ideal, neither more nor less. The idea that her male ideal will be able to satisfy all of a woman's needs is so firmly lodged in her mind that it takes a *very strong sexual influence* to color her attitude toward men *sexually*, something that, in principle, should be entirely possible when her sex need develops during and after puberty.

172. *The Ideal Image as Basis for the Choice* The more a woman's ideal is limited to his appearance, walk, carriage, speech, gestures, etc., the easier it will be to awaken her sexual need to its full capacity. Young girls most likely fall for men like film stars and cowboys. In an older woman the contact need is dominated by the desire for security, care, understanding, self-respect, and similar objectives. These wants take precedence over earlier superficial requirements. Here is a distinct difference, at least quantitatively, between man's and woman's sex manifestations. The majority of women are reacting only to men who principally arouse their emotional needs, whereas most men may feel sexually attracted to any woman who can awaken their sexual need.

173. *How the Woman's Full Sexual Need Is Aroused* While a man immediately from puberty is fully aware of his active sexual instinct the above-named components of a woman's need for contact dominate her consciousness to such an extent that she is practically satisfied if these components are met. She has, as a rule, no actual need at this time for sexual intercourse. One generally says that a woman has to be *aroused sexually* before she becomes fully aware of her sexual need. This is mainly done by means of caresses. The curtain will lift from her eyes and she will suddenly see the man before her who so overwhelmingly aroused her longings. The man and her sexual need in all its shades, hitherto entirely concealed to her, are now being revealed in all strength.

174. *"The One and Only . . ."* Poets have sung of the lovers who, as two halves, must find and fit each other, if they are to know the full meaning of being a complete human being. That is very fine, and it is rather easy to imagine women with such a collection of intense, strong and richly developed needs that to them there seems to be only *one* man who can possibly by the *right* one. Yet it is not so easy to imagine a man having his life completed by only one "right" woman.

In practice it seems to be as follows: It is beyond doubt that a woman may be aroused sexually by a man whom she was not previously particularly fond of, but through this experience she may feel herself attached to him with very strong ties of sympathy. However, generally a woman may be aroused sexually only by those men who, in her opinion, primarily are able to satisfy her dominant need. These are men who, at any rate to a certain extent, come up to her ideal image. Such a man may frequently just by a glance, a word or a casual touch arouse a state of strong sexual excitement in her while the casual touches and even advances of other men may awake a pronounced dislike and disgust. A wise woman physician, who understands other women very well within this particular field, wrote to me: "It is by no means true that a woman, as her sexuality gradually develops, feels attracted to men as males in general. No, she reacts to certain men only."

175. *She Is His—Irrevocably and Forever* A woman who has become conscious of her full sexual need directed toward a definite man has made her choice—if indeed it can be called a choice. For instead of using her will power in acting she may fling it to the winds. How irrevocable and final the choice a woman sometimes makes has been revealed to me by many of the sex during personal consultation. One of them has written down her impression: "Everything in a woman is drawn toward the beloved. Her entire being *wills* only him. There is a strong sex urge in many women. It points with the directness of a magnet to that one man!"

176. *Women and Sexual Intercourse* A woman may have just as strong, though more slowly aroused and hardly as fre-

quent, an urge to have intercourse as a man. This is a normal condition if her sexual needs has been awakened. We must only note that she does not, like most men, feel an urge to sexual intercourse in general. She longs for intercourse with a definite man who has been able to satisfy her sexually. To the sexually awakened woman the realization of intercourse becomes indeed only a question of circumstances. It may often turn out to be a matter depending upon the personal attitudes of the parties to the sex morals prevalent, or prescribed by society. We shall later consider the subject of intercourse between engaged couples.

Here I shall only make this observation about woman's voluntary giving herself to a man. On one hand it is dictated by how heavily social sex morals influence her—those sex morals imposed by society. On the other hand, this influence is opposed by her sex need and by the more or less easy access afforded her in overcoming the moral barriers. If there are no artificial barriers, or if they are overcome by the woman's fully developed sex need, then the question of sexual union will be but a question of opportunity. It is as simple as that. The woman's whole body then reaches out to the beloved. Whether she knows it or not, she is ready to abandon herself to him without waiting.

5

LIVING TOGETHER

Chapter 16: SEXUAL NEED AND SEXUAL INTERCOURSE

177. *An Introductory Remark* As an introduction to this chapter it is unfortunately essential to direct attention to the fact that living together sexually is not the same as having sexual intercourse. The difference is evident in the terms—there is a difference between "having intercourse" and "living together." And the difference becomes most salient if we submit these concepts to a closer investigation.

178. *What Are the Characteristics of Sexual Intercourse?* Sexual intercourse only presupposes that when the commanding need of it arises a creature of the same species, but of the opposite sex, will be available to satisfy the need. Male dogs, for example, seem indifferent to which female is involved. It is such considerations on the part of the "customer"—though he may not be conscious of it as a rule—that form the basis of by far the greater part of what is termed prostitution. On the whole, sexual intercourse refers to relations of a distinctly fleeting nature, both in time and meaning.

179. *What Are the Characteristics of Living Together?* Living together sexually is quite another matter. It presupposes a *selection* of the sex partner. At the same time, more practical, economic considerations may influence or dictate the choice. Consequently, living together sexually, both in respect to duration and meaning, takes on a distinctly *permanent* character. It gradually grows to comprise numerous needs with their still more numerous forms of expression, of which sexual intercourse represents only a part, although an indispensable part.

180. The Three Stages of Living Together Sexually To permit a detailed investigation of the matter of married life (sexual living together) we must have a general view of the phases through which it is normally expressed and the basic knowledge of the terminology necessary to describe them. The following should, therefore, be read with particular attention.

1. *The allurement stage* is the period during which contact is made. This approach stage is activated by interior and exterior influences; conscious ideas, desires, and ideals originate and are directed toward persons of the opposite sex. At this stage the need of contact is the dominating urge.

2. *The sexual excitation or tumescence stage* in which the approach is continued more directly in the form of love play, both partners generally participating. That brings the nervous system into a certain pleasurably tinged unbalance, while the sex organs at the same time are becoming swollen by the increased flow of blood.

3. *The relaxation or detumescence stage* follows the stage of excitation. An excitement climax is reached in moments of very intense sexual excitement called the *orgasm*. The stage of detumescence replaces this exciting phase. This detumescence is characterized by a marked relaxation, a most restful feeling in body and soul, accompanied by a distinct well-being. At this phase the detumescence need is dominant.

181. Conditions of the Allurement Stage The generally more passive contact is mostly up to the woman. The active part or pursuit is commonly carried on by the man. Together this serves to bring the two sexes in contact in a general way, and, later on, to bring a particular individual in touch with a particular individual of the opposite sex. This presupposes a choice.

The individual wants, as father or mother for her or his as yet unborn children, another individual of the same general outlook and standing. Where sex life has become regulated by social precepts—as is the case in every community that acknowledges marriage—it is of definite importance that each party chooses as a life partner a person to whom he is not drawn exclusively by a sexual or mating urge. The partner should also be the one with whom he is in fullest understanding, and with whom he will share life for better or worse even far into old age. The allurement stage, therefore, may correspond to the *love choice*.

182. Conditions of the Sexual Excitement Stage During the erotic stage the sex organs become conditioned in preparation for the performance of the sex act. Both these organs and the nervous system are brought into a state of unbalance of so special a nature that striving to re-establish balance becomes an *irresistible urge*.

It was formerly popularly believed that a sexual need could be satisfied as soon as it had entered upon the active phase. This is a great mistake which many men have discovered for themselves, and for which some feel quite ashamed. There is no reason to be ashamed, however. One should not be misled by what we observe in our richly fed domestic animals, or what we might read concerning the leisure classes or other people who have not enough to do.

The sex needs of these groups of people have become abnormally dominating because, having so much leisure the sex urge gains a greater interest and influence with the opportunities afforded. To a person living a healthy, natural life with plenty of work the need for sexual outlet is not always so urgently present that it strives for satisfaction. And in any case, satisfaction cannot be obtained by a brief, superficial excitement. Men and women usually differ considerably in preparing for intercourse. Many men are able from the summoning stage to proceed directly to the sexual act, but the ordinary procedure, at least as far as the woman is concerned, is that there must be a more or less prolonged interval between the two phases to enable her to take her proper part in intercourse, and make her long for its completion. And this, the *second* phase of sexual union is precisely the *stage of erotism* corresponding to the *love play.*

183. *The Conditions of the Relaxation Stage* The relaxation stage following orgasm is partly responsible for the reproduction of the species, and to a degree provides assurance that the greatly heightened urge to regain equilibrium that grew out of the erotization stage will be satisfied. The reproduction of the species is assured by the fact that the relief obtained by the man is directly linked to the ejaculation of his seminal fluid. In addition, the relief ensured through the relaxation stage of the more and more intense emotional and physical need is experienced as an overwhelmingly poignant feeling of sensuousness, or well-being, that is characteristic of the *orgasm.* It may be explained that the need, that steadily had been growing during the preceding phases, is met in the form of a relief, which seems to come at one sudden climax. And it is the orgasm, the climax, which brings back mental and physical balance.

Chapter 17: THE ALLUREMENT

184. *The Urge to Show Off* It is common knowledge that adolescents like to show off their strength, skill, or other talents. This is often exhibited in an exaggerated manner, by running, hopping, jumping, dancing, performing athletic feats, boasting of imaginary exploits, by whistling, singing, taking undue risks or displaying courage. This urge to show off, this *strutting*, particularly in boys who want to make an impression on girls, in the opinion of modern psychologists, is a forerunner of the self-conscious, fastidious, relatively methodical display of his person in the young adult man, and of the charming, flirtatious, coquetry in the young woman, when in love.

185. *Being in Love, and the Decision to Do Something about It* We have seen how love manifests itself in puberty. As a rule it is more universal, less distinctly directed, on a special person of the other sex. I have never seen or heard what was for me a completely satisfying definition of love. One might perhaps say that love is a biologically conditioned idea or consciousness that a certain person can satisfy a great number of emotional and physical needs. If the couple share this consciousness their love is *happy;* if the consciousness is not mutual, their love is *unhappy.*

186. The Three Senses in the Allurement Stage   In the allurement stage three senses are specifically involved and active. They are, smell, hearing and, above all, sight.

187. Odors (Scents) as Lure   In the animal world it is generally the male, rarely the female, that has recourse to odors as a means of calling a partner. Many animals have special *scent organs,* glands which secrete odors. This, for instance, is true of certain butterflies whose scent organs are located on the abdomen with many scent hairs on the legs and thighs. Similar scent organs are found in beetles and bees. Some insects have odoriferous scales which fall off and spread scent around when males ready for mating rub their wings against each other. Among the red deer, the female has a small visible scent spot on the back of its front leg. At every step she leaves a scented trace to lure and guide the stag. In polecats, martens, and foxes the odor glands are placed near the tail. The musk deer gives forth an odor which members of the opposite sex of this species can smell at a distance of almost two miles.

188. Human Odors   Each individual has his own particular scent or odor which may affect other people as being either attractive, neutral, or repulsive. It is this individual scent which makes it possible for a dog to track down a criminal if it has sniffed something with which the man has been in contact, as an article of clothing or some other things he has touched.

189. Artificial Scents, Perfumes   Perfumes can only be viewed as substitutes for natural odors, as supplements to them, or to cover them up. They are used partly from the desire to imitate or to reinforce the natural odor of the body, yet may be employed because one wants to cover up his body odor.

190. Lure Affecting the Sense of Hearing The sense of hearing, too, plays a not insignificant role in the sex call. One can cite, as an example, the change in the male voice at puberty. The male voice has a greatly stimulating effect on woman. Yet the opposite effect has also been observed: a woman's voice may excite a man sexually. In mammals the voice is used as a means of sexual lure during the "heat" or "rutting season," different animals having their own special call. This call is heard by the coveted member of the opposite sex and has a stimulating effect on both male and female. The repetition of these calls at stated intervals, in the opinion of many scientists, is the origin of rhythmic singing.

Rhythmic repetition of the same note has a very suggestive and fascinating effect and serves the urge of attraction as a means of allurement, charm, and seduction. This might be the basic explanation of the intensely erotic effect produced by singing and music. The lovesick yelping of a dog, the lascivious purring of cats, the roar of the lion, and the crowing of the rooster. All these sounds are the equivalent in the animal world of the human love song.

191. *The Human Love Song* The voice exercises a formidable attraction in the human race too. Not only in singing, but through the spoken word. The triumphant ring of a voice, the smooth flow of speech, a resonant male voice, a woman's frail cry; words of admiration, love, and flattery; words of comfort, cheer, and pity; tears and laughter and promises; sighing in all its shadings, everything that can be spoken, wept, laughed, or sighed is used in the service of love and lure.

192. *Lure through Sight* However, the most essential sense is that of *sight*. Sometimes sight is called the essential aesthetic sense, also in regard to human love lure. This is not entirely correct. Beauty does not necessarily exercise lure, although to most *men* it means a good deal. But *women* sometimes choose outstandingly ugly men, and, in most cases, these men are greatly beloved by their wives. Even though the sense of sight as a rule plays the most essential part at the first meeting, it loses its prevailing significance rather quickly as the lure continues.

throughout the ages, it has been considered sexually alluring. In our own age where fashion demands that women look as natural as possible, the use of cosmetics remains as widespread as ever. Make-up usually has a sexual effect only in the very earliest stages of the summoning. During the actual love play when the sham can be seen at close range, it often has a repulsive effect on a man. He wants to kiss and caress a woman, not a painted doll. A study of women's love of colors, as illustrated in her clothes, would fill volumes. In her conception of the importance of color appreciation each woman reveals to some extent whether she has good or bad taste, or possibly no taste.

Chapter 18: LOVE PLAY

197. *The Three Senses at Play in the Sexual Excitation Stage* The love play corresponds to the excitation stage. This stage, in addition to using the senses of the approach stage, principally calls upon the following three senses: Smell, taste, and touch of which touch is by far the most significant.

198. *Touch in the Service of the Sex Need* The definition of love given by the philosopher Spinoza is still a valid one, according to the viewpoint of some present-day psychologists. Spinoza said: "Love is a certain titillation accompanied by the idea of an exterior cause." Inasmuch as the sense of touch takes in the biggest area it is, for that reason alone, *a priori* the most important of the senses that are active in the erotization stage. The nerve ends of the sensatory organs of the skin are very similar to the organs of voluptuous sensation located in the head of man's penis, the woman's clitoris, and in the corresponding nerve end organs of the external labia majora and the red borders of the human lips. On the strength of that, one may better understand some authorities who maintain that the sexual act is primarily a skin reaction. In reality the human skin may be regarded as one large organ of voluptuous sensation in the service of the erotic stage, the strongest accentuation of feeling corresponding to definite parts, among which the genital organs are the most prominent.

193. Significance of the Sense of Form On considering the unfolding of the sex urge, it seems that the feeling for form and joy at fine shapes prevail. It is generally supposed that when a young man looks at a girl's legs he follows them up in imagination to her sex organs. This is not always true. What he expresses when he looks at female limbs is more often the joy he feels at the shape of the leg, especially the calf. Women's figures in general attract men sexually, just as masculine forms have a similar effect on women.

194. Appreciation of Form and Figure Is Subject to Changing Fashion Female forms, in particular, have erotic influence, and in addition to the sex organs and the legs, this is also true of the breasts, hips, and buttocks. In the human species the female breasts develop at puberty. In animals they increase in volume only near the end of pregnancy and before the young are weaned. In our modern civilization the sight of female breasts always will provoke a certain degree of sexual excitement in a man. The erotic effect of female breasts, however, varies greatly; it is a matter of different customs. In many primitive peoples this effect does not seem to be felt, and women are not considered immodest if their breasts are exposed.

195. Fat Buttocks In addition to the breasts, the hips and buttocks often affect men powerfully. This is particularly true of primitive peoples, as, for instance, prehistoric European races and present-day African tribes. The Hottentots regard exaggerated, extremely fat buttocks as one of the most coveted signs of beauty in a woman.

196. The Importance of Color Appreciation In many animals the appreciation of colors plays an essential role in provoking sexual excitement through sight. In monkeys ready for mating the parts around the genital organs shine in all the colors of the rainbow. This produces a decidedly exciting effect on the opposite sex. In several savage tribes numerous and magnificent tattooing are considered very effective at the come-hither stage of sex relations.

Women have always used make-up, and at different periods

199. *The First Intentional Touch* There is no difference in quality, only in quantity, between touches of various kinds. It has been said, therefore, and not entirely without justification, that the first intentional touch of the beloved person's skin is already an initial sexual union. From the chaste movement of stroking the loved one's hair to the violent tempest of the passions the difference is, in reality, only one of quantity, not of quality.

200. *The Differences between Excitation and Reaction to Excitation* When we say "threshold of excitation" we mean the margin of an irritant or stimulus below which it is not effective. Some persons are strongly susceptible to excitation, and they have, therefore, a low threshold of excitation. Others, less susceptible, have a high threshold of excitation.

Sexual excitation—which has been compared to itching as well as to tickling—is subject to practically the same reactions as tickling: when the threshold of excitation has been reached, the effect is evident. But once the threshold of excitation has been reached, the effect is not dependent upon the strength of degree of the irritant. On the contrary, a very strong degree of excitation may well result in a state which was not at all intended. In other words, strong excitation may defeat its own purpose. Therefore, what the reaction to a certain excitation will be like depends first and foremost upon the interior condition of the organ in question. And it is by no means essential that there should be a quantitative correspondence between the excitation or the irritant and the reaction to the excitation or the activity it releases.

201. *Fields of Excitation or Erogenous Zones* On the body of both men and women there are a number of places particularly sensitive to caresses. These places are the so-called fields of excitation or erogenous zones. The body of both the man or woman is physically prepared for intercourse through nerve response signals sent out from these very sensitive areas of excitation when they are caressed. The most highly sensitive areas are found where the skin and the mucous membranes come together, as the lips, around the anus, in and about the female sex organs, and the nipple of the female breast.

202. *Erogenous Zones in Women* As mentioned before, the apertures or different types of openings of the body belong in this category: eyes, ears, nose, mouth, and the sex organs proper. In the sex organs the vagina and the uterine opening are very sensitive. In many women the breasts, and particularly the parts immediately surrounding the nipple, also frequently respond erotically to touch, and the nipple itself may become erect. In most women the hairline, the neck, the interior side of the thigh, and the buttocks are also among the important zones of excitation. Above all, the touch and full excitation of the clitoris plays a great part in preparing the woman for completely giving herself in the sexual embrace.

203. *Erogenous Zones in Men* Man who hasn't the same need of being aroused in preparation for sexual intercourse as woman, does not possess as many definite zones of excitation as woman. However, in most men there are particular parts of the body which they particularly delight in having caressed. As in the woman, it may be the neck, the hairline, the inside of the thigh, the buttock, and the various body openings. In many men it is more especially the genital organs, the penis head, the roots of the penis, or the scrotum.

Chapter 19: SEXUAL INTERCOURSE, COITUS

204. *The Sexual Act* Sexual intercourse often causes young people much anxiety. As a rule, the young men are more nervous about the experience of their first intercourse than their boastful attitude leads one to believe. Most young women look to the day when it shall take place with some dismay, perhaps even with a feeling of repulsion, and fear.

205. *Love Must Be Mutual* Countless marriages have failed because they were built on a physical passion, which, as a rule, was based on the man's terrific urge for release. It resulted in violent efforts on his part to arouse and to conquer the woman. Both must be in love. Innumerable women have become unhappy because they thought that their partner's sexual desire would develop into *love*. This hoped-for transformation seldom takes place. For the desire in a man is aroused with amazing ease and cannot at all be trusted. And in addition, it is on this point that most men are rather sensitively critical. If a man feels that the woman appeals only to his physical desire and responds to that, he may very well exploit the opportunity thus afforded, but he may well be lacking in respect or despise her afterwards. When a woman permits a man to leave the stage of initial approach and start in on the excitation stage, the love play, characterized by caresses, then the first great natural step has actually been taken toward the fulfillment of sex life, which is intercourse. It is not always true, however, that a woman who gives a man a kiss may also eventually give herself to him completely.

And in a similar way, many *men* of certain social groups prefer only petting, i.e. love play without the natural physical conclusion in intercourse. Thus the Kinsey Report states that 88 per cent out of all the American men interviewed petted, and that 28 per cent of these achieved orgasm thereby. For a woman, however, petting will in the long run always be felt as something incomplete. For her it is a substitute, the only mitigating factor being that, through this incomplete form of sexual gratification, she does not lose her virginity, and at the same time does not run the risk of becoming pregnant. But should such a central reservation be involved one may, as a rule, take it for granted that the partners really do not *love each other*. Thus the ethical condition for intercourse must be this: that they be married and really love each other completely.

206. *The Practical Conditions for Sexual Intercourse* The ideal sexual intercourse also depends upon very practical conditions. The most favorable condition for intercourse is for the partners to be alone and undisturbed. To have ideal intercourse they must have plenty of leisure. Seclusion is particularly significant in affording the woman, through preparatory love play, the necessary time to attain the peak of sexual excitement. The man should preferably be well rested, otherwise erection may fail completely.

207. *The Prelude* This is the love play at its height, nearing culmination. It is a true and very striking description to speak of it as "play." Play is an activity where one happy experience follows naturally upon the other.

208. *Insertion of Penis* The secretion of lubricating mucus from the big glands of the male vesicles and the mucous glands of the woman generally become active during the love play. The entrance to the vagina and the tip of the penis are therefore already moistened or lubricated in such a way that the penis may be introduced without strain. At the same time the increased blood stream which swells the external female genital organs has caused the vulva to open somewhat. As the entrance to the vagina lies far back in the vulva, the penis cannot, as a rule, be introduced unless the woman spreads her legs.

209. *Positions for Sexual Intercourse* No definite position for sexual intercourse can be prescribed. The numerous variations described in certain literature, in my opinion, only serve to excite the reader's curiosity in a rather base, shallow way. These accounts do not reveal anything which every couple truly in love cannot find out for themselves sooner or later. It might be added that such descriptions are only limited selections from hundreds of different procedures current the world over. One position for intercourse is no more "correct" than another.

In most civilized countries, the position most frequently adopted is this: The woman lies on her back with legs spread out, perhaps with a pillow under the buttocks to facilitate insertion of the penis, perhaps with her knees drawn up and flexed so that they approach her shoulders. In that case it is essentially the man who performs the copulatory movements.

210. *Orgasm* Imaginings and sensatory impressions through sight, hearing, taste and touch may have caused an erection which takes place through the effect of the sexual center on the erection center at the base part of the spinal chord. By increased flow of blood and decreased circulation the spongy tumescent organs have become filled and this has caused the penis to grow to about twice its original length and swell to three or four times its original volume. When the penis is introduced into the vagina, man's and woman's most sensitive erogenic zones come into direct contact: the erected penis touches the external labia and the walls of the vagina, and if there is complete correspondence between the size of the penis and the vagina the glans will eventually touch the cervix of the womb close to the uterine opening. If, after intromission, the woman stretches her legs and closes them, the penis ridge will excite the woman's clitoris and the tumescent organs surrounding it.

The excitation is felt like a penetrating voluptuousness or sensitive delightfulness which they seek to increase by new movements whereby the sensory organs are further affected and the sensual pleasure grows still more intense. This extremely pleasurable sensitivity reacts on the erection centers and on the adjacent ejaculation center. During the continued love play, through the heated blood, the enthusiasm called forth by the love act and the consciousness that one loves and is loved in return, the man's spermatozoa are ejaculated together with the other secretions of the seminal vesicles and the prostate gland into the vas deferens. Simultaneously, a number of muscles in and around the man's genital organs contract in a few rhythmical jerks and eject the seminal fluid with considerable force.

This ejaculation bringing about relaxation, the climax of the man's sexual enjoyment, is the *orgasm*. If the woman's curve of excitation has followed the man's she will reach her orgasm at the same time he does. Already during the movements of intercourse by contracting the vaginal muscles, she has been able to get a firmer hold on the penis in slight movements. As the orgasm is attained, extremely pleasurable, sensuous, convulsive contractions of the muscles of the uterus as well as of the vagina come about, and she feels her entire pelvis close around the man.

211. *The After-play*   The after-play is an essential part of sexual intercourse. It takes longer for the orgasm of the woman to "fall away" than in the man, and consequently, the man who interrupts intercourse immediately after his own orgasm will not, in a normal intercourse, afford the woman the complete enjoyment of her orgasm. After the orgasm both partners feel a wonderful physical and mental relaxation as an intense, beneficent exhaustion after a strong exertion. Indescribable peace descends on both of them. The harmony is now as perfect as it can be when both feel united in soul and body as one single being. If they feel like it, they may continue the love play for some time yet, only more tenderly, and more quietly than before, and they may, both together or separately, achieve another orgasm. Most frequently, however, the blood which filled the sex organs retires rather quickly, the penis losing its erection. As a rule both fall asleep and for some hours enjoy the soundest, most trusting and peaceful sleep imaginable.

To round out this chapter I would mention that the convulsive contractions of the vaginal muscles, which take place during the orgasm, in very infrequent cases may be so persistent that it becomes difficult to withdraw the penis (in which case it is called *penis captivus*—the captive penis) until some time has elapsed.

6
HYGIENE OF THE COUPLE'S SEX LIFE

Chapter 20: **BODY CARE IN SEX RELATIONS**

212. *Care of the Male Sex Organs* Keeping the sex organs clean requires the greatest care. Underneath the foreskin *smegma* may easily collect. It consists of particles of dried secretion from the tiny sebaceous glands under the foreskin that are in constant activity, together with the residue of the lubricating fluid formerly mentioned and of sperms. Such impurities may cause tiny tears and scratches in the thin skin that covers the glans and thus provide entry for venereal germs. A man must cleanse his penis daily, and if he is not circumcised, he should push back the foreskin and wash the glans and the inside of the foreskin.

213. *Care of the Female Sex Organs* Women have a still greater number of more active glands, than men. The women's glands constantly secrete matter both in the internal and the external sex organs. Therefore, the female genital organs require still greater care than the male.

214. *Cleansing the Vulva* The urethra has its outlet in the vulva where a residue of urine may be present and spread an unpleasant odor. From the vagina an acid fluid is secreted into the vulva that may moisten the skin and underthings; also, a great number of sweat and sebaceous glands in and around vulva secrete various pungently smelling substances. A woman should, therefore, wash her external genital organs daily. A wash cloth or sponge reserved for this task exclusively should be used together with hot water. If nothing else can be had tepid or cold water will suffice. The wash cloth or sponge should always be used from front to back. This direction in washing is recommended in order to prevent anal impurities from being carried into the vulva which is separated from the anus only by a very short area of skin, the perineum. Mothers must teach their daughters this personal cleanliness and in that way washing of the vulva will become an automatic procedure in a woman's daily toilet.

215. *Keeping the Vagina Clean* As mentioned above the vagina is always teeming with tiny organisms whose job it is to keep it clean. Douching is, therefore, as a rule superfluous, *and should only be done on the advice of a physician* as it may otherwise do more harm than good.

216. *Douching of the Vagina* If the vagina, however, is particularly affected and appears sore and red (which may be the case if vaginal inflamation is present) or if the woman has a great deal of sexual intercourse, the secretions may take on the nature of a *discharge*. This need not always be regarded as a disease, however. But it may become advisable or necessary to douche the vagina. If such douching is to achieve its purpose and carried out in a manner to prevent any injury it is essential that great care is taken in selecting appliances for it, as well as the kind of solution one wants to use. Another important point is to be careful *not to overdo*. A woman should never take douches more frequently than the quantity of discharge present makes it necessary.

217. *The Hand-bulb Syringe* A syringe consists of a rubber bulb with a nozzle that can be unscrewed. As a rule, it is equipped with a small safety collar designed to prevent the syringe from being inserted too deeply into the vagina. The simpler the design of a syringe, the easier it is to keep properly clean. If it has the occluding collar, and if the nozzle is about the size of a finger, thus ensuring that it cannot be inserted too far and perhaps injure the delicate posterior parts of the vagina, a hand-bulb syringe usually can be considered harmless. Models with a rather pointed nozzle and without the occluding collar are definitely not to be recommended, for they may constitute a risk to the genital tract. The hand bulb is rather expensive to use, because the bulb being of rubber is not very durable. One particular inconvenience about the hand-bulb syringe is its small size which does not permit sufficient douching, wherefore it is necessary to refill it. That means it has to be taken in and out several times, generally at the cost of cleanliness. Hand-bulb syringes with a pumping device are rather complicated and, probably for that very reason, are not widely employed.

218. *The Douche Bag* Use of the so-called douche bag has a number of advantages over the syringe. The douche bag consists of three parts: a bag, or container, a long rubber tube, and a nozzle of glass or ebonite about as large as a finger. The average size container holds from about two to three pints which is sufficient for one douching. It should be placed high enough for the water to flow through the tube at a suitable pressure. A small clamp is put on the tube or you curve it and hold it with two fingers. In a sitting posture the woman brings the nozzle up along the posterior wall of the vagina deeply into it to ensure that the whole vagina is well flushed. Care should be taken to let the liquid flow slowly and gently. After the douche the bag or container must be carefully cleaned, the nozzle scalded and wrapped, or placed inside the container until it is to be used again.

219. *What Quantity of Fluid and What Temperature Is Suitable for a Douche?* To rinse and thoroughly cleanse the vagina will take two or, better still, three pints.

The temperature must correspond to the body temperature. If you fill one third of the container with boiled water and then add the special douche preparation of the other two thirds a suitable temperature will be obtained. *Hot* douches are used only in special cases.

220. *Composition of the Douche Liquid* As a recommended rule the douche preparation should be as mild as possible. If the vaginal discharge is moderate and not complicated by any particular disease, the main purpose of the douche is to cleanse. If one wants to add some kind of disinfectant it must be a mild one, in acidity preferably corresponding to the natural acidity present in the vagina.

221. *Douching with Pure Water* Many women take their douche with pure water, heated to body temperature in the manner indicated above. That is a purely mechanical cleansing process comparable to an ordinary shower bath. However, pure water by itself is not to be recommended, as it may act as an irritant. A very basic mixture right for the vagina should contain a pinch of kitchen salt.

222. *Douche with Physiological Salt Water* Kitchen salt used for ordinary cooking is really sodium chloride. All body tissues and fluids contain a small quantity of sodium chloride (0.9 per cent). Vaginal secretions are also slightly salty, and thus for douching one to two teaspoonful of kitchen salt should be added to about two pints of water. Such a solution is called *physiological salt water*.

223. *Adding a Touch of Acid* Since the vaginal secretions produce a slightly acid reaction because of their contents of lactic acid bacteria it seems quite logical that a weak acid solution can be added to the douche. This possibility is something women have been familiar with for centuries. If, for instance, vinegar acid—a weak acid closely related to the lactic—is used, a suitable quantity will be one to two teaspoonful of ordinary table vinegar for about two pints of water. If lactic acid—another weak acid—is used, one tablespoonful of a 33⅓ per cent lactic acid solution should be added to about two pints of water.

224. *Adding a Brew of Camomile* Camomile is one of the mildest disinfectants in existence and excellent to mix in the douche water. The camomile extract may be prepared at home. Generally speaking it must be weaker than a mixture of camomile tonic for drinking. More concentrated manufactured preparations are also available at the drugstores. Printed directions for use come with each package and should be followed faithfully.

225. *Douche Mixed with Special Disinfectants*   A disinfectant acts to fight an infection by injuring or destroying the infecting organisms, which are, as a rule, bacteria. Only in case of a markedly inflamed condition in the vagina, where disease-spreading propagation of micro-organisms must be halted, is there any reason to use stronger disinfectants. There are many such disinfectants and under the direction of an experienced physician they serve their purpose well, but they have no place in the daily hygiene of a healthy woman. These preparations are often widely advertised and sell at high prices, but a woman using such solutions has no guarantee that they suit *her* special case. On the contrary, it may be dangerous for her to experiment herself. Women should therefore refrain from buying and using disinfectants of that category except on doctor's orders. Most of them are obtainable only by prescription.

Chapter 21: HYGIENE OF SEXUAL LIVING TOGETHER

226. *How Often Is It Considered Natural to Have Sexual Intercourse?*   Let me say at the outset: In really happy marriages this problem does not exist at all. The love play comes about as a natural result of the mutual attraction between husband and wife. It is terminated by intercourse when the occasion offers—sometimes frequently, at other times, rarely. But the question of how often a couple should ordinarily have sexual intercourse is a question that persons seeking advice in sex matters frequently ask their doctors. Experience has shown that there is no over-all valid reply. It depends upon how the sex need of the husband and wife manifests itself; when, and how frequently, it stirs.

227. *Man's Desire for Sexual Intercourse*   As formerly described, the sex need is nearly always astir in the male, both as an approach and contact need as well as the desire for relief through intercourse. In many men the urge for intercourse may be felt once or several times a day. In others, weeks, months, half a year, may pass without the sex need making itself felt so strongly that it has the nature of a desire or need for sexual intercourse. As by far the greater percentage of man's total ejaculations—particularly those of married men—take place in coitus, the frequency of the total ejaculations represents a certain standard of the man's desire for coitus. Kinsey has determined that the frequency of ejaculations in 77.7 per cent of the men examined varies from one to six to seven a week while the ejaculations of the remaining 22.3 per cent are rarer or more frequent. In many cases the frequency of the male need of coitus would seem to be rather a matter of habit. However, the age of the man plays also no small part.

228. *Woman's Desire for Sexual Intercourse* For centuries the old wives' tale has circulated that women had no sexual desires. As demonstrated before this statement is utterly erroneous, and it has been one of the privileges of our century to establish that a normal woman has normal sex desires and craves normal gratification in a normal coitus.

229. *What the Ancients Suggested* In former days few men asked the opinion of women. It was, therefore, as a rule the ideas of man that prevailed. In the classical Greek epoch the sage, Solon, said that ten days constituted a suitable interval between two sexual acts. Mohammed said eight days. And the later developed rhythm system recommended that in most cases intercourse twice a week would be suitable.

230. *The Present-day Norm* Kinsey has, through his examinations of American marriages, found that the frequency of sexual intercourse recedes smoothly with the advance in years. His investigations disclosed that men at the age of twenty have sexual intercourse with their wives about four times a week, at the age of thirty about three times, and through the ages of forty to fifty it is about two times a week. Before the age of sixty has been reached, about 6 per cent have ceased having any sexual intercourse at all, and the average frequently is only about once a week. In those marriages where the husband usually makes the decision the rhythm of intercourse twice a week is found to be, by and large, characteristic of the present era in the United States.

On the other hand some women, probably due to hormone conditions, feel particularly strong sexual desires several times a month. At any rate, it is a fact that many women consider sexual intercourse once or twice a month a suitable, normal rhythm. If that is the way the wife feels, it is natural for the husband to endeavor to be fully aware of it, and to observe those periods and approach her at these times. That will afford the maximum chance for building up a sexually harmonious marriage.

231. *Is It Harmful to Repeat Sexual Intercourse After a Short Interval?* The reply to this question is that intercourse may be repeated—literally—as often as the partners desire and the man can. The subsequent ejaculation or ejaculations as a rule take a longer time in coming about than the first one. The man's capacity for quick repetition of orgasm diminishes with the advance in years. According to Kinsey: an average 20 per cent of men at the age of fifteen have one or more orgasms besides the first one; 15 per cent at the age of twenty; about 8 per cent at the age of 25, however, about 9 per cent at the age of thirty; and only 6–7 per cent already at the age of thirty-five. However, in most men the capacity for erection is somewhat diminished after the first ejaculation, and in most women the sex urge is satisfied when they have reached an orgasm. There are, however, also frequent cases where the erection reappears shortly after the seminal fluid has been ejaculated, and when both partners then feel a strong desire to repeat the act with another orgasm, there is no physical or any other reason why they shouldn't.

During the first ejaculation so much seminal fluid has gone that not much remains for the next. It takes at least about ten hours for the testes to fill up a man's seminal depots, so that a *normal* ejaculation of sperms can be repeated. While the new orgasm which the woman enjoys may be far more sensuous the second time or later, the man's sensuous sensations will generally decrease proportionally with the quantity of seminal fluid ejaculated. By his repeated ejaculation the sensations tend to become localized in the genital organs proper rather than sweep over him in the intense, intoxicating ecstasy that accompanies the first orgasm.

232. *Diminished Sex Need* There are extremely harmonious marriages where neither partner has any particularly strongly developed sex need and where sexual intercourse occurs only a couple of times a year. If that is the case, it is normal for them. Kinsey reports a case of a physically normal and healthy man who for a period of thirty years had ejaculation only once. Brain work is noted for its restricting effect on sexual desire. Work which takes up a great deal of one's thoughts (and this, for example, not only includes the mental activity of the man of the house, but also the bustling housewife's daily management of her home) will therefore, at certain periods, tend to diminish the sex need or relegate it to a secondary place. The same is true if one is physically exhausted, requires sleep, etc. If the woman's need for sexual intercourse is essentially less than the man's this often may be related to the fact that she does not habitually attain an orgasm.

233. *Heightened Sex Urge* On the other hand, the sex urge may be very strongly increased both in men and women without calling for the epithet "morbid." I know men who are capable of having intercourse no less than twelve times in twenty-four hours. Havelock Ellis describes a case where the husband felt a desire for sexual intercourse as many as twenty times in twenty-four hours, and Kinsey reports the case of a man, a learned and capable lawyer, who through thirty years had, on an average, thirty ejaculations a week. A husband's exaggerated sex urge may often prove injurious to the wife, causing her to undergo much suffering. The contrary may also be the case, namely, the wife who most frequently and/or strongly feels the need of intercourse. Schopenhauer, as a matter of fact, takes it for granted that the sexual urge is present at all times in woman to such an extent that she quite naturally feels inclined to satisfy two men with normal sexual desires. Many women have declared to me that it is true for them that their sexual urge actually may be that strong. However, these women could not imagine exchanging their marriage partnership for membership in a cooperative such as the philosopher Schopenhauer suggested. According to this it is a fact that many women—far more than one would imagine—have a sex urge very much stronger than that of their husbands. When this is the case, it may truly be said that they do not have sexual desires naturally satisfied to the extent in which such desires are present.

234. *Exaggerated Sexual Intercourse* By the term exaggerated sexual intercourse we mean that a man and a woman have intercourse more frequently than is truly normal to him or to her. This brings about a marked debility, fatigue, sleepiness, lack of vitality, and a feeling of tedium. In the man this condition sometimes brings about the irritation of the prepuce and pains in and around the pelvis and its muscles. In the woman it frequently causes a soreness of the outer and inner labia or in the vagina. Persons with proper self-control indulge in sexual intercourse only at those times when both partners know that they can abandon themselves to complete and fresh enjoyment.

235. *Illness and Other Circumstances Influencing Habits of Intercourse* In certain countries persons suffering from *venereal diseases* are forbidden sexual intercourse by law. If a person suffers from *other illnesses of the sex organs* each case will depend upon the measures recommended by the physician. There may be cases, for example, where one of the partners—due to some other type of contagious disease—does not wish to expose the other partner by intimate contact. The question of the advisability of having sexual intercourse may also arise if one of the partners has an illness that may influence his or her condition unfavorably.

7
DISTURBANCES IN A COUPLE'S SEX LIFE

Chapter 22: WHAT ARE THE CAUSES OF DISTURBANCE IN A COUPLE'S SEX LIFE?

236. *Introductory Remarks on Apparent and Real Causes* When persons who have disturbances in their sex life at last decide to ask the advice and guidance of a physician, they have, as a rule, had ample time to think of the cause or causes of the difficulties. As a rule the individual has found them in the other party, which is rather human thought not always in conformity with the actual facts obtaining. But even if such cases are left out of consideration, the apparent causes which people have discovered for themselves often prove to be the false ones. If, for instance, a man states that he is incapable of satisfying a woman because he has too early ejaculation, the cause of the premature ejaculation remains to be found. The cause may very likely be found in the woman. Perhaps a woman reveals that the cause of her unhappy sex life is the man's caresses which she dislikes, and which prevent her from becoming sexually satisfied. The reason why he behaves as he does and the reason why she dislikes it—causes which may simply originate from a variety of possible social differences—remain to be found. This brief account shows the great significance of tracing these deep and actual causes. The biological and the psychological research of the last decade has aided materially in making such an investigation more relevant than ever before.

In this connection should be mentioned a large-scale investigation, initiated in 1938 by Dr. Kinsey, American professor of zoology, which will be completed in less than a generation. The goal of the full research is to obtain the highest possible amount of detailed information concerning the variations in human sexual behavior. The method used first to gain this information was through the thorough interviewing of 100,000 American men and women. The first results were made public in 1948, published in *Sexual Behavior in the Human Male*, the so-called Kinsey report, which was based on inquiries using a very intensive polling technique.

Previous to the preparation of the report about 12,000 individuals, about half of which were men and the other half women, were interviewed. The report itself gives information of the sex life of 5,300 white American men, each of them having answered about 300 questions, some of them answering an additional 220 questions.

Kinsey has divided the data from the individuals investigated into their various age groups, groups of married, unmarried, etc., and the material in these divided groups was subdivided from a social point of view with the consideration that the number of years of education was to be the best standard. Thus there are three main groups given with 0–8, 9–12, and 13–more years of education, which, in broad outline, correspond to grade school education as representing the educationally lowest group. The high school education was a representative factor of the middle group, and university education was one characterization of the educationally and, accordingly, in Mr. Kinsey's view, socially highest group. The sexual habits, and, accordingly, the sexual moral concepts, appear also to differ widely among individuals in these social groups. The results indicated thereby that 85 per cent of young men from the grade school group, at the age of 16–20, had intercourse before marriage, while only about 75 per cent of the high school group and even only 42 per cent of young men of the university group in the same age class had intercourse before marriage. On the other hand, petting was practiced to such an extent among men of the university group who had not married before their thirtieth year, that more than 61 per cent of them attained orgasm through petting, while those with grade school education rejected this intense petting as being immoral and generally only indulged in love play as an introduction to intercourse. In the highest educated group it was, if anything, considered normal to be naked during intercourse—89 per cent were naked. In the case of the lowest group, however, nakedness was by many considered quite repulsive. In the highest group an aversion prevailed against two persons drinking from one and the same glass and the passionate kiss was looked upon as one of the most elementary and important links in love play. However, in the elementary school group there was no objection against using joint eating and drinking implements, while the passionate kiss was considered abominable. Factors such as those mentioned above often play a great part as real causes of a couple's unharmonious sex life. Thus it will always be necessary to have one's attention drawn to the difference in the social conditions of the parties concerned when trying to advise the troubled parties. The mere knowledge of the fact that the tendency of "birds of a feather flocking together" is operating in this field of human activity, is sufficient basis for a better understanding of each other's reactions. With such understanding the first step toward harmony in sex life is already taken.

237. *What Are Inhibitions?* Earlier we explained that a reflex means a manifestation of life brought about by an external or internal influence without the intermediate action by a conscious decision. The reflex path consists of, first, the nerves that lead to and away from the reflex center, and secondly, the center itself. Various conditions in this reflex path or reflex arch may, however, cause a reflex to become stronger or weaker or, as we say, to become inhibited. The inhibitions are of particular interest to us here. Certain reflexes, mainly conditioned reflexes, that follow the reflex path or arch, may be inhibited by the mere fact that they are made to work too often in rapid succession. Therefore, it is believed, the nerve cells in the reflex center get tired. Moreover, it is a matter of common knowledge that a reflex process, such as breathing, may be inhibited by a message from the cerebrum. Altogether, the brain seems to have a constantly restraining (inhibitory) influence on the reflexes of the organism. This view is partly substantiated by the fact that reflex move-

ments are much more marked when a person is asleep than when he is awake. All self-control is really based on such so-called psychic or *mental inhibitions*. At the same time they may give rise to various disturbances in a couple's sex life, as we shall see in the following. *Physical inhibitions* also occur. It is, for instance, a well-known fact that the erection reflex may fail during coitus if disturbed by outside influences, such as noise.

238. *The Ego and Its Attitude Type* We are born and we die as individuals. We also live as individuals. Even if two human beings are quite well suited to each other in respect to social conditions, habits, interests, and tastes, they are, however, widely different: each has his personal individuality, each his particular Self with particular reactions attached to it. It is this very fact: one ego facing the other ego that creates the deepest richness in a couple's life but it is also this fact that gives rise to the deepest and accordingly most serious lack of harmony.

The little baby discovers gradually the difference between the ego and the non-ego, first through the experience of pain and the observance and the sensation of its own movements. Soon further experience with the memories of previous events are added, and constantly new recognitions of its own functions and needs. Thus over a period of years a conception of his own self takes form in the individual: "That is the way I am, My own Self, my Ego."

The Ego is constantly subject to outside influence. In this connection it should be remembered that "outside" influences need not solely refer to environment. These may equally well include influences that originate in the mind of the individual. However, these influences have not become, or, have not *yet* become part of the self which up to now is considered by the individual as his real self. Thus, for instance, when the sexual need makes itself felt for the first time, it is definitely an "outside" influence in relation to the self, and this often leads to a harsh, defensive war until one is finally forced to acknowledge that the sex need must be adopted and recognized as an integral part of the self. Here lies the *psychological* explanation of the fact that adolescents at the onset of puberty are torn and drawn in many directions at once.

It was Jung who first clearly demonstrated scientifically how human individualities by means of a special test method may be divided into two main types, namely: *the objective type* and *the egocentric type*. A person's attitude type may be determined by so-called *association tests,* to the effect that the person in answer to a word (the association word) replies with the first association, i.e. association of thought, consequently with the first word that *immediately* occurs to him, the reaction word. The test is repeated with a long series of association words. For instance *the objective type* may generally reply to the association word "rain" with the reaction word "water" as his first association; further: wedding—marriage certificate; accounts—figures; and world-famous—Edison. *The egocentric type* responded, on the other hand, to the same association word for instance as follows: rain—nasty; wedding—New Year's Eve (the person's own wedding day); accounts—irritating; and world-famous—wonderful. These examples clearly demonstrate the traits characteristic of the two different types of attitude of the Ego. The factor of conflict of the two markedly different types of attitude lies also, as a rule, in the quite simple fact that the one simply *does not understand* the attitude of the other.

239. *Tolerance and Intolerance* Through the numerous influences to which a person is constantly exposed, and upon which he takes his stand, it is revealed that the *Ego is really evolving,* changing all through the person's life. In other words: one gets to know oneself better and better and is sometimes surprised, on the basis of one's conception of one's own self so far, at "so that it is the way I am." I am not the same I was ten years ago, twenty years ago, indeed, hardly quite the same as I was yesterday. When a person recognizes this and at the same time recognizes that the Ego of other persons is likewise undergoing changes, the person's appraisals will result in *tolerance* of other people's opinions and remaining ego-content. This also is usually accompanied by a marked *skepticism* as to any *one* type or person being absolutely and irrevocably right and permanent. Tolerance as a *conscious* phenomenon is based on appraisal, and first and foremost on the appraisal of the person's own self. If it is not conscious tolerance, we call the unconscious attitude *indif-*

ference. *Intolerance* is often thought to spring from ethical, religious, or other complexes in the self. However, intolerance is really always due to a lack of recognition or to an inadequate appreciation of one's own self or of other's self or—most frequently—to both, which is a sign of psychic immaturity.

240. What Is Understood by Mental Maturity? A person is said to be psychically mature when he has attained a thorough knowledge of his own self-content and knows how to appreciate it in relation to that of others and at the same time is aware that he is constantly changing. The psychic maturity does not occur at any definite age. In rare cases it may occur early in adolescence, or several years before the person's twentieth year. Generally it is not attained until at the end of adolescence, and will then most frequently fix the time for its termination. Many people will never attain it, or perhaps not until their hair becomes gray.

241. *Egotism* An individual, whose actions are only determined by his own needs, consciously making the needs of others secondary, is called an *egotist*. Egotism is in its nature a form of intolerance and always a sign of mental immaturity in the person. Thus egotism is also a general trait in all children; originally it is a countermeasure against the refusal of the all-powerful adults and bigger or stronger children to fulfill their needs. The examination of adults whose conflicts are due to their egotism has also shown that their egotism is invariably the result of a feeling of inferiority and outright fear of otherwise not being able to gratify their needs. In this manner egotism is the result of a complex. Egotism is by far the most frequent cause of disturbances in a person's sex life. Egotism and a harmonious sex life are an impossible combination.

242. *The Importance of Character* If a person's appraisals are not marked by logic, with the consequence that his attempted actions also lack logic, we speak of the person having a *vacillating*, or *weak* character. If the contrary is the case, the person has an *integrated*, or *strong* character. And, finally, as the appraisals harmonize with the general, or the appraiser's own morals, one talks of a *good* or *bad* character. Numerous couples' unharmonious sex life is due to the fact that one of the parties —or both parties—on the basis of his or her own conception, finds that the character of the other party is bad. In cases where both parties are of the same opinion as to what is good and bad character, the course of conflicts that might occur will, in many instances, depend upon which of the combinations—a strong-good character, a strong-bad character, a weak-good, or weak-bad character—each of the parties has. For the physician or marriage counselor who is attempting to gain an understanding of couples' problems it is often of great importance first to determine what possible combinations of character are present in the specific case.

243. *What Is a Complex?* Most people consider complexes as *always* being disagreeable. And these people usually believe that if you have them, you must get rid of them as quickly as possible. This conception is a misunderstanding. An essential factor in the general attitude of the individual (or Ego) is a series of what are, as a rule, strongly emotionally colored ideas or appraisals of everything that meets the Ego from the outside. It is just these types of ideas which are called complexes. A girl may, for example, have the complex that she can only be happy if she gets married to a certain man. This is one example of what is called a *desirable complex* or an *ideal*. Or a young man may, for example, have this complex: that he, when the opportunity presents itself, will be unable to attain an erection, and, therefore, must avoid sexual intercourse. This is one example of a very unpleasant complex. It may in this case be called an *undesirable complex*. This complex may ultimately have this effect: when the time for intercourse arrives he is actually incapable of attaining erection, even if there is nothing organically wrong which might prevent erection.

244. *Conflicts and Repressed Complexes* Complexes are such fixed components of the Ego that a conflict may arise if the conditions compel the person to abandon his complexes. For example, some sort of conflict will arise if the girl cannot get the man she desires so strongly. And a conflict will be involved

should our young man marry some day despite his fear of intercourse. And another example: a source of conflict may be a woman who has the complex that she will not have any children. She may be concerned because of her figure, her work, or fear of childbirth. She may prefer to remain childless because she is afraid her husband will tire of her, or pay less attention to her, or for a wide variety of other reasons. This woman marries a man who loves and wants children in his family. The only way to solve the conflict is either by the husband giving up his insistence on their having children or by the woman shedding her complex. This second possibility may occur through the husband convincing her that those fears or anxieties that are at the bottom of her complex are groundless.

A complex is frequently *unconscious*. A psychoanalyst is the only person capable of uncovering the presence of such a complex before steps can be taken for its removal. A special form of unconscious complexes are the *repressed complexes*. These repressed feelings are repressed complexes—strongly emotionally tinged ideas which the person does not consider as fitting in with the rest of his Ego. Therefore, it is this type of complex which he has attempted to ignore. Repressed complexes may be the cause of a series of mental sufferings, which are jointly called *neuroses*. These neuroses represent the most frequent area of examination of the psychoanalysts and frequent area of treatment for the psychotherapists. A few examples from practice concerning disturbances in a couple's sex life: A young wife was unhappy in her marriage without being able to point to any special reason for being so. Her reaction to the free association test word "career" was "disaster." It was later determined that her husband devoted himself so exclusively to his work that he neglected her. Her disappointment in this situation had developed into a complex. The nature of her complex can be described as strongly colored with displeasure. But since the importance of her Ego did not permit her to admit that she was being neglected, she repressed the complex. Her complex thus developed into a neurosis.

Another case of a concerned husband: A wife came to admire her husband greatly for his cleverness in making money. However, he later happened to show wrong judgment in general transactions. His own realization that he actually wasn't so clever after all became a fixation with him, a complex fixed in his consciousness. In the resulting fear of losing his wife's admiration he repressed the complex. The man endeavored to convince himself that he had not been stupid, but had been the victim of bad luck. Maintaining this reasoning in discussions with his wife his repressed complex developed into a typical "inferiority complex." This inferiority complex became the cause of the impotence that brought him to the physician's consultation room.

245. *Alcohol and Sex Life* Alcohol has a strong effect on the organism because it is absorbed into the organism much more quickly and easily than other carbohydrates. Alcohol changes the body's entire sugar metabolism. The rate of sugar metabolism is closely connected with the sympathetic and parasympathetic nervous systems. Therefore, the consumption of alcohol will greatly influence the activity of these two nervous systems and through them that of the somatic nervous systems. Symptoms of a slight alcoholic influence will be some release of *inhibitions,* and through a large consumption of liquor the *reflexes* themselves for the time may be lost.

It is not uncommon that many women, who otherwise have difficulty in obtaining an orgasm, reach it rather easily if slightly under the influence of liquor. This is often true of those women who really feel an aversion for intercourse. In cases where the woman herself wants to have intercourse and accompanying orgasm, despite her fears, a little liquor may sometimes be directly recommended. This recommendation may apply to cases of impotence due to inhibitions in the man. In both cases the effect of the inhibitions is undesirable or directly harmful. Removing the effect of the inhibitions with liquor, in this respect, proves beneficial.

However, this beneficial influence is quite like a drop in the proverbial bucket compared to the dire consequences of the use of alcohol when it reduces and, eventually, completely abolishes the *normal* inhibitions. This actually means that a person who is really under the influence of liquor is not able to control himself as he would have been if he were sober. While under the influence of liquor people may do things that fill them with dismay and horror when they recover from its effects. Then it may often be too late to avoid the consequences. When you consider that proper understanding, exactitude, care, and the ability to think are based on the functioning of normal inhibitions it becomes clear that using liquor indisputably increases ruthlessness as well as indifference and stupidity. And all this applies even more to the field of sex than to any other field. Both in man and woman drunkenness often obstructs the activity of the sex centers so strongly that it will be difficult to bring about sexual desires. The male's capacity for intercourse may also be considerably diminished by the influence of alcohol. As a matter of fact, the same thing may be observed in individuals who are chronic alcoholics.

What is really dangerous, after all, is liquor taken in small quantities, for these limited amounts weaken the normal inhibitions without the person losing his mental decision and physical capacity for action at the same time. That is the dangerous situation. Innumerable unwanted pregnancies have been the result of one or both parents being under the influence of liquor at the moment of conception. An English physician who investigated the social importance of venereal disease has revealed that about 80 per cent of the patients who consulted him about venereal diseases had been under the influence of alcohol at the time they exposed themselves to the disease. Drinking is one of the most serious hazards to the ideal development of a couple's sex life for reasons such as these as well as the fact that the habit so often leads to moral decay if not kept within the bounds of moderation. How much liquor an individual can hold before he may be said to be under alcoholic influence varies greatly in different individuals. It also depends upon the state of the organism at the moment of consumption. If taken on an empty stomach its action is much stronger than otherwise.

246. *Purely Physical Causes of Disturbances in Sex Life*
If we have described the psychological causes that may disturb sex life in such detail in the preceding sections, the reason is, as mentioned above, that also in cases where psychological reasons are not the root causes of the sexual disturbances, they generally complicate them even if sexual disturbances are due,

initially, to purely physical causes. There are many such causes.

One of the purely physical causes is the so-called *focal infection*. The theory of focal infection has been the subject of much controversial discussion ever since it was first advanced by an English physician, Hunter, in 1900. The essential feature of the theory can be stated quite simply: Infectious matter for one reason or another is confined in one of the cavities of the body, particularly in connection with infections of the teeth, the tonsils, and the sinuses. From this focal point bacteria and their viruses may be spread all over the body. As a result various ailments may appear, the presence and origin of which could not otherwise be explained. The ailments referred to are chronic rheumatism, heart trouble, kidney diseases, and certain diseases of the nervous system.

Some physicians, moreover, hold the opinion that certain other illnesses and some of the disturbances in a couple's sex life may be due to focal infection. Among the ailments that will be mentioned in this book are inflammation of the Fallopian tubes as a result of appendicitis; inflammation of the uterine mucous membrane; inflammation of the foreskin; impotence; and masturbation. Certain difficulties attendant on nursing a baby are also sometimes ascribed to focal infection. The treatment of such infections is largely directed toward clearing up the seat of the infection, whether by dental surgery, removal of the tonsils, douching of the sinuses, etc.

It is still too early to give a verdict as to the real importance of the focal theory. Yet all over the world many well-known scientists are working to discover whether focal infection can be discounted as the cause of the disturbances here under review.

Chapter 23: IMPOTENCE

247. *What Is Understood by Potence and Impotence?* The word potence denotes an ability to do something. The word impotence denotes a corresponding lack of ability and is almost exclusively applied to the sphere of sex and originally—in ancient Rome—meant the inability to control one's passions and was thus an expression of licentiousness and unbridled passions.

In our day the words have the following meanings: *Potentia generandi*, which is the same as fertility, means the ability to beget children, and *potentia coeundi* (ko-eundi), the ability to have intercourse. *Impotentia generandi*, the same as sterility, means inability to beget children, while *impotentia coeundi*, means inability to have intercourse. Inability to beget children may occur both in man as well as in woman and will be dealt with in detail in the chapter on sterility. Inability to have intercourse may likewise occur in both man and woman. However, the word impotence, when used by itself, generally refers to a quite specific condition, *i.e. the man's inability to carry out intercourse due to lack of erection.*

In some cases the impotence is evident in this way: the erection present at the beginning of intercourse rapidly goes down and thus prevents the man from keeping up the copulatory movements as long as required to attain an orgasm. In other cases there may be no penis erection at all, with the result that the penis cannot be inserted into the woman's vagina, and there is no attempt at intercourse.

248. *Natural or Physiological Impotence*   This is the term that fittingly describes the failure to have erection immediately following one or more acts of intercourse in rapid succession. It expresses a relaxing of the tense blood vessels leading to and in the sex organs. This relaxation may be due to that fact that the sex center or the erection center, or both, are no longer as sexually responsive as before intercourse. The sexual act thus reaches its climax through the relief and ensuing relaxation of a number of complicated reflexes. A reflex of complex character may tire, and the more complex it is, the quicker it tires. This is due to biological reasons, as mentioned earlier. This reflex fatigue may serve as an explanation of the natural impotence after intercourse. However, the matter is not yet clearly defined in all its aspects.

249. *Impotence Due to Disease or to Violent Injury*   If the sex glands or the nerve centers or ganglia through which the reflexes are transmitted are diseased or injured in some way, it affects the reflexes responsible for the over-all sexual excitation of the organism and in addition those reflexes in the spinal cord that are especially responsible for erection also can be affected, and the result may be impotence. This, therefore, takes place in some diseases of the spinal cord. Certain poisonings may also cause impotence. This is particularly true of opium, morphia, cocaine, bromine, carbon monoxide, and, not infrequently, alcohol. Various infectious diseases, such as grippe, when it is of long duration, and several other diseases affecting strongly the general condition may also cause impotence. In a certain form of diabetes impotence is often an early symptom of the disease. Diseases in the penis (a pronounced contraction of prepuce,) may also cause impotence. Impotence occurs, of course, when the penis suffers severe injury or is completely severed.

250. *Impotence Due to Insufficient Sexual Excitation*　If the sexual excitation or desire, brought about in the usual manner, as through sight, touch, etc., is inadequate, erection will not occur. Therefore, in the given situation, impotence will result. This occurs in many marriages. Paradoxically, one of the causes of a husband's ensuing unfaithfulness in such a case may really be ascribed to his faithfulness. For through his faithfulness he may grow so accustomed to his wife's sexual intercourse, that, finally, there is no air of fascination any more. That this is true is proved by the fact that such men are generally excellent partners in extramarital ventures.

If impotence comes about during intercourse, it may be due to a lack of contact excitation. This may occur in cases where the man, over long periods, has used a condom, or if the vagina—as may happen after difficult childbirths or in women approaching middle age—has become so limp and large that it is able to afford the penis only a small measure of excitation. Sensible female gymnastics after childbirth might help to prevent such vaginal conditions and, in that way, contribute to doing away with this form of impotence.

251. *The Woman's Part in the Dual Responsibility*　In some cases it may partly be the wife's own fault if her husband grows so accustomed to her sexual charms that he becomes impotent. Such a woman has not fulfilled her part of the marriage bargain. In contrast, a woman who throughout the years, with constantly renewed freshness, is able to impress her man, remain attractive and arouse his passion, has fulfilled a very essential part of the dual responsibility. It is really a question of the wife's being able to renew herself.

252. Alcohol and Impotence It was described earlier how complete and utter *intoxication* may lead to marked inability to have reflexes. It was pointed out that those rather special reflexes essential in carrying through intercourse, particularly the erection reflex, may also cease. In these cases the resulting impotence will be due to the influence of liquor. This may also be one of the results of *chronic alcoholism.*

Slight intoxication may cause inhibitions or repressions to disappear partly or completely. For this reason moderate intake of liquor may sometimes produce a liberating effect on those forms of impotence that are described as *inhibited impotence.*

253. Inhibited Impotence, Also Called Emotional Impotence Inhibited, or emotional impotence occurs when inhibitions, particularly those originating in the brain, interfere with the normal functioning of the erection reflex. Such barriers may be of widely differing origin and are frequently based on complexes. According to Kinsey these inhibitions are the cause of practically all cases of impotence in men below the age of fifty-five.

Many men during their adolescence have had an attitude toward sex life, especially toward intercourse, of which strong traces remain in their mind. They may have had the idea that sex was something impure, sinful, ugly, or repulsive. Others have grown out of adolescence with notions that the sex act is ridiculous or unaesthetic. Or a man may have been disappointed at a former intercourse or attempts at intercourse. The result is that when he faces a natural intercourse, his mind may be so strongly inhibited by his memories that his penis erection fails. Perhaps, in other cases, erection may be achieved only to disappear again, with the result that the intercourse cannot take place. Such a man is impotent because of his inhibitions. In still other cases the woman involved may suddenly say or do something that awakens a notion in him that the intercourse is undignified, ridiculous, or unaesthetic, the resulting inhibition causing impotence.

If a mother is overtender and emotional toward her sons, or a father to his daughters, a psychological fixation may originate. Such a fixation in the sons in relation to the mother, or in a daughter in relation to the father, is called the *Oedipus complex*. These complexes not only exist in the terminology of the psychologists, unfortunately, they actually occur in real life. This imaginary sex relation may become a grave barrier to the unfolding of a normal sex life and, insofar as the man is concerned, may become the underlying cause of impotence, he himself being entirely unconscious of such a complication.

A special form of emotional impotence is caused by *fear*. A slight fright may be enough to lose an erection completely at the time the man thinks he hears some one approaching; or he is suddenly seized with fear that he may catch a venereal disease; or he becomes afraid of causing an unwanted pregnancy, and so on. Many men think that their impotence is due to their having lived "a little too hard." But this is an entirely wrong conception. A man does not become impotent because of having lived "a little too hard." On the other hand, just his fear that this might be the reason may cause his impotence.

The mere fact that the cerebrum is the center of thought activity in the brain may affect adversely a man's capacity for intercourse. We may hear that while persons of leisure may have intercourse daily if they so desire, manual workers are capable of it only at a few days' interval, and office workers at still longer intervals. Pointing in the same direction is the observation that office work—if strained beyond the limit natural to the individual—produces impotence.

254. *Impotence Due to Impotence!* This title is the most concise statement of still another origin of impotence. For example, a man has been impotent during intercourse. Such a thing which may occur on one occasion may have happened from time to time to literally every man, and no particular significance should be ascribed to it. However, the next time this man is about to have intercourse, he fears that he will again be impotent. Such anxiety is linked to the fact that the inability to carry through the intercourse—in which, as a rule he himself has taken the initiative—is felt by him to be a great humiliation or disgrace. I think it may be stated without exaggeration that if a woman ridicules the inadequate man in that unfortunate situation he will probably never approach her again. It means that much to a man, particularly to one having sensitive pride or being jealous of his honor. In any case such a man may lose his self-confidence; a very forcible inhibition develops which is almost absolutely certain to reappear on the next occasion when he is confronted with a similar situation: he *fears* he will be unable to achieve the intercourse and so he cannot! That is the definition of "impotence due to impotence."

However, such a man can spare himself all his anxiety! First, he should know that such a form of impotence may happen to any man occasionally.

255. *Treatment of Impotence* If lasting impotence should set in, the person must consult a doctor. The treatment consists in administering either *androgenic substances* or *chorion gonadotropine* or both, and sometimes sedatives. Many forms of impotence require psychotherapy and that is by far the most effective remedy. In any case, medical treatment, as such, is only of limited value if it is not accompanied by the guidance required for the removal of the whole complex of underlying psychological disturbances.

In those more tragic cases when the penis has been severed accidently modern surgical techniques have been of remarkable value.

Finally, it should be mentioned that the psychological treatment, in certain cases, may be supplemented with *mechanical* treatment. This is generally understood to be the support of the penis during sexual intercourse by means of a little apparatus called an *erector* of which there are several types.

Chapter 24: TOO EARLY EJACULATION

256. *What Is Understood by Too Early Ejaculation?* Ejaculation takes place very quickly after the beginning of intercourse between animals. In the case of the very manlike chimpanzees, for example, the release occurs ten to twenty seconds after the penis is inserted in the vagina. According to Kinsey in perhaps three fourths of men ejaculation occurs within the first two minutes, and in a significant number in less than one minute or even ten or twenty seconds after intromission, through intensely psychological and physical influence during the love play even occasionally before the penis is inserted into the woman's vagina. Thus an *early* ejaculation is not abnormal. On the contrary, a man who in any other situation reacts quickly and strongly is considered a particularly well-qualified man. The term "too" early ejaculation is also one of only limited justification. "Too" early is used in relation to the occurrence of the female orgasm in each particular case. In respect to this tensing of the moment of beginning one might with equal justification speak of a too late female orgasm. However, there are often such great differences that they give rise to serious conflicts in the sexual life. In common usage, this means that a man has a too early ejaculation if he is unable to delay its occurrence until the woman—provided she is normal—can achieve orgasm.

257. *What Causes Too Early Ejaculation?* At the beginning of the sexual life together too early ejaculation is a very ordinary occurrence. Mutually satisfactory adaptation does not take place until the woman—as is generally the case—gradually develops the ability of achieving earlier orgasm simultaneously with the man, who purposely accustoms himself to delaying his orgasm. He should be able to accomplish this through contraction of the muscles around the rectum.

258. *Treatment of the Too Early Ejaculation* The best existing treatment for the too early ejaculation consists of sensible information concerning the physiological process itself and the adjustment that must be made by the partners. During the second or later acts of intercourse carried through immediately after the first one the ejaculation generally occurs after a longer time than the first coitus. Thus a quick repetition of the intercourse may, in some cases, be recommended. The advice may frequently apply both to the man and to the woman.

Chapter 25: ABOUT THE SATISFACTION OF WOMAN

259. *Simultaneous Orgasm*   The male and female excitation are identical, except for the postlude or after-play. In effect, if man and woman begin the love play *simultaneously*, the excitation curve of both will follow an identical course, ascend together, and reach the orgasm simultaneously. The love play may begin, perhaps, by a look that reveals that their thoughts are directed toward belonging to each other. However, such closely matched action occurs only in truly happy marriages with a thoroughly harmonious sex life.

260. *The Unawakened Woman*   In the past there has been much talk of the *unawakened woman*. She actually does not exist. A woman generally needs awakening before she becomes conscious of her passion. When people talked of the unawakened woman they meant that woman had to undergo a regular training sometimes for several months, before her sex urge reached its full intensity. At the present time, however, it is known that woman's sex urge is clear and direct from the very moment she meets the man capable of arousing it.

261. *The Unsatisfied Woman*   It is estimated that nearly half of all women have never attained an orgasm in their married lives. This is unfortunate when one realizes that the cause of this failure is ignorance. Such women must have surely felt their husband's orgasm and perhaps experienced a certain vicarious satisfaction that they were able to give him pleasure. Later they may have acquiesced and resigned themselves to the feeling that it had to be that way, while the situation weighed on their minds as a profound disappointment. "Was that really all?" may have been their thought. Because of ignorance half the women who have regular sexual intercourse have not felt, do not know, what the orgasm, sexual release, is!

262. *A Serious Obstacle to Happy Marriages*   We must all help in removing that ignorance which is one of the most serious hindrances to sexually satisfactory marriages. We must establish the fact that every woman not only has a possibility, but also a right to obtain sexual satisfaction, orgasm, in her marriage. First of all, it will give *her* life an entirely new quality, and the husband also will be happier in the knowledge that he is able to satisfy his wife. For the woman the important thing in this respect is that she be willing to follow the husband's lead in his love play, reacting in some perceptible way immediately when he starts it. And what is needed in the husband is the exercise of his self-control. He can best use his self-control in keeping up the love play until the wife is ready. Furthermore he should endeavor to approach her at those times when she is most susceptible to love. For many women this consideration by the husband is the most essential element in the whole matter. It is his duty to find out about these periods and remember them. He should, in addition, endeavor to find out about her most important zones of excitation.

263. *Sexual Neuroses* When the husband has ejaculated, and thus obtained his orgasm his penis generally shrinks and becomes limp. As a result he most often will have to interrupt intercourse rather soon after, or he will not be able to continue it in such a way that he can carry the woman further forward toward her orgasm. The harsh fate of the unsatisfied woman is therefore this: that while the husband may fall asleep quickly after having achieved his release, she is lying there beside him wide awake, her senses tense, a prey to her waking dreams, and perhaps bitterly considering herself as nothing but an instrument, an accessory, for his use. She may regard him as a ruthless egotist, who thinks only of his own pleasure. In time, such a wife who repeatedly has been brought on to a high pitch of sexual excitation without obtaining release may develop a *sexual neurosis*. This disturbance is responsible for the majority of calls from women patients who seek the advice of nerve specialists in sex matters. It must be considered of the utmost importance that such couples be given sensible and correct guidance on how to go about achieving married bliss. In many cases a repetition of intercourse, as soon as possible after the first one, will put everything in order. The conditions then, as a rule, will be such as to render it more difficult for the man and at the same time easier for the once ungratified woman to attain orgasm.

264. *The Highly Sexed or Erotic Woman* The excitation curve of the highly sexed or erotic woman ascends more steeply than that of the ordinary woman. She generally reaches her orgasm considerably before the man and may reach it one or more times during intercourse before the man attains his, and then even follow his orgasm. This is probably due to the fact that such women are already, in imagination, deeply involved in the love play before it actually starts. Such women are frequently extremely happy in marriage.

265. *The Easily Satisfied Woman* Some women are erotic in the sense that they react very quickly to their husband's caresses and therefore reach an orgasm promptly. They then remain somewhat inactive, and do not, as a rule, obtain another orgasm simultaneously with the husband.

Chapter 26: **FRIGIDITY**

266. *What Is Frigidity?* The term frigidity really has two meanings. In very few cases women may be without potential sexual desire, as a result of a lack of hormones or other deficiencies causing a type of infantilism. This is called frigidity by nature. Frigidity by nature is always preceded by other, very obvious signs of infantilism; thus sexual coolness is but a symptom among others. Therefore, frigidity by nature necessarily will have already been detected before sexual relations are established.

Generally, however, the term frigidity is used to denote sexual coolness, and the large majority of so-called frigid women should properly be placed in this second category. The women who come to me for advice concerning their sexual coolness very often incorrectly believe they are suffering from frigidity by nature.

267. *Sexual Coolness* Frigidity then, generally, means *sexual coolness.* The sexually cold woman will remain entirely passive and insensitive during intercourse. She does not derive any benefit or pleasure from intercourse at all; most often she feels only loathing. Already at the early stage of approach the man often arouses her distaste; she shows no understanding during the love play stage and may oppose it. She may be angered by the man's caresses which she often regards as salacious and offensive. She fears the sexual act as something revolting and often faces it with defiance, as it seems to her to be not only repulsive senselessness, but also a cruel dishonor. The man usually is not able to comprehend why she meets him with such cold scorn when he turns to her. This may be quite difficult for him as among sexually cold women there are a great many who by their looks, manners, and general behavior produce a particularly exciting effect.

268. *What Causes Sexual Coolness?* Unfortunate circumstances in development may cause sexual coolness. The young woman may not have been ready for sexual intercourse when it was forced upon her. She, therefore, reacted coldly. Sexual coolness may also be due to certain inhibitions. Perhaps the young girl has been told or has heard so much about how disgusting sexual intercourse was supposed to be from limited or detailed accounts given as a rule by well-meaning mothers, aunts, or other relatives, who themselves may never have experienced or understood the meaning of the whole thing. In this manner she developed: fright, disgust, or repulsion were instilled in her attitude toward sexual intercourse. There are quite a wide variety of other possible reasons; the first attempt at intercourse may have been so badly bungled that she felt no inclination for a repetition. She perhaps did not get the man she had set her heart on, and decided to remain faithful to him in her longings and thoughts when she entered into a "marriage of reason" which, of all marriages, is the most unreasonable. She may place an arbitrary limit on her sexual desires from misguided religious or ethical ideas, or from fear, or because her partner proves to be psychologically so very different from her, or because quarrels and misunderstandings mar their married life.

Self-gratification or masturbation is regarded by some as a frequent source of sexual coolness. Such an idea is based on a false interpretation of what sexual coolness really is. The woman who habitually satisfies herself and finally only reacts by excitation of the clitoris, is very far from being sexually cold. She actually may be just the opposite. She may only be unable to obtain release through a normal intercourse.

269. *Treatment of Frigidity* Even in the few cases where frigidity is frigidity by nature and, therefore, is due to *some defect in physical development, infantilism,* good results may sometimes be achieved through therapy. Since it is the development of hormones which is deficient we have, therefore, a distinct guiding line as to what treatment should be adopted. In those cases success depends upon starting the treatments as early as possible. Sexual coolness, may sometimes have something to do with certain changes in the ovaries (degeneration through tiny cysts). However, this point of view makes no provision for what treatment should be applied. In most cases, therefore, the therapy of sexual coolness can only consist in giving sensible advice and guidance to the couple. The particular psychological guidance depends on each individual case. Such guidance should be given to the husband as well as to the wife.

Chapter 27: GENITAL SPASMS— VAGINISM

270. *What Are Genital Spasms?* Genital spasms, also called vaginism, is a relatively rare complaint manifesting itself by the violent contractions of the vagina as soon as any attempt at intercourse is undertaken. The contractions are so marked that it is impossible for the penis to make its way through the convulsively closed vaginal opening.

271. *What Causes Genital Spasms?* In very rare cases the genital spasms may be caused by a real, mechanical obstacle to the insertion of the penis: a tear that hurts, a particularly narrow vaginal entrance, tender remnants of the hymen, etc.

A more frequent reason is masturbation practiced over a long period results in the vulva and the vagina becoming extremely sensitive. Also ailments in the internal abdominal organs may be the cause of genital spasms. However, the great majority of cases are of a nervous nature. This type may be due to early notions about intercourse being something painful; previous experiences may also have provoked fear of intercourse. As additional causes of these spasms we may mention the wife's aversion to the marriage partner and fear of an unwanted baby.

272. *Treatment of Genital Spasms* Vaginism is a very unfortunate condition. In rare cases surgery may be necessary, in other cases it may be relieved or helped by mutual understanding between husband and wife. And one intercourse, normally carried out, may do away with the condition forever. Genital spasms always require treatment by a physician when they appear. Sometimes it is considered necessary to keep the married couple separated for some months to permit the exaggerated fear to vanish. In other cases certain forms of psychotherapy, including exercises in relaxation, eventually supplemented by methodically executed dilatations, may bring about a successful result more rapidly. In case of a very difficult vaginism it may become necessary to have recourse to artificial insemination. After the baby has been born the genital spasms will usually have disappeared.

Chapter 28: DISPLEASURE AT INTERCOURSE (DYSPAREUNIA)

273. *What Is Dyspareunia?* In some rather recent medico-scientific literature there is a certain tendency to define *dyspareunia* as especially painful at intercourse. Such a definition is not wholly correct. Dyspareunia means any form of displeasure at intercourse without indicating any particular reason for it. It occurs in two forms. *Primary dyspareunia* means that the woman has never felt any pleasure or satisfaction in sexual intercourse. As a rule the deeper reason is deficient sexual development. *Secondary dyspareunia* means displeasure at intercourse experienced by persons who formerly had felt enjoyment during sexual intercourse. The causes for these conditions are many and differ widely.

274. *Dyspareunia in Men* Primary dyspareunia occurs mainly in deficiently developed individuals who have no special interest in the female sex. These men may have this condition because of poorly developed sex organs and rare, deficient, or no erection. It is rather the exception for such persons to get involved in sexual intercourse and thus risk sexual disturbances. They generally remain bachelors or perhaps slip into marriage more or less against their will. There is a possibility that hormone treatments may be of some benefit in such cases.

Secondary dyspareunia, on the other hand, occurs rather exclusively in men who were previously able to have intercourse, but who, after several unsuccessful attempts, refrain from trying again, because they fear they may not be able to complete the undertaking.

275. *Dyspareunia in Women* If primary dyspareunia occurs in women the majority of them are deficiently developed sexually, frequently having a poorly functioning hormone sex system and infantile sex organs. These women are often poorly fitted for having children. Hormone treatments may sometimes be recommended in these cases which largely correspond to frigidity due to deficient sex development.

Secondary dyspareunia in women may be due to varying causes. The most common reason for their displeasure during intercourse is that these women have repeatedly been disappointed in having failed to attain release through orgasm, or they have not experienced the orgasm in the way they had been yearning for. Common causes are also found in emotional disappointments that have called forth a feeling of disgust with the male sex in general, or diseases in the genital organs that make intercourse painful. Finally, when a mother is nursing her baby, dyspareunia may occur, but this form of dyspareunia normally disappears as soon as the child has been weaned. If any treatment is needed or possible, it should consist of psychotherapy.

276. Ten Reasons Why Women May Refuse Sexual Intercourse On the basis of what has been presented in preceding sections concerning a woman's normal sex life and its disturbances, the most common reasons why a wife refuses to have intercourse with her husband may now be enumerated as the following:

1. She is sexually cold.
2. She does not love him.
3. She fears pregnancy. This is a frequent reason, particularly when economic difficulties are present, complicated by ignorance of other means of birth control than continence. It may be, though, that reasons of conscience prevent a wife from employing such means.
4. She is reluctant about having intercourse because the husband too often fails to satisfy her.
5. Intercourse is painful because the hymen is tough or not entirely opened up, or because of an organic fault in the genital organs, or because of an inflammation in the external or internal genital organs.
6. When she had her first intercourse her male partner showed a lack of consideration, in ruthless brutality for example, which she cannot forget.
7. She suffers from inhibitions, whose origin is rooted in faulty sexual education.
8. She experiences displeasure during intercourse because she is nursing her baby at the time.
9. She is displeased at intercourse because her sex need at the moment is at its periodic ebb.
10. She is tired.

Chapter 29: HATRED AND JEALOUSY

277. Hatred and Its Causes It is not our intention to make a thorough analysis of hatred, however tempting such an undertaking might be. All we want to do is to present a basic foundation for the understanding of the nature of hatred. This is essential inasmuch as hatred, or suppressed hatred, plays an overwhelmingly great part (hitherto rather often not considered) in the disturbances of the couple's sex life as such, and in married life in general.

It has been found that such disturbances may be remedied in a great many cases if the partners can determine the origin of the hatred that is almost always discovered in their relationship. This justifies us in concluding that in many cases such disturbances could be prevented. They could be prevented if people—before they get engaged or marry—could be properly informed and thus be given an opportunity to probe into this matter of hatred.

We have already pointed out that a feeling of hatred may take root in an individual if the person's need meets with opposition that makes its satisfaction impossible. This is particularly true when it is the need of self-assertion and self-respect that is at stake, because the individual considers such frustration offensive. Infringement on a person's ordinary need of comfort may also incite hatred.

Every offense creates a need for compensation, and this need clamors for satisfaction. *Hatred* is such a need, and we get a very good idea of its nature by observing the manner in which this need seeks to obtain satisfaction. It may be achieved through interior or exterior reactions.

Inwardly hatred may mask itself in many different disguises: as aversion or anger, or both, in the presence of the hated person; as annoyance or fury at his success and, conversely, as a spiteful relishing of his failure; or as fear of his renewed success, and hope of his complete defeat.

Outwardly, hatred may also reveal itself in a great number of reactions. Some of them are typical *defense reactions*, such as avoidance of parties or other social gatherings in which the hated person will participate, and demonstrative departure from a party when a meeting with him cannot be avoided; cancellation of subscriptions to periodicals in which the hated person's writings may appear; withdrawal from membership in their common political party, etc.

The other type of outward reactions are typically *aggressive reactions*. When meeting the hated person one tries to lord it over him, maybe start a fight; one resorts to deceit or trickery of every description, directly by trying to put obstacles in his way, and indirectly, for instance, by slander. The hater, on the whole, quite often with complete disregard for his own comfort and even at the risk of his life, demonstrates his passion for hurting or destroying the object of his hate. That, as a matter of fact, is the basis of *sabotage* in its widest sense. Sabotage in varying degrees is extremely frequent in human relations and can be found also in the animal world. Among human beings it starts right back in the kindergarten, continues through the school and workshop, to business life and professional circles, in the conduct of war, and in marriage which we mention last here, because it is the most important to remember. Concrete examples of manifestations of hatred are superfluous, I believe.

278. *Hate Hinging on Love* Within a couple's sex life and, apparently, most often where the sex partners are not married, all forms of hatred may crop up. The love of an individual may be prosaically defined in part as a biologically conditioned consciousness that a certain other person is capable of satisfying a number of one's physical and emotional needs. If it later develops that these needs cannot, after all, be satisfied, a hatred—hinging on love—may develop as a result of the thorough disappointment, unhappy love, contempt or loathing. The dissatisfied partner gradually comes to regard the other partner's sexual approaches as unpleasant or even repulsive, and may come to hate the other on that score. Love also may change into hate by one partner offending the other's need of self-assertion or self-respect, or both. This form of hatred, however, definitely tends to change back into love again, particularly if both partners realize what is at the bottom of it, and both seriously endeavor to reach an agreement on how to rid themselves of it.

279. *Jealousy* The hatred directed toward a person who has attained a reward coveted by oneself, is called *jealousy*; if the reward that both endeavored to obtain is the love of another person, the jilted suitor's hatred is called jealousy conditioned by love. The basis for such jealousy is the hater's need of self-assertion. It also may possibly be because the person has been offended when he was evaluated and found lacking in something. The manifestations of jealousy are exactly the same as those of any other form of hatred. Evidence that the underlying cause is some offended need can be found. It is usually traced to the circumstances in which a man, afflicted with a marked need of self-assertion, self-respect, and a feeling of ownership, gets especially furious if he believes his monopoly at intercourse has been lost. Woman's jealousy, on the other hand, seems to hinge largely upon infringement of her need of belonging to her man, and of her need of security. For this reason a wife, as a rule, does not make such a show of jealousy toward a person her husband sleeps with as toward a person with whom he entertains a friendship on the basis of genuine understanding.

As will be apparent from this, all forms of jealousy are based on an infringement of the need for self-assertion. The transgression, however, need not have any direct connection with the person against whom the jealous feeling is directed. If, for instance, a man's need for self-assertion has been infringed upon on some previous occasion—perhaps for an entirely different reason—without obtaining some type of satisfactory compensation, a residue may be retained in his mind in the form of an *inferiority complex*. This complex comes to represent a special kind of jealousy, perhaps the most common of all. It indicates that the jealous man has so little self-confidence that he constantly fears another man will take his beloved away from him. As in all other feelings of inferiority there is a great deal of vanity in this jealousy which most frequently is unjustified. A man suffering from such a complex must, therefore, realize that his peace of mind will be restored when he properly considers the reasons his wife loves him: she may not love him for his intelligence, or because he is handsome, rich, or anything else—qualities in which others might very well surpass him—but simply because he is the way he is, because he is himself. The man, furthermore, should be proud if others admire his choice, which reflects on his judgment and discrimination. On top of that, his jealous actions may themselves justify behavior which previously had not been contemplated. Thus unfaithfulness in the husband or wife may be for the first time seriously considered only as a result of the suggestions provided by the jealousy displayed by the other party.

8

MARRIAGE

Chapter 30: CHOICE OF A MARRIAGE PARTNER

280. *Importance of Choice* Both husband and wife must love, honor, and respect each other. Sexual attraction alone is not enough, as we have mentioned several times in preceding sections. The physical attraction that at times may seem to them to be overwhelming, often has a tendency to disappear after marriage. On the other hand, many a young woman has shed bitter tears because she married a man who was deeply attracted to her but could not arouse and satisfy her active sexual need.

281. *About the Age for Marriage* The partners should not only be physically fit and properly developed; they should also be mentally mature, with a good sense of tolerance and having a definite character. These conditions will not generally be fulfilled until the man is about twenty-five, and the woman about twenty years of age, even though there are great variations on either side. By far the majority of marriages are entered into shortly after these ages.

282. *Getting Acquainted* Certainly the most important preparation for marriage is getting to know one another well. One who endeavors to determine the actual cause of most unsuccessful marriages usually finds that it is rooted in disappointment.

And what is disappointment? It is the feeling that one's expectations have not been met. Therefore, the extremely important function of the engagement period is to provide the opportunity for the couple to really know each other well. My advice to any engaged couple is "be yourself!" In this I say: "Neither of you two should—for fear of jolting your partner's sensibilities—hide those basic opinions you may hold, whether moral, ethical, religious, social or political, or of any other nature. And to get to know each other's views on sex."

In respect to sex the couple must above all ascertain whether they have the same *attitude* toward sex life, since a marriage partner's avoidance of sexual intercourse *may* be considered sufficient cause for a separation.

283. *About Intercourse Between Engaged Couples* In this matter the partners must be thoroughly convinced that they are compatible. To be certain of that they must know whether they can satisfy each other sexually, in intercourse. However, by education and inclination I must admit that I personally tend to hold the view that intercourse should not take place before the marriage ceremony. This is my personal position, although I am acquainted with and respect all the arguments in favor of premarital relations (as, for example, that real love asks for no *guarantees*). It is not rare for a young woman to come to me for a consultation, asking to be measured for a diaphragm for use when she is married. If, upon examining the young woman, I find that the hymen is unbroken, I call attention to the fact that it will be very difficult to take the measurements with the hymen still in place. If I add that, in some people's opinion, the first intercourse should take place without the use of any kind of contraceptive, many of the young women receive it with genuine relief and joy, declaring that that was the way they had always wanted it to be.

And yet I consider it my duty to say this: By far the majority of the innumerable married couples whom I have queried on these matters, the greater number told me that they had had sexual intercourse before the wedding. I found, moreover, that among the happiest of these married couples the fiancé had loyally left the supreme decision to his girl.

Each person must take these words of mine and ponder them in his own way. They are very revealing in regard to happiness in marriage. The question of sexual intercourse or no sexual intercourse between engaged couples depends entirely on the moral standards of the couple involved.

Statistics show, however that 43.5 per cent of all first-born children are conceived before the wedding. It should be noted also that Kinsey's investigations disclose that 85 per cent out of all married American men state they have had premarital intercourse.

284. Prenuptial Medical Examination Vast efforts are devoted to the outward preparations for marriage. Considering this it is strange that only a few states seem to care much whether the young couple is physically sound and healthy, and able to fulfill the bodily requirements of a married couple. Nothing, however, would be more logical than, in addition to the other legal documents already required for contracting marriage, there was added a medical certificate on the general health of the marriage partners. Such an examination should place special emphasis on the good condition of their genital organs and specify that they were free from symptoms of any dangerous *communicable* diseases.

285. Hereditary Taint Modern research on heredity reveals grave warnings against thoughtlessly entering into the state of matrimony. For in choosing a marriage partner it must be borne in mind that one does not just marry that particular person, but in reality also marries his or her kin. Insanity and mental afflictions may be hereditary and lie dormant although they may not have shown up for several generations. Certain forms of epilepsy are hereditary, as well as certain nervous disorders, diseases of the eyes and ears, of the blood, and several other diseases. A number of physical malformations are hereditary too. I do not recommend that a partner must break the engagement because it is found that the other may eventually transmit some hereditary taint to the offspring. But the matter ought to be thoroughly discussed and investigated *before* the wedding. Love must stand its test in relation to these hard facts, and the test should be made before marriage in order to limit potential misfortune as much as possible.

286. *Endogamy* Among many peoples the custom of endogamy has prevailed since time immemorial. Under such a practice persons of *different* race, people, tribe, hereditary caste, class or religion, are *forbidden to intermarry*. The Chinese do not marry with surrounding uncivilized tribes, and not even the common religion, or a common fatherland, can erase the deep antipathy an Arab feels toward a Turk; a Kurd toward a Syrian Nestorian, or a Magyar toward a Slav. Marriages between Lapps and Swedes are very rare and are regarded as dishonorable to both. It is equally rare for Lapps and Norwegians to intermarry, and it hardly ever occurs that a Lapp marries a Russian.

In antiquity, Athenians and Spartans were not allowed to marry foreigners. The Romans were forbidden marriage with barbarians. Such ties were punishable by the death penalty. The historian, Tacitus, gained the impression from his study of the Teutons that they too abstained from marrying into foreign tribes. In southern Mexico one formerly was only permitted to marry within the native *rancho*, and the Hottentots always married members of their own *kraal*.

In Wales, in olden times, marriage could be contracted only between members of the same clan. The Hindu caste system is known for its severe endogamic precepts. In Rome patricians and plebeians could not marry each other until the year 455 before Christ. The old Germans (Teutons) punished a freeman who had sexual intercourse with a bondwoman; and a freewoman who was guilty of a corresponding offense had to pay for it with her life. In Germany, as late as the thirteenth century, a woman who had sexual intercourse with her bondman lost her freedom.

It is evident from these examples that endogamic precepts are based on lack of mutual respect and understanding. Such practices will some day lose their remaining importance when the human race shall have advanced in altruism and common tolerance. This will occur when civilization gradually—in spite of periodical backsliding—succeeds in narrowing the gap that divides nations and different social classes from each other.

287. *Exogamy* This term is defined as marriage between members of two different families or clans. Violation of the accepted practice was strictly punishable, as in the cases of endogamy mentioned in the preceding section. Exogamy has never become quite as widespread as endogamy, and none of the many attempts to explain its origin seem satisfactory from a scientific point of view.

In old Bogotá, in Colombia, men and women from the same town were not allowed to intermarry because they were all held to be brothers and sisters. A brother, however, might very well marry his own sister, provided she was born in another town. In Australia the native population is divided, on the one hand, into resident hordes and subdivisions of hordes; on the other hand, into clans, comprising individual members of the different hordes. There a man is forbidden to marry a woman within the same horde or subdivision of a horde.

Numerous African and East-Indian tribes are not permitted to marry within the population of the same town. In certain parts of Russia a man always chooses his bride from a strange town, and even in regions where this is not the case, the bridegroom is called by a synonym meaning "stranger." Greenland Eskimos consider it peculiar and blameworthy if a young man and a young woman who have grown up together and served in the same foster family want to marry. And according to the Arctic explorers, it is considered most correct if the respective marriage partners come from different home towns. The interdictions against intermarriage between relatives existing in modern times must be regarded partly as a residue of ancient exogamic precepts, partly as the result of hereditary considerations. There is a hereditary risk that the offspring of too closely related persons may be inferior in quality to that of unrelated persons or of kindred ones more distantly related.

288. *To Whom Is Marriage Forbidden?* A particular loathing of *incest*—sexual intercourse between close relatives—seems to have been very widespread throughout the ages. But the conception of who was to be considered a close relative was subject to wide variations. Cambyses and other Persian kings married their sisters, and in the Book of Genesis we read that Abraham married his half sister and considered this relationship legal because they did not have the same mother. In most civilized countries marriage between first cousins has been forbidden practically up to modern times. In France, for cousins to marry it was necessary to obtain the consent of the authorities, in Italy that of the king. However, in the great majority of countries marriage between cousins is now permitted.

289. *Choice of a Parent for One's Children* This is a matter of great importance in selecting one's marriage partner. I have already mentioned a little concerning it in connection with the question of hereditary taints. But let me add a few words to the young man and woman in love who are considering marriage.

Young man! Remember that the girl whom you want to marry will be the mother of your children! Do not give them a mother who is merely good looking and otherwise superficial, vain, and selfish! Will she be capable of making a good home for your children? Will she be able to bring them up in such a way that they will become good, happy, honest people?

And you, young woman, who contemplates marriage! Is your sweetheart the kind of man you wish the father of your children to be? Would you want your children to model themselves on him? Is he such a person that you could say to your children: "If you want to make me happy, try to be like your father!" If it became necessary, would he work and deny himself in order to give your children the start in life that is their right?

One may put these questions to oneself without fear. True love will be able to reply to them with an honestly meant Yes, and this is part of the proper preparation for marriage.

Chapter 31: **MARRIAGE AND SEX LIFE**

290. *Like "Law and Right"* Many will ask: Isn't marriage and sex life the same thing? Can there be a normal marriage without sex life, or a normal sex life without marriage? It is not at all easy to answer this question. That is probably why more has been written on this subject than on anything else in the world. And one has the impression that the discussion will go on. "Marriage" and "sex life" are not identical. They must be considered in the same light as the term "law and right." Law and right are not the same. If they were there would be no reason to call them "law and right," although one has the same inclination to think of "law" with "right" as of "marriage" with "sex," and *vice versa*.

291. *Marriage and Sex Life Are Closely Linked* Married life is intimately bound up with sex. The greatest sex activity occurs within the framework of matrimony. The fervor and intensity of sex life in marriage is quite superior. But it presupposes acknowledgment of the binding, lifelong character of the marriage tie. Only where both partners accept full responsibility, mutually working at the happiness of the *couple*, wishing to share not only the joy of life, but also its sorrows, do the personalities of husband and wife develop. The teamwork for home and children, therefore, naturally increases their mutual regard and trust; only when these conditions are present is there existent right soil for developing the *deepest emotional understanding* and the *highest sexual happiness*.

Says the Bible: "For this cause shall a man leave his father and mother, shall be joined unto his wife and they two shall be one flesh." It is further written: "What therefore God hath joined together let not man put asunder." On the basis of these two quotations matrimony has been proclaimed a mainly religious institution. This has been maintained purely on a basis of interpretation. In the two quotations just mentioned there is nothing whatever to indicate that they refer to matrimony in the sense we deal with it here.

Two people who love each other without being married, when they have declared to each other under responsibility to God that they will henceforth consider themselves as joined together without benefit of the clergy, might be entirely justified in sheltering under the Bible words: "What therefore God hath joined together let not man put asunder." Even though excellent Christians stimulated by the best intentions have published books and championed viewpoints maintaining that marriage is a religious institution, one cannot help thinking of what these quotations *really say.*

292. *Matrimony as a Social Institution* No, matrimony is a purely social measure. The interest of the churches in marriage has not been a matter of consistent policy during the course of centuries. Historically, marriage is a civil, purely social institution intended to legalize sexual ties in their social and economic aspects and to provide security for the offspring.

293. *The Medico-hygienic Significance of Matrimony* Marriage being a social institution, it has become subject to customs and conventions, a number of which are far removed from love and its being. A great number of marriages called "marriages of convenience" are the outcome of adherence to such conventions, considerations of business, respect for traditions and wishes of parents, etc. If, as a physician, I find it practical to give a brief survey of the various forms of marriage it is in order to best elucidate a number of medico-hygienic conditions in relation to matrimony. These conditions, in conjunction with the *love* present in a marriage, will determine whether it is going to be a success or not. Frequently neither bride nor bridegroom knows anything about these matters which may cause friction and unhappiness and which could be avoided if one is forewarned.

Chapter 32: DIFFERENT FORMS OF MARRIAGE

294. *What Is Monogamy, and What Is Polygamy?* *Monogamy* is a form of marriage in which one husband has one wife, and one wife has one husband. *Polygamy* refers to a form of marriage where one husband has several wives (*polygyny*) or one wife has several husbands (*polyandry*). With a few exceptions, Western civilization has always recognized monogamy as the only legitimate form of marriage.

295. *Not Polygamous, but Polyerotic* In offering a defense for polygamy in the form of polygyny the argument usually presented is that man is polygamous by nature, in contrast to woman who is generally monogamous. Both statements, however, are equally erroneous. In reality, man is not polygamous. Normally he is not interested in, or inclined to have, several homes or to divide his house into sections each with a wife and her children. The misunderstanding is, perhaps, largely due to people failing to distinguish between the terms *polygamous* and *polyerotic*. For there can be no doubt that innumerable men are polyerotic—in that they are sexually attracted to more than one woman and desire, or at least are not disinclined, to have sexual relations with more than one of the female sex. In exactly the same way there are women—fewer in number perhaps—who at certain times feel sexually attracted to men other than their husbands. When women—in contrast to men—curb their polyerotic tendencies, not permitting them to be expressed, it is undoubtedly partly due to the traditional convention that "decent" women do not "behave like that." Yet their principal inhibition stems from the fear of getting unwanted children out of wedlock. To this latter consideration comes the related fear of the consequences which might involve her position, particularly in relation to her husband.

296. *Practice of Polyeroticism* It is not correct to say that many men and women, although living in monogamy, really practice polygyny or polyandry. What they actually practice is polyeroticism. In societies where polyandry for women or polygyny for men is legitimized by law, man's polyerotic tendencies are afforded a natural outlet within these matrimonial forms.

But this situation does not exist in a society that accepts only monogamy. In such societies polyeroticism also flourishes, but not openly; it flourishes secretly.

A doctor's profession in our day and age often comes close to being that of a father confessor. From my experience I cannot help coming to the conclusion that married faithfulness occurs only in a minority of cases. Faithfulness would seem to exist under two circumstances; first, in those happy marriages where the partners understand each other, and are rather instinctively or by intimate knowledge of sexual behavior capable of fulfilling each other's sex needs completely within the range of monogamy. In this circumstance polyeroticism, of course, would not interest them. Faithfulness seems to exist under the second circumstances among couples who disapprove of unfaithfulness in marriage for ethical, religious, or other—perhaps purely practical—reasons. Included in this category may be couples who realize they are not happy together.

297. *Causes of Polygamy and Polyeroticism* The principal cause of polygyny and polyandry, matrimonial forms that have been practiced in many different tribes throughout the ages, is connected directly with population problems. Either there were more women living in a certain area than men, or more men than women.

Many people believe that polygamy was the original form for marriage. Such a view is not correct. The evidence that has been advanced to support this theory cannot stand up against the arguments of science. Exactly the opposite condition actually prevailed. Polygamy seems to presuppose a certain degree of culture, including a limited inclination to jealousy. And it is a fact that polygamy does not occur among the most primitive savages.

In families practicing polyandry the relationship is generally solved by the wife (wives) belonging to all the brothers, the oldest brother holding the position as privileged husband. In India there are areas in which polyandry is carried on where the number of men in the community exceeds that of the women, and with polygyny where there are more women than men.

One of the basic causes for *polyeroticism* is the *forced periodical self-restraint* of the male. Certain women menstruate for one or two weeks, which may mean an essential limitation of sex intercourse. Another frequent cause is that "he falls in love again." The wife may have neglected to keep herself fresh and pretty. She may have forgotten that she must have the same exciting effect on her husband and be as attractive to him as before they were married and during their early times together. She forgets that he must really be wooed anew every day. Or perhaps, in his humdrum everyday existence, the husband may have forgotten that it is up to him to keep bright and burnished the aura of their first enthusiastic love, not only as the "lord and master." He should be as the brilliant comrade, the chivalrous knight from the engagement days whom the wife expects to receive with open arms every evening when he comes home from work.

In communities of former days *children* were considered a symbol of prosperity and respect. Children continue to represent the best social security the parents may have in countries that have no old-age pensions.

The word *proletarian* is derived from the Latin word *proles* (offspring) and originally meant that a proletarian was one who served the state by begetting children. In long periods of history, particularly in young communities, in ancient Israel's New Zion, as in modern Canada, and in the cabins of African villages, the desire to have many hands to help with the work, by begetting numerous offspring, has tended to further and condone polygamy, and particularly polygyny. In this connection it is characteristic that the Mormon state of Utah was founded in a *pioneer* country.

298. *Historical Basis of Monogamy* In the hunting age of human history woman's labor was not worth very much. By his hunting the man was responsible for both food and clothing for his family. At this historical stage monogamy was predominant. Later, when agriculture became the dominant activity, the wife and children came to represent a valuable labor force, and polygamy had its flowering.

Abstinence in sexual intercourse during pregnancy and the period of nursing is no longer considered necessary. Following the rather general introduction of the bottle feeding of babies the nursing period has been shortened or breast feeding eliminated entirely in some cases. In this manner and other ways civilization offers women the chance of maintaining their good looks and youthful appearance much further into middle age than ever before. Parents' desire for children is less marked, and to have a lot of children is no longer an absolute aid in the fight for survival, rather the contrary. In the present day people have friends in addition to their relatives, and other yardsticks for measuring riches and esteem than numerous children. The widespread use of domestic animals, household utensils, and machinery has greatly reduced the necessity for the wife to contribute her work.

The emotion of love has become a more subtle thing, with the result that the passion for a particular person is more intense. In civilized communities more attention is now paid to the feelings of the female sex, and this emancipation of women has opened up possibilities for their achieving economic independence which in many cases has freed them from the necessity of marrying in order to live.

299. *Ethical Basis of Monogamy* In the preceding sketch of the historical development of monogamy several ethical viewpoints have already been mentioned. In addition, there is a number of principles championed by monogamy's most zealous defenders. These say that no one man has a right to take several wives as long as some men can't even get one wife. It is maintained that polygamy is but an expression of licentiousness given a legitimate guise. Polygyny is considered a practice which works an injustice on the female sex. *Forced monogamy* as a Christian principle dates back to the early Christian communities where monogamy was the only form of matrimony that was recognized. The Church of Antiquity on the whole—to a great extent on account of a literal belief that the Day of Judgment was near—looked skeptically on matters of sex and regarded unchastity as about the worst sin. The church at that time held the female sex in limited esteem and professed a loathing of sensuality.

300. *The Monogamous "Feeling"* The undisputed revived growth of monogamy is undoubtedly due, primarily, to a genuinely monogamous feeling apparently present in the human being. Even among savages intense passion for a particular individual of the opposite sex is not unknown. Therefore, even in communities where polygyny is permitted, one may observe very definite examples of consistently practiced monogamy. In various forest tribes in Brazil, marriage is monogamous. The same was true of several extremely primitive Californian tribes.

Among the Karoks, for example, not even the chief was permitted to have two wives. Every man, however, could have as many slave women as he was able to take care of, yet it was considered most blameworthy if he had sexual intercourse with more than one. Among the Veddahs (in Ceylon) and the natives of the Andaman Islands monogamy is upheld very strongly. In many places illicit sexual intercourse is regarded as a capital sin. In several Indian tribes both polygyny and the practice of having concubines are forbidden, and in many places in the peninsula of Malacca polygyny is not known to have been practiced. There were many regions in Australia where polygyny was unknown until the Europeans arrived, influencing the natives' practices. Monogamy cannot be said to be a practice of sexual relationship limited to human beings. Apes, for example, are also monogamous.

301. *An Australian Group Marriage* In certain parts of Australia special group marriages are found. The tribe is divided into classes of which all brothers in one class are considered as married, *a priori*, to all daughters of the other class and, consequently, are not allowed to marry anyone else. In one class the brothers may be called, for instance, *Ipai*, and the sisters *Ipata;* in another respectively *Kubi* and *Kubitha*. All Ipai are then considered to be married to all Kubitha, and all Kubi to all Ipata.

302. *Schopenhauer's Tetragamy* The philosopher Schopenhauer formulated his so-called tetragamy (marriage of two men and two women) on the basis of several assumptions: The number of men and women in the world are about equal. Women function as reproductive beings for only half of their allotted life-span during which time they are man's partners in the pleasures of the senses. What woman's sex capacity lacks in *duration* is amply made up for by her being able *during that period* to satisfy two or three men without sustaining any harm or injury. Within monogamy she is only given the chance to exploit 50 per cent of her sex need and receives gratification of only half of her further desires. To regulate this condition Schopenhauer proposes that two men share a woman while she is still young. After she has lost her bloom, they shall again share a young Number Two for the rest of their days. The philosopher considered that the advantage of this arrangement was that both women's material needs could be taken care of. Also he held that every young man, as he sets out on his career at a time when he is least proficient in world wealth, would be responsible for the upkeep of only half a woman and possibly only a few small children. Later, when his financial situation may well have improved, he would be responsible for one, eventually two women, and many children. Schopenhauer believed that if an arrangement of that nature is not adopted, men during one half of their lives will carry on illicit sexual relations, and during the other half would be "cuckolds." As a result, the women would also be divided into two groups: the cheated and the cheats. In conclusion he said: "He who marries young will later be saddled with an old wife, and he who marries late first gets venereal diseases and thereupon gets his brow decorated with horns! The woman must either sacrifice the flower of her youth to an already jaded man, or later discover that she is no longer a fit partner for a man still in the force of his age."

303. *The District Manor in Oelseby-Magle*   Schopenhauer's eighteenth-century plan of tetragamy has some very obvious limitations and will probably never be completely realized in practical life. Nevertheless, in a modified form, it was actually practiced in nineteenth-century Denmark by a number of civil service employees.

In Denmark clergymen were and still are salaried by the State, being servants in the State Church. It was then customary for a young minister, for instance, in order to obtain a good livelihood to be obliged to marry the widow of his predecessor. When she died he married a young wife, who, after his death was taken over by the new parson together with the vicarage and the living. This practice, however, died out about a hundred years ago.

Chapter 33: ORIGIN OF MARRIAGE

304. *Stealing the Bride (Rape)*   A very ancient form of making a marriage, if not actually *the* most primitive, was rape, stealing the bride. I have mentioned that a strong aversion

to too close intermarrying is predominant in very primitive peoples. This attitude, added to the frequently encountered difficulty of finding a wife within one's own tribe without gratifying her relatives, would be the main reason for gaining a bride by rape.

305. *Purchasing the Bride* Among most primitive, agricultural peoples the man is obliged to pay a price for his bride. In many Australian aboriginal tribes the custom of a woman-barter has prevailed: a woman from one family is simply exchanged for a woman from another family. All over the globe was the old, still more widespread custom that the young husband must literally work for the father-in-law until he has paid a suitable compensation in labor for his bride. Thus, in Central America, Peru, China, and Japan it was customary to pay the woman's father or family some remuneration with a certain number of cattle. Illustrative of this is the fact that our word for pecuniary is derived from the Latin word *pecunia*, which originally meant cattle. The purpose of such a sum or compensation was partly to compensate the girl's father for his estimated loss in labor by giving up his daughter, partly to refund him the money or care he had spent in raising her. Women were regarded as valuable property at that time. Loss of property had to be compensated; sometimes it was even considered a *duty* for the father to claim such compensation.

The higher castes of India were pioneers in abolishing the purchasing of brides. In very ancient Greek and Roman civilizations only limited traces were retained among the plebians. The patricians, on the other hand, had long ago abandoned the custom. In the Scandinavian countries, however, the old custom of buying the bride was kept until the countries had been Christianized about the year 900.

306. *Exchange of Gifts* As purchasing of brides became obsolete or was abolished, the practice was replaced in many places by an exchange of gifts between the two families involved. In other places, the purchase sum changed into the dowry. But in that case it was the wife who received the gift, either as a dowry from her father, or as a wedding gift from her husband.

307. *The Dowry* The new attitude toward giving and receiving money for the daughter in marriage with its debasing quality resulted in the gradual abolition of buying and selling the bride. The old practice changed into the exact opposite form: viz., presenting her a *dowry*. Originally, the dowry represented a type of compensation for the not entirely abolished practice of bride purchasing. In times when women were more numerous than men, it also represented an inducement to one of the few available bachelors to take a daughter away, and might be regarded as a regular prize. In other instances, it might serve to show that the father would participate in the expense of maintaining the home of the newlyweds. In ancient Greece, and in Rome even more so, the presentation of the dowry actually signified that the marriage was legal. This was in contrast to living with concubines who did not bring any dowry. Dowries might amount to very large sums. In Greece, for instance, at the time of Aristotle, the total value of dowries had mounted to the point where no less than two fifths of entire Sparta belonged to women. Right up into more modern times legislation in certain European countries provided that the bride's father must pay the wedding expenses and furnish the young couple's home. In Latin countries the dowry or *dot* still plays so great a role that fairly recently a rich peasant would not accept a small farmer's daughter for her son because she could bring no dowry. Not until the present century has the tendency to regard *love* as the essential thing in a prospective marriage become so widespread that the question of dowry is losing its importance.

308. *Secret Marriages* In the Middle Ages a marriage in Scandinavia according to ecclesiastical and secular law was considered to be legal if the partners had mutually declared that they would marry each other. No public act was required other than the necessity for only two valid witnesses testifying to the arrangement. This accord—the "pledging of troth"—stated that the partners were hence married and sufficed in making the union legal.

If, however, the accord declared that the marriage would not take effect until a later date, it was considered to have been definitely contracted from the moment sexual intercourse had taken place. In that case the pledging of troth entailed the exclusion of any of the partners having sexual intercourse with another person, and eventual offspring were regarded as "born in wedlock." This latter stipulation was also valid in case of a secret pledging of troth, i.e. a troth which had not been publicly proclaimed, also called a "secret marriage." Not until 1799 was the pledging of troth finally abolished.

309. *The Wedding as a Condition for Sexual Intercourse* Measured by the long yardstick of history, the wedding as a condition for sexual intercourse is a modern innovation, less than 150 years old, unknown when our great-grandparents and great-great-grandparents were born. Thus, sexual intercourse between engaged couples—apart from the latest 150 years—has always been a common practice in Denmark. When countless persons in this day and age maintain that it is the free and voluntary consent of the partners that determines the matter, such an attitude is certainly not as radical a departure from custom as they believe. But it should never be forgotten that the pledging of troth which in former days entitled a couple to initiate their sex union meant: *that* the relationship was monogamous, *that* neither partner should have any other sexual tie, *that* the relationship was a binding one, and *that* eventual children were to be considered as having been born in wedlock. To reintroduce the pledging of troth as an act just as valid as the wedding ceremony would, therefore, only be an attempt to put back the clock of history.

Pledging of troth never was analogous to "trial marriages" or "companionate marriages," for those are relationships that can be regarded only as loose ties since they lack the condition of respect for promises made if any such have been made at all.

310. *The Wedding Ceremony* The official wedding ceremony in its present form differs in various countries according to the religions prevalent in them. However, all wedding ceremonies have several things in common. The ecclesiastical or the civil authorities, or both, *publicly proclaim* the legality of the marriage.

Chapter 34: EARLY MARRIED LIFE

311. *The Wedding Night*   The term "wedding night" means the first day or night that sexual intercourse or an attempt at intercourse takes place. This event in particular occupies the young woman's thoughts and often fills her with fear.

There is no reason to be afraid. The anxiety and fear are generally due to well-meaning mothers who, in hushed distaste and in ambiguous allusions, have talked and yet not talked about this event. Perhaps these mothers themselves have rather trying memories of their own wedding night. The basic reason, however, more often is that in their pettiness and lack of insight they really enjoy being exciting and do not properly consider that their attitude might do harm to the daughter.

312. *Breaking of the Hymen (Defloration)*   If the hymen is intact it will generally break at the first sexual intercourse. This is felt as a tension in the hymen by the woman when the penis is pressed into the vaginal opening. In many women the hymen gives way under the pressure in the course of a few minutes, and either dilates, stretches, or breaks easily. The only sensation felt directly is the cessation of tension in the tissue.

There is no question of bursting or splitting of the hymen. In some women very limited bleeding may occur. This, however, generally stops immediately. It is also a very rare occurrence that the vaginal opening is so narrow that intercourse cannot be fully carried out during one of the earliest attempts. If the hymen is *very* tough a small surgical operation easily solves the difficulty.

313. *The Initiation*   If the couple have had sexual relations prior to the wedding night the challenges involved are not as great or the same as those encountered by couples who have had no experience. Then the wedding night is truly a woman's initiation into her married life: she becomes a wife. If the two love each other, and if during their period of engagement she has known how to call forth his affection and protective urge rather than merely excite his sexual desire, then he will certainly realize that on this first night he is undertaking a great task. He will know that now she gives herself to him body and soul. The woman who marries a man without first having tested his real love and tenderness adopts a too carefree attitude in marrying him. But if a woman knows that he loves her and is overflowing with all the fine things he wants to do for her, then he will know how to make the bridal night what it should be to her: the initiation into her woman's life. The wedding night is a great test for a husband. He must prove that he does not think of himself only, but of her, his loved one, and of her happiness; and if they love each other she may be quite sure that he will prove it to her.

314. *The Husband's Responsibility on the Wedding Night*
The husband must know that the first night may make or mar their marriage. The bride has come from her own circle, from her childhood home and family. At the wedding reception she may have listened to any number of toasts perhaps emphasizing again and again that she is entering upon a new and decisive phase of her life. The bridegroom must realize that the wedding night is the introduction to their married life together and that if this introduction turns out to be right, he thereby enters upon the truly intimate happiness of his own life. The wedding night may require great self-control on the part of the husband, but if he is aware of his task he will know what to do. Then the old idea of the priority of "a husband's rights" will not be present in his mind and, consequently, not hers either. Whether or not she has looked to the bridal night with fear and trepidation she will never forget his care and tenderness on that first night, but will love him for life. And when she feels that the solicitude for her is uppermost in his mind then fear, anxiety, and strain will disappear as the morning mists vanish before the rising sun, and neither he nor she will ever completely know afterwards how they became mates in body and soul.

Chapter 35: MARRIAGE IN PRACTICE

315. *The Great Expectations* The primary object of this book is to offer a guide to couples in the practice of a happy marriage. My greatest misgiving when I decided to write really was this: The more one emphasizes the ideal aspects of marriage the greater will be the expectations thus aroused and the possibility of disappointment. The risk that these expectations will not be met thereby increases also.

The expectations linked to the idea of marriage in a modern civilized community—where the marital union is generally preceded by infatuation—are exceedingly great. The faults and imperfections that unfortunately are part of all of us and which daily married life soon reveal, are not seen in the building brilliance of the initial revelation of love. The aspect of imperfections is swept away by love's passion. Her lover's courtship convinces her that she is the ideal woman in the eyes of the ideal man. And she, therefore, endeavors to live up to the ideal man she thinks he is. The man, of course, is affected in a similar way; he endeavors to measure up to the ideal woman by being the ideal man. All this makes it quite simply and yet overwhelmingly certain that never were two people more ideally suited. If outside circumstances do not make it absolutely impossible, marriage is regarded as the only natural thing. Being in love is like that; it makes expectations soar!

When the couple, with mature and deliberate purpose, have endeavored to get to know each other well, expectations are, as a rule, still at a peak. He shows her greater courtesy, consideration, esteem, care, and admiration, in short, more chivalrous homage than any man has ever done before.

She, in turn, shows him tender solicitude, considers his habits, shows admiring respect of his opinions, indulgent yielding and loyalty that cannot fail to be signs of a happy future. In the light of disillusions found after marrying some will stamp their previous courtship behavior as false—but from my knowledge of a very great number of marriages I maintain that it is quite *genuine*.

Added to all this comes the sharing of the new sexual experiences, and the expectations they arouse.

316. *The Happy Marriage* That a marriage is happy means that the expectations the parties had when engaged are met on all essential points, and possibly surpassed on others. That, in brief, is the secret of a happy marriage.

The great majority of couples will soon discover that their happiness is a thing that has to be reconquered every single day. That requires a conscious effort on the part of both husband and wife. This is inherent in the fact that marriage is the most concentrated form of communal living that exists. Therefore, to a most definite extent, it demands three things that are of the utmost importance in community living: 1. learning to adapt oneself, and to compromise; 2. to be a good companion; 3. to be considerate. Marriage has also been called a school, and that is a very striking comparison. Like education, marriage has a general over-all aim and purpose, but both school and marriage are more concerned with *the methods* by which the aim and purpose may be realized.

The immediate purpose of marriage is to meet the expectations linked to it. At the same time, through the social demands it makes, it affords each partner an opportunity to draw richly on the other's personality and opinions and, by the same token, a chance of escaping from the primitive and narrow egotism of *Self*.

317. *How to Keep a Marriage Happy* As to the methods of attaining the embracing objective in marriage, *the first years* generally determine whether the marriage will be happy or not.

Here are a few purely practical hints as to what husband and wife may undertake in other respects to keep their marriage happy.

1. Have your own home.
2. Tell yourself every morning that *once* you were very much in love and that your original, innermost, tender desire every day—*today, too*—is to make the life of your marriage partner richer and happier.

3. Be cheerful and show mutual good will and understanding, not least when the budget comes up for planning.

4. Thank each other, also, for little trifles and services that have become part of a daily pattern.

5. If you have differences of opinion then *immediately* show your willingness to compromise, and after that, live up to your decision loyally.

6. On the whole, show mutual loyalty. Keep your promises. If you have children you must loyally permit your marriage partner's decision on both small and large things to stand, if it was made before yours, even though you do not approve of it.

7. Be loyal in the company of others. Face interference by relatives (or outsiders) with an unshakable, united front.

8. At *all times* avoid nagging and bickering.

9. Never let a day pass without clearing up differences—forgive, and ask forgiveness.

10. Build your home on some religious conviction.

If, for the first 365 days of married life, a couple adheres to these principles and puts them into practice—*and it can be done!*—their marriage will probably be secured! Secure, and happy!

318. *The Unhappy Marriage* The unhappy marriage starts essentially the same as the happy marriage. Generally there are the same conditions, the same possibilities and, what may become the vital point, *the same expectations.* As mentioned before, it is the first year that sets the general direction. The first little quarrel that is not resolved and forgiven by both may remain in the mind as a gnawing disappointment. Gradually, as the disappointment becomes an infection, the mind becomes incapable of seeing anything but the unfulfilled expectations. The cause of the disappointment may be sexual, or general, or on some minor point.

Sometimes people come to a doctor for consultation about these problems with a list of accusations almost as long as the total of the marriage partner's qualities. It may be the sexual expectations that have suffered a grievous setback whereas all the other expectations have been satisfactorily met. Or the contrary may be the case. Much insight and great psychological sense are required to salvage such marriages and help them to a new start. In the great majority of cases the attempts at salvage are successful. Medical and psychological measures generally correct the faults. In very special cases, however, there remains nothing for the marriage consultant to do but to advise divorce.

Unfaithfulness is the most frequent cause for divorce.

Kinsey's investigation has revealed that from 30 to 45 per cent of married men have intercourse outside marriage. Furthermore, his investigations show that conjugal unfaithfulness within the lowest social group occurs most frequently during the younger years but later becomes less frequent. The facts are the reverse within the highest social group.

Divorce courts in the United States granted two million decrees in 1947. This figure, however, was considerably smaller than that of 2,285,539 for 1946, the first actual post-World War II years. A comparable jump in the divorce level occurred in the year following the first World War. However, in the years since 1887 (the first year statistics are available) the percentage of divorces in the country has been rising steadily, from 8.7 per cent to the 1947 relation of 13.9 per cent. The underlying basic cause for divorce is the fact that before entering into matrimony the partners did not fully realize the *fundamental requirements* for a happy marriage, nor were they able to understand them as these requirements gradually dawned upon them. Such lack of understanding is found to be the most consistent cause of separation. The husband and wife must truly love each other. That is the first and the most essential quality of marriage. And most successful marriages are lifelong.

9

SEX LIFE OF THE UNMARRIED

Chapter 36: YOUNG PEOPLE BEFORE MARRIAGE

319. *Early Youth* This period is of the greatest importance for the young man and woman. Above all, this is the time they develop and mature and must find themselves. Through comradely association with young persons of the opposite sex they must also try to find their own place in relation to sex.

Early youth may be a wonderful time, one so heralded by the poets. For most people it remains—in retrospect—the most radiant and richest period of their lives.

The insecurity of puberty has been replaced by the assurance of youth. You discover the joy of getting to grips with your work and mastering it. Comradeship with other young people shapes you, and friendship gives you strength and depth.

320. *Sexual Abstinence Before Marriage* To most young people sexual abstinence is the natural course, until the day they marry the person they love. Abstaining from sexual intercourse is not physically harmful. On the contrary, to many young people it may prove to be a very valuable factor in character development inasmuch as such restraint puts self-control to severe tests. The question of self-gratification or masturbation which the young person (if not before, then usually at this time) must face is a problem of wide scope. A special section of this book, therefore, is devoted to it.

321. *Chances for Early Marriage* In modern Western civilization a man cannot, as a rule, marry until he has reached a rather advanced age. It is generally imperative that he acquire a number of necessary skills if he is to be able to offer social and economic security to a wife and children. A man who marries at twenty-one is considered to have married early. And even at that, he has to live through a period of several years in which his sex need is fully developed and makes itself felt, without being able to permit himself to let it have normal satisfaction in marriage.

In the main, the problem has hitherto been a specific *male* problem, hardly existing for the female. It is true that more boys are born than girls—the proportion internationally is 106 to 100—but in all countries through many generations, probably due to hereditary ailments in connection with the male sex, boy mortality has been so much more marked than girl mortality that hitherto there has been a surplus of women, particularly of young women. However, statistics from more than one country show that this condition is undergoing a radical change.

Chapter 37: THE UNMARRIED YOUNG MAN

322. *The Frank Young Man* As far as he is concerned things fall into shape rather fortunately. He knows that there are not only differences but also points of likeness between men and women. He considers young women as comrades and treats them accordingly. He has the courage to be his own natural self. He is big enough to realize that sex is not meant to be something temporary, but a lifelong relationship. And that guides him in his behavior with girls. He is courageous enough to avoid an *early* engagement.

323. *The Shy Young Man* But for the majority things are not that easy. Many young men—many more than one would think—are actually shy in the company of girls. The young man's bashfulness generally results from his being self-centered, and even vain. I would say to this type: You may be *unassuming* and modest, yes, that commands respect. But don't be bashful. Women are inclined to look up to a man, just because he is a *man*. Thus the more self-assurance he shows, the more they seem to look up to him.

324. *The Over-aggressive Young Man* The over-aggressive young man is often not the "big shot" (nor so much at ease) he appears to be. He actually may have an inferiority complex, which he attempts to hide. This type usually brags of his latest "conquests," whether or not they actually occurred.

One of the characteristics of *flirting* is that both parties know they are playing on the borderline of promiscuousness. If the over-aggressive young man should go for a frank and apparently good and intelligent girl, he ought to know that she may be deceived by his outward behavior toward her. Should he try to have affairs with very young, inexperienced girls, he must realize the great responsibility he takes on.

Chapter 38: THE UNMARRIED YOUNG WOMAN

325. *The Frank Young Woman* What characterizes her behavior is her expectant attitude. She knows it may be long until the right one comes, but she also knows that when he does come sex life will reveal itself with might and force. With this attitude she also knows that to bring about such a transformation she must wait till the *right* man comes.

This knowledge gives her that straight-forward look, and protects her better than the warnings of a thousand mothers and aunts. While observing and listening to the young men in her circle, in her own heart she keeps her ideal high. In her way she is able to distinguish between those young men who mean something to her and those who do not.

326. *The Modest Young Woman* Sexual modesty is generally regarded as being more ethically valuable than the opposite: sexual immodesty or shamelessness.

In the same way that shamelessness denies the *ethical* factors in sex life, so modesty seeks to gloss over the existence of the *physical* factors in it. In this connection it must not be overlooked that sexual modesty in principle generally stems from one of two basic sources: a deficient sex development (infantilism) or from a type of education that represented sex life as something unclean. Modesty in certain cases is actually a conscious or unconscious cover-up for an exaggerated interest in sex matters. It is not unusual either to see the most modest young woman fall for the over-aggressive young man! In practical life, however, modesty in spite of its failings, is valuable, because it may *protect* the young woman. And if she can only give it up when the *right* man comes, she is not so badly off. And neither is he.

327. *The Frivolous Young Woman*   On the other hand, there is unfortunately a host of immodest, shameless, promiscuous flirts whose talk is centered on sex, do heavy necking, and abandon themselves to men for the sole reason that the *men are male*. It is in such women that the young man will meet his deepest disappointment when he is ready to bestow his love with honor and respect. These girls are either ignorant or stupid; no one taught them that desire without mutual love leaves a woman with a terrible sense of emptiness and loathing, and makes the man, consciously or unconsciously, feel contempt for her who offered herself too freely.

Chapter 39: THOSE WHO NEVER MARRY

328. *Unmarried People in the Older Age Groups*   The different factors involved in marriage depend upon so many racial, moral, ethical, aesthetic, and other conventions that there will always be persons who never get married. The causes are many and infinitely varied. Beneath these causes there is often a great human tragedy. For example, one person may have formed his or her ideal, but never met it. Another lost the sweetheart and cannot imagine anyone else. A third loves one who is already married or is not able to return the love, for some other reason.

A fourth is afraid of marriage; a fifth did not meet anyone who wanted him or her; and a sixth did not want the one he or she could get. Certain women and also certain men see in their work something bigger and better to live for, and renounce the idea of marriage. Some women—to their everlasting regret and chagrin—waited too long for *him* to propose; the reason may have been that she was financially independent and successful while he was poor and perhaps fearful of taking the first step.

329. *Natural Celibacy* There are two groups of human beings in which celibacy (the voluntary unmarried state) can be regarded as *natural*. First, there are persons who are born without, and grow up without, sex needs. Many eminent women belong in this group; although rare, some men are properly placed in this category, less than one man in a thousand. For all of these persons celibacy is the natural state. This may be the proper place to establish that a person without sex needs as a rule differs from his or her fellow beings only on that one point. All other emotional and intellectual qualities may develop freely in such persons, and what is more, in many cases they develop in a less egotistical direction than in persons with normal or highly developed sex needs.

Secondly, there are persons—although they are rare—who, urged by a deep inner experience, devote their lives so much to serving an idea and to living up to their vocation that for them everything else—sex needs and sex relations included—is devoid of interest. To them too, celibacy becomes a logical and natural state.

330. *Unnatural Celibacy* Modern psychoanalysis, however, has revealed a form of celibacy characterized as *unnatural*. This form is always the result of a sexually abnormal or "deviated" mind; thus a markedly homosexual person will often feel that he or she has no alternative other than celibacy. The great majority of this group, however, is formed of persons who shun all sexual relationships because they got a wrong start in sex matters.

Psychoanalysis shows, for instance, that a man may be afraid of women or that he had been educated under a system that considers anything to do with sex impure. Such individuals may throughout their entire life carry on a severe and cruel battle within themselves in the effort to suppress temptation and keep "impure" thoughts and luxurious images away. That is the origin of the motif, so often used in art, about the temptations of the monk. The minds of such persons are split. They are driven by their—frequently very strong—sex urge which attracts them to women, while at the same time they suffer indescribable spiritual agonies merely by being in the presence of a woman. It is pitiful to reflect that if such a self-tortured individual were married to a healthy and normal woman he would very likely be released from all these battles and scruples and would also achieve a happy and harmonious sex life.

331. *Sublimation* There has been much scientific speculation as to what happens to the energy normally spent in satisfying the sex need, in people who do not have any sexual intercourse. In actual practice, such persons often possess eminent capacities in other fields. In this connection the question of a "refinement" or *sublimation* of the sex need has come up. The term means this: As the special need for a physical release through sexual intercourse is suppressed other component parts of the total sexual need may become greatly accentuated. Thus, for example, a need for domination or protection, which may have formerly been quite secondary, now provides the individual with a satisfaction which serves to maintain his unique psychophysical balance.

332. *Spinsters* Why is a spinster frequently the object of scorn? This is the general attitude among a large percentage of people who estimate the value of women so exclusively in their capacity of wives and mothers. But isn't that quite wrong, a dated, and also an illogical way of thinking? These same people are generally the least likely to appraise the value of a man exclusively in relation to his function as husband and father.

Many women have proudly rejected men because they found them too unmanly; others did not get the man they loved, and these chose spinsterhood. I will admit that there can be something helpless about a spinster and perhaps that has contributed to create the impression of something pitiful and slightly ludicrous about her. She may frequently be queer or eccentric and testy, it is true, acid and contrary, angular and awkward and knotty in her exaggerated spinsterishness.

Let us not forget, however, that among the spinsters of the world there are great and noble women, some of real stature, women who carry their heads high, conscious of their worth, women who were not willing to give up their independence, for they considered independence a treasure not to be renounced. They have chosen to be alone, and they *are left* alone, but at the same time they grow strong in their unapproachable citadel. As their treasure of independence draws cumulative interest it grows steadily. Some of them develop into highly eccentric individuals, but others grow to be proud, yet humble, personalities, women whose characters men often admire the most.

Chapter 40: NONMARITAL SEX RELATIONS

333. *Facts to Be Faced*   Nonmarital "affairs" are generally condemned. Yet extramarital sexual relations are almost as widespread as nonmarital ones among unmarried couples.

According to Kinsey 85 per cent out of all men have sexual intercourse before marriage. His investigation of American men also disclosed that 30 to 45 per cent of married men—varying with different groups of age and social standing—have relations outside of marriage.

Very often external circumstances present an obstacle to two people marrying, although the relationship between them in private amounts to marriage. In their relationship they both know they love each other, that knowledge which alone authorizes two persons to declare themselves husband and wife, and whether it is secret or not, becomes a matter of secondary importance to them.

334. *If She Gets Pregnant*   There are enthusiastic champions of modern secret marriage who argue that such a marriage may be just as good as an officially registered union, as long as

the relationship is: 1. monogamous, being between two people alone; 2. intended for life; 3. and that both partners are fully aware of their responsibility. However, the principal object of the marriage ceremony officially proclaiming that this couple will now found a family probably is to protect the woman and the possible children. On that score some solid thinking should be done and defenders of the unofficial marriage should realize this: in our present social order a woman runs great social and economic risks by entering into a sex relationship with a man to whom she is not legally married. It is the risk of becoming pregnant. Precautions may be taken by both partners against such a possibility considered at the time undesirable. Nevertheless, she does run the risk. *Both* must know that it *may* happen; she may become pregnant, and they must both realize that *if* she does, she cannot legally attempt to be a party to an abortion, as she may endanger her own life. So, if pregnancy occurs, the couple should marry properly if they can. They should in every way share the live responsibility, in doing all they can to protect their child, and, if possible, draw their life closer together than before.

In this case too, the only *realistic,* essential condition is that they love each other. If this is true of the man, then he will do his very utmost to shoulder the responsibilities of the baby and herself—*she* may be sure of that. And if they do not love one another in the best way, he still should realize that he should not turn his back on her and take his irritation out on her with recriminations, or vanish without caring what becomes of her.

335. *Sexual Promiscuity*   This expression is a term applied to a person who may have sexual intercourse with more than one person. In practice sexual promiscuity frequently means that sexual intercourse is carried out promiscuously within a large or small circle of persons of both sexes. Prostitution is a special form of promiscuity.

336. *Prostitution*   Indiscriminately engaging in some form of sexual relations for which one partner receives money or payments in some other similar form, is called prostitution. According to Kinsey almost 70 per cent of all American men, and 37 per cent of married men, have had connection with pros-

titutes on one occasion or more. In many countries there are special houses of prostitution, *brothels*, where the prostitutes carry out their professional service. In other countries official prostitution and brothels are unlawful. Nevertheless, prostitution goes on more or less openly, as *street prostitution, bar or hotel prostitution,* and *home prostitution.* The last form is practiced under cover of some trade or profession.

Happy love by its very nature is the absolute contrast of prostitution. Men who seek prostitutes are deserters of real love, and for a woman prostitution is the most degrading profession that exists. The unmarried man who seeks a prostitute has already taken the position that sexuality and love can be separated, and later on when he approaches marriage it will be very difficult for him to experience fully genuine love with a fine healthy woman. Moreover, association with prostitutes constitutes a risk to a man's health. In a very high percentage of cases prostitutes are found to have one or more venereal diseases. What their condition may mean we shall consider in the next to the last part of this book that is devoted to venereal diseases.

10

FERTILIZATION, PREGNANCY, CHILDBIRTH

Chapter 41: PROCREATION

337. *Twofold Purpose of Sexual Intercourse* For thousands of years men have been aware of the relationship between sexual intercourse and subsequent pregnancy. The various pleasures involved have been known for a still longer time.

However, more scientific knowledge about the nature of begetting and conceiving was not acquired until 1850 through the investigations of Du Barry, and this immediately gave rise to a discussion about the purpose of intercourse. During the decades preceding the first World War, in which a narrow moral attitude prevailed, every intercourse that did not have pregnancy for ultimate objective was regarded as immoral.

The reaction against the old attitude often resulted in licentiousness. Another effect which came to exercise the widest influence was the change in attitude expressed in the popular literature all over the world. This literature seemed to proclaim the triumph of exactly the opposite view toward the shattered traditional position; sexual intercourse was described and vaunted by these writers as an act containing its goal in itself. This conception has characterized great segments of the generation now in, or about, their fifties.

But the new generation, modern youth, has reacted against this. It is characteristic that the generation now between fifteen and forty quite realizes the great importance of sex enjoyment to married happiness.

338. On the Origin of Life At the time of Aristotle the ancient Greeks thought that all species of small animals, not merely very primitive organisms and tiny insects but even mice and such like, might generate spontaneously from mud, dirty rags, and other impurities. This idea went unchallenged through the periods of European antiquity, and the Middle Ages and still later.

As late as 1859 the French Academy awarded a contest for an essay—won by Pasteur—on the subject of whether animate matter may generate or be generated from inanimate matter. Even today some people continue to believe that lice and itch mites are spawned by dirt. It was not until the human egg was discovered that information about its fertilization and other points of human reproduction could be propagated, properly formulated, and presented to the general public. This awareness on the part of the public occurred an amazingly short time ago. The existence of the human egg was first observed (beyond any possible doubt) by Von Baer in 1828. When Benjamin Franklin proved that lightning was an electrical phenomenon and Franz Schubert composed his immortal *lieder* no one had as yet seen a human egg.

339. Origin of the Stork Fable Among certain primitive peoples the concept of virginity is unknown. Marriages are arranged long before the partners reach the age of puberty. It is the practice among some Australian tribes, for example, to contract marriages when the girls are eight years old. Mating may begin even earlier, in play between boys and girls. As a result, such primitive peoples regard intercourse only as a pleasure. Pregnancy and birth are considered miracles, unassociated with intercourse. They believe that pregnancy starts when the first movements of the fetus are felt—about four or five months before birth. It does not occur to the primitives to consider any connection between a sexual act—that may have taken place four or five months previous—and the pregnancy.

However, primitive peoples are always inclined to link things that occur in close succession or simultaneously as immediate cause and effect. In many tribes, therefore, the child's totem is determined according to the place where the mother felt the fruit of her womb stir for the first time—be it near a tree, a plant, animal, or a stone. The idea involved is this: the *spirit* of the tree, the plant, the animal, or the stone at that very moment of the woman's discovery takes up its new life in the woman. An anthropological account of these matters has been given, among others, by the Dane, Frederik Poulsen. The Aranda tribe believes that the child spirit lives in stones and, no bigger than a grain of sand, this spirit enters into the woman through her navel. Among other tribes the people believe that eating the fruit of certain trees results in pregnancy. Still other groups are of the opinion that pregnancy comes about through the noise of the wood of a special "fertilizing tree," shaped into a musical instrument called a *churinga*. From antiquity comes the account of how the virginal Io was made pregnant by the Greek god Zeus merely by a touch of his mighty hand. The old Peruvians believed the rays of the sun could make a woman pregnant. Thibetan myths have it that demons beget children by touch too, and the birth of Buddha was said to have been caused by the ascetic Dukula touching the ascetic Lady Parita's navel with his right thumb. In India childless women seek the blessings of their womb by following in the footsteps of Buddha. The familiar custom of throwing a shoe after newlyweds when they drive away is the last innocent vestige of that ancient belief. The idea of a "fertility tree" has survived right up to our own times. This concept survives as a symbolic act among South Slav peoples whose brides are given apples to put in their bosom. The Greeks of our own day let the bride eat a pomegranate.

In various parts of Germany the belief in the existence of babylands—located in bogs and deep wells—has survived, and a great many variations of the belief are found in a large number of fairy tales. Not so long ago in Nierstein-on-the-Rhine people were told that the children came from an old linden tree at the foot of which there was a well leading to the babyland below. In India it is the ibis bird, and in the Germanic countries it is the stork that supposedly acts as the agent between human beings and babyland. The stork trustingly builds its nest on roof tops, but seeks its food in the bogs where the tiny child spirits live! The old Norse peoples called the stork Abedar, meaning "Bringer of Children." When it was disclosed that the stork brought the little babies there was originally no intention of deceit; they really believed what they said. The actual moral "deceit" only began in the eighteenth century rococo period and grew even stronger during the following century.

340. *Paternity and Determination of Blood Type* It is easy to determine who is the baby's mother; for it is, of course, the woman who bears the child. But to determine who the father may be is often a matter of dispute. In different lands and at different times opinion on that subject has been subject to strange customs and traditions. One of the most extraordinary customs about fatherhood is probably found in the so-called *fratrogamy*, meaning brother-marriage, as practiced in some South Indian tribes. The woman has sexual intercourse with all brothers in a family, yet the child's real father is considered to be the brother who in the seventh month of her pregnancy gives her a bow and some arrows. That act makes him the father of all her subsequent children, until another brother gives her a new bow and arrows. Death does not alter the relationship in any way; a man is considered as being the father of legitimate children, even if the children have been born years after his death. Roman law established as a general rule: *Pater est quem nuptia demonstrant*, i.e. the husband is considered the father of the child.

Recent research on heredity has finally thrown a clearer light on these problems, for now it is possible to employ the blood-type paternity test. This test can determine whether a certain man—whom the woman designates as the father of her child—may possibly be its father, *or* cannot possibly have fathered a certain child of a certain mother. On this basis, however, it is not possible to make sure whether a certain man is the *only* man who could have fathered a certain child of a certain mother. In devising new methods for determining paternity spermatozoa tests may sometimes prove to be of importance. The increasingly frequent use of *insemination* in most recent times has given rise to a series of problems of law. These legal questions are in connection with the fatherhood, partly concerning the donors and partly concerning the rights and duties of the child, both mutually and as against the mother of the child and her conjugal partner, if any, and the community. These are problems which most existing relevant law has not foreseen, and upon which, therefore, no stand can be taken.

Chapter 42: HEREDITY

341. *Hereditary Elements, Genes* All the qualities a living being has inherited from its parents are called, with a comprehensive term, the *aggregate characters, hereditary type*, or *genotype.*

The totality of an individual's qualities of every nature—i.e. genotypic plus later qualities acquired by direct environmental influence—is called its *phenotype*. The *genotype*, or the aggregate of inherited potentialities, may be compared to a mosaic of separate hereditary tendencies, each corresponding to a fragment of the mosaic. Such a fragment, *one* hereditary quality, is called a *gene*. The genes are considered very big molecules, not visible to the naked eye. But we know that they have some relation to the *chromosomes*—colorable, threadlike, generally spiral-shaped structures that are present in all cell nuclei. We also know that the parents' qualities are transmitted to the offspring through the medium of the chromosomes.

342. *The Chromosomes Merge When the Egg Is Fertilized* When a child possesses qualities partly stemming from the genes of the mother and partly from those of the father, this mixture is due to the fact that when the egg was fertilized the chromosomes in the mother's egg cell with *their* contents of *genes* merged with the chromosomes in the father's sperm cell with *their* contents of genes. The combination thus achieved does not change when the cell divides later, but *every pair of chromosomes* in the child's body will always, for the rest of its life, contain the original maternal and paternal genes in their original mixture.

343. *Number of Chromosome Pairs* The number of chromosome pairs varies in different species of animals and plants, but it always remains constant within the individual cell nuclei of one organism. But since the number of chromosomes in a cell does not run into a very high figure, the so-called *chromosome-number* is identical in many different animals and plants. However, they are not capable of merging, or of substituting for each other. The chromosome-number in a human being is forty-eight, consisting of twenty-three pairs of so-called *autosomes*, plus one pair of sex-chromosomes.

344. *Indirect, Mitotic Division of Chromosomes, Karyokinesis Before Fertilization* Fertilization cannot occur simply by the merging of two ordinary cells—i.e. cells with the normal chromosome number, one male and one female. In that way the chromosome number would constantly double and would not remain constant, unaltered through generations. Therefore, previous to fertilization a division of the number of chromosomes both in the male sperm cell and in the female egg cell takes place, thereby reducing their number by 50 per cent.

In the sperm cells the maturity division takes place at a preliminary stage, occurring immediately before the sperm cells are ready to do their fertilizing. Therefore the sperm cells contain only twenty-three single *autosomes* plus a single special sex chromosome. In the egg cell, the mitotic division takes place directly after the sperm cell penetrates into it; the process is probably set off by the entry of the sperm cell into the egg. Like the sperm cell the egg cell then contains twenty-three single autosomes plus a single special sex chromosome. After their mitotic divison sperm cells and egg cells get the same name. They are both called *gametes*.

345. *Sisters and Brothers Do Not Develop Alike* In the *maturity division* is a form of *mitosis*, each chromosome-pair dividing in such a way that one chromosome with its *genes*, stemming from either the father or the mother of the individual to be, is drawn toward one attraction sphere. The other chromosome with its genes goes to the opposite attraction sphere—if it is a sperm cell. If it is an egg cell, it is ejected. When twenty-four chromosome *pairs* are about to divide like that, every imaginable combination of the total forty-eight individual "paternal" or "maternal" *chromosome-partners* may result.

To illustrate: Imagine 24 couples dancing in a hall; at a given signal the two partners that form each couple must separate and go to opposite ends of the hall. How then will the crowd at one end of the hall be composed? Well, *theoretically* it may consist only of men of various types, as: tall and small, fat and thin, bearded and unbearded, men with brown eyes, men with gray eyes, or with blue eyes; cheerful men, intelligent men, hot-tempered men, thrifty, cross, spirited, flat-footed, rich, well-to-do, poor men, and men in modest circumstances; pale men and garrulous men, tired men, dark men, reactionary men, and stamp collectors, etc. . . . And at the other end of the hall we will find all the different ladies: obese and slender, dumb or shrewd, beauteous ladies and joyous ones, ladies with flowers in their hair, ladies whose lips are sealed, red-haired, long-legged, emancipated ladies, etc., etc. That is just *one* potentiality.

Suppose, however, a single one of the men changes places with his partner, then the crowd at each end would immediately be of a different pattern. And it would change still further if yet another man should change places with his partner. And think of the difference if the first couple changed back again! The number of potential patterns is very high. With twenty-four couples the crowd at one end of the hall may be combined in 16,777,216 (2^{24}) different ways.

In exactly the same manner there will be 16,777,216 potential variations of the distribution of chromosomes in the sperm cell or the egg cell after the mitotic division. Inasmuch as it is the different *genes* in the individual chromosomes that determine the child's heredity, it will be realized that two egg cells fertilized by two sperm cells will practically never have a chance of coming out alike, i.e. in exactly the same pattern. This means, therefore, that it is almost impossible that children of the same parents—apart from *twins from one egg*—can ever be identical.

346. *Sex Chromosomes* Sex chromosomes are definite chromosomes that contain the hereditary tendencies, *genes* that will determine whether the offspring will be male or female. It is often possible to distinguish these sex chromosomes from the other chromosomes—i.e. autosomes—in the organism. This is possible because the autosomes are smaller than the sex chromosomes, and the fact that the two chromosomes making up one pair of sex chromosomes are of unequal size.

347. *Sex-determining Chromosomes in the Egg Cell* In order to illustrate these matters more clearly it is customary to use the symbol XX for the sex-chromosome pair in a woman because the chromosomes in it are identical. Every cell throughout the female organism contains twenty-four chromosome-pairs, namely twenty-three autosome pairs and one XX sex chromosome pair. When the egg cell—that consequently also contains these chromosomes—comes to its mitotic division this transformation will occur: immediately prior to merging with the chromosome of the sperm cell, the divided egg cell will consist of twenty-three *single autosomes* plus one *single X-chromosome*. This egg cell was the result of the mitotic reduction of the original XX-chromosome pair.

348. *Sex-determining Chromosomes in the Sperm Cell* In contrast to the cells in the feminine organism, *every cell* in the male organism contains, in addition to the twenty-three ordinary autosome pairs, a special sex chromosome pair symbolized as Xy, indicating that the two chromosomes in the pair are *not* alike.

At the mitose, while the sperm cell is developing, these two special sex chromosomes divide in their unique way. Half of the finished sperm cell gets this combination: twenty-three ordinary *single* autosomes plus one *single* X-chromosome. The other half of the finished sperm cell gets this composition: twenty-three ordinary *single* autosomes plus one *single* y-chromosome.

349. *What Determines the Baby's Sex?* According to modern concepts the genes that determine the sex are not exclusively linked to the sex chromosomes. The sex will also depend upon the *balance* between one gene with a *male* stamp which in human beings is found in the autosomes, and *a more dominant* gene with a *female* stamp that is contained in the X-chromosome.

As described in the sections immediately preceding this one, the mitotic-divided egg cell ready for being fertilized contains twenty-three single autosomes that then carry the male factor, plus one single X-chromosome with—as we just said—a predominating female stamp. If this egg cell now is fertilized by one of the sperm cells (which similarly contains twenty-three autosomes with a male stamp plus a single X-chromosome gene with a female stamp, constantly growing smaller and more predominating), the merging will result in a fertilized egg cell with twenty-three autosome *pairs* plus one XX-chromosome pair. It is true that this fertilized egg cell also contains among the autosomes, genes with a male stamp, but the double dose of female sex genes in the XX-chromosome gets the upper hand. This will result in the egg developing into a girl baby—in accordance with its *genetic sex determination,* as the term goes. If, on the other hand, the egg cell is fertilized by another possible type of sperm cell (that in addition to the twenty-three male autosomes giving a male stamp, contains one y-chromosome, but *no* X-chromosomes with a female stamp) then the double presence of male genes will have a unique composition. After fertilization these male genes will predominate over the single presence of female genes originally present in the egg cell ready for being fertilized. The fertilized egg will then have a certain female stamp, it is true, but according to the genetic sex determination it will develop into a baby boy. All these circumstances serve to explain why there is no such thing as a 100 per cent male or a 100 per cent female. Herein lies the explanation of certain bisexual phenomena and of the concepts of heterosexualism.

350. *The Sperm Cell Alone Determines the Sex* The conclusion we draw from the above then is that every egg, after having been fertilized, is capable of developing into either a boy or a girl. Moreover, *not until* the sperm cell enters the picture with its added contents—*either* an X-sex chromosome *or* a y-sex chromosome—will it be determined whether the child is to be born a girl (X-sex chromosome) or a boy (y-sex chromosome).

351. *Equal Number of Boys and Girls* At the mitotic division of the sperm cells there is exactly the same number with

X-sex chromosomes as with y-sex chromosomes. There are, therefore, exactly as many finished sperm cells with an X-chromosome ready for their job of impregnation as those prepared with a y-chromosome. In view of the above-mentioned conditions of sex determination there is the same number of chances for the fertilized egg to develop into a boy as into a girl. Since, however, actually more boys are born than girls (the proportion of 106 to 100) it has been suggested that this might be due to the fact that the boy-giving sperm cells, which contain the somewhat smaller y-chromosomes, might have greater capability of spontaneous movement than the girl-giving sperm cells with their heavier X-chromosomes. The sperm cells stand a better chance of winning the race to the egg and fertilizing it.

352. *When Is the Baby's Sex Determined?* It is inherent in the circumstances of sex determination that the baby's sex is fixed at the very moment of fertilization, in reality at the precise moment when it becomes clear whether it is the sperm cell with an X-chromosome or a sperm cell with a y-chromosome that will be the first to reach the egg cell and penetrate into it. At that moment the whole sex of the child is decided and nothing can be done to alter it later.

353. *Influence of the Parents on the Baby's Sex* It will be clear that parents are unable to exercise any directed influence on the development of the child's sex. As we just pointed out, the sperm cell with an X-chromosome is considered to be heavier than that with a y-chromosome. For parents to have any chance of influencing the sex of their future baby, it would be necessary, if, for instance, boys were preferred, to find a way to obstruct the progress of the heavier X-chromosome-bearing, girl-producing sperm cells, or to increase still further the speed of the lighter y-chromosome-bearing, boy-producing sperm cells. In that connection some scientists have suggested that by introducing a small quantity of lactic acid into the vagina its acidity would be increased, and under those conditions it might not be outside the realm of possibilities to give the more spontaneously-moving y-chromosome-bearing, boy-producing sperm cells a headstart.

However, these matters still remain to be investigated in much greater detail.

354. A Woman Who Can Bear Girls Can Also Have Boys If a wife bears several girls, but no boys, it is not her "fault," but rather the nature of the husband. Years ago, a husband was entitled to throw over his wife if she brought forth only daughters. Even today many a husband tacitly or openly blames his wife if she continues to bear girl children. But our present scientific knowledge has disclosed that the husband is the cause from a chromosome point of view, which is what matters in this connection. It does not lie in the egg cell contributed by the wife, for that was capable of developing into a boy as well as a girl, but in the husband's sperm cells and, to a certain extent, perhaps also under favorable or unfavorable conditions they meet in the female organism.

355. *Chromosome Division and Cell Division After Fertilization* After the egg has been fertilized the new cell instantly begins to divide. Every chromosome now splits *lengthwise*. For a brief moment there are three times as many chromosomes as before. After the lengthwise cleavage each "set" of divided chromosomes is attracted to one of the cell's two poles and the cell continues to divide itself into smaller cells. Since the chromosomes have split lengthwise the genes that are supposed to be arranged in the chromosome rather like pearls on a string, have also been distributed in such a way that two sets of chromosomes and, consequently, the two new cells resulting from the cleavage have become exactly alike. These two cells are constituted exactly like the original cell in regard to chromosome composition. This principle of mitotic division is the basis of the growth of the whole organism, and explains that every single cell in the female organism contains an XX-chromosome pair, and that every single cell in the male organism contains one Xy-chromosome pair, with the exception of the sperm cells ready for their task of fertilization.

356. *What Is Eugenics?* Eugenics is a science dealing with conscious efforts to "improve" or "refine" the race. As far as human beings are concerned the general objective dates back to antiquity.

In improving the breeds of domestic animals veterinary science makes use of a wide variety of available means. A distinction is generally made between *positive* eugenics and *negative* eugenics, also called preventive or prophylactic eugenics.

357. *Positive Eugenics* In his *Republic* and in *Laws* Plato suggested a series of "ideal" plans for human stud farms with a complicated system of control, a matrimonial lottery, destruction of babies, and abortions as eugenic measures.

The vast majority of people in our day and age find these plans most unattractive.

However, the matter deserves some brief mention because in this connection Plato has taken a rather important element of heredity into consideration, namely the possible mingling and shifting of qualities that may result from crossbreeding, emphasizing that marriage should be entered into only if it would benefit the country. A young man who is too hot-tempered and excitable should aim at becoming the son-in-law of calm, stolid people, he says, and as a general rule, those who would marry should seek alliances with individuals whose temperaments are suitable for blending in a complementary manner.

358. *Negative or Preventive Eugenics* The goal of negative, preventive, or prophylactic eugenics is the attainment of an improved race by taking such measures as would prevent individuals with undesired qualities—manifestly due to heredity —from reproducing their kind.

Chapter 43: FERTILIZATION

359. *The Unfertilized Egg* As mentioned before the unfertilized egg is caught in the Fallopian tube and immediately launched on its way toward the uterus by the vibrating cilia or hairs inside the tube. At this stage the egg is surrounded by a slimy film. Fertilization takes place when it is met by a sperm cell that manages to penetrate through the film.

360. Sexual Intercourse Is the Normal Method of Fertilization In the human being the possible opportunity for the intimate contact between the sperm cell and the egg is brought about by intercourse. During intercourse an average of 345 million sperm cells are ejaculated into the vagina. These sperm cells immediately set out on their quest for the egg, rapidly traveling toward the interior of the uterus and further up into the Fallopian tube. Whether the woman attains an orgasm or not during intercourse has, it is believed, no influence on whether the egg is fertilized or not.

361. If Sexual Intercourse Cannot Take Place Various circumstances may be involved which favor employment of so-called artificial insemination. This will be explained in detail in the section about birth control or fertilization control. This is, however, the place to say a few words about fertilization that may be effected in spite of male impotence at sexual intercourse.

362. Fertilization in Spite of the Husband's Impotence In the various causes of impotence where the man's testes and other necessary glands are in good functional order, it is possible to try to obtain his sperm cells and forthwith deposit them in the wife's genital tract so as to give the married couple a chance of having children in spite of all. The different causes of impotence have been mentioned earlier.

363. Fertilization in Spite of the Wife's Impotence at Sexual Intercourse Moreover, we described that genital spasm (vaginism) might constitute practical impotence in the woman at taking part in intercourse. In view of the fact that vaginism occurs mainly in women who have not previously given birth to a child, and that it is generally corrected after childbirth, it might be fair and reasonable to have recourse to artificial insemination —if the condition has proved ungovernable by every other method—and thus bring about pregnancy and birth.

364. The Steeplechase of the Spermatozoa Immediately a veritable steeplechase is on between the many sperm cells. The first obstacle of any importance is the vaginal mucous plug in the cervix of the womb. This natural obstacle may only be forced when the *hyaluronidase* of the sperm cells has dissolved the vaginal mucous plug. Through the Fallopian tube the sperm cells have to fight their way and overcome the contrary movement, the lashing moving cilia. Only those sperm cells which are capable of making their way through these obstacles reach the egg. Thus the future baby's fight for existence as far as one half of it is concerned—the sperm cell—actually has started before it has met the egg cell—the other half.

365. *The Last Spurt* The egg cell, finally, is surrounded by a great number of sperm cells which push and poke into it, then recoil a little the better to attack again, and then go for it with all their strength like tiny torpedoes. What makes the egg cell weaken and select one of them, at last "making up its mind" to take in one, has always been a mystery. Now it is believed that the solution of the riddle lies in the hyaluronidase, carried along with the sperm cells, which, through the thrusts of the sperm cells against the mucous film of the egg cell dissolves this film in the places where it is struck by the sperm cells.

366. *The Sperm Cell Penetrates into the Egg* For suddenly, on the surface of the egg, a minute protrusion appears, like a pout, in the direction of one of the sperm cells. An opening appears in the egg through which the head of the victorious sperm penetrates. Thereupon the film of the egg closes again and simultaneously the whole surface of the egg thickens and toughens, making it impossible for any other sperm cell to enter.

367. *Actual Fertilization, Fusion of the Pronuclei* The whole sperm cell does not penetrate into the egg. The tail breaks off and the head, containing the pronucleus of the sperm cell, continues toward the pronucleus of the egg cell. While the approach is under way the last mitotic division of the egg takes place.

The nucleus of the sperm cell and the biggest of the divided nuclei of the egg cell complete their fusion. Following this the fertilization has definitely been achieved.

368. A Miracle Has Happened The fertilized egg—from now on called the *zygote*—at once starts its cleavage and at this point our *understanding* of what happens further is only theory. It is possible to explain that a cell may divide and become two cells of the same kind, but it is impossible to understand and impossible to explain scientifically how this single cell, the zygote, in the course of nine months can develop from an embryo into a brand-new human being with all its *different* kinds of cells: muscle cells, sinew cells, nerve cells, epidermic cells, blood cells, kidney cells, etc., nor can we explain the development of new sex cells that in their turn will help continue the species, bringing forth new generations.

Chapter 44: PREGNANCY

369. Cleavage of the Zygote The fertilized egg, the zygote, splits by so-called *cleavage*. First it divides into two cells, these divide into four, the four become eight, and then sixteen, and so on, always doubling, and as we know, this soon results in an astronomical figure. Originally, these cells are probably alike in every respect.

370. Twins from a Single Egg At this early phase the zygote may sometimes split into two cells, each of which develop into an independent zygote. When two embryos develop from the same original zygote they often come to resemble each other in mind and body like peas from the same pod or like "two drops of water." They are the so-called *single-egg (uniovular) or identical twins*, which are always of the same sex because they contain the same sex chromosomes. The basis for this close similarity is the fact that having come from the *same* egg cell and the *same* sperm cell they contain the same *genes*, thus having the same aggregate hereditary tendencies, in each of the innumerable cells of their organisms.

371. Other Twins, Triplets, etc. Twins, triplets, even quadruplets, may also result if several ripe eggs happen to be present in the Fallopian tubes and become fertilized by different sperms. In such cases the babies need not be of the same sex, inasmuch as some of the sperm cells may be X-chromosome-bearing (which will result in a girl), while other may carry y-chromosomes (resulting in a boy). Statistically represented, one in every eighty births results in twins, and of twin births every four or five are single-egg twins. Triplets occur once in every 6,400 births; most triplets are made up of single-egg twins and an independent embryo. It is rare for all of the three embryos to have developed from the same egg, or from three different eggs, each fertilized by a separate sperm cell. Quadruplets are so very rare in human births that the phenomenon is considered unique and outside the range of systematic research. Quadruplets are born probably in every 512,000 births, while births of quintuplets occur even more rarely.

372. *The Transportation of the Zygote (Fertilized Ovum or Egg) Through the Tube* It is not known for certain how long it takes for the zygote to proceed through the Fallopian tube. Some investigators consider the duration is three or four days, while others believe the journey takes about ten days or more. The zygote is carried along by the lashing movements of the hairy cilia lining the interior of the Fallopian tube.

373. *Tubal Pregnancy, Extrauterine Pregnancy (Ectopic Pregnancy)* The diameter of the Fallopian tube at its connection with the fundus of the uterus is somewhat narrower than near the ovaries. This variation or narrowing due to former infection may obstruct the passage of the zygote (fertilized egg) through the tube. Fertilization is generally supposed to take place at the outer extremity of the tube, quite near the ovary. During the first part of its passage through the tube, the zygote divides, but does not grow, unless it should happen to be obstructed and attach itself to the mucous membrane of the tubal wall, in the same way as would normally occur in the uterus, absorbing nourishment from the tubal membrane. In that case we have a so-called extrauterine pregnancy, a *tubal pregnancy*.

374. *Tubal Abortion and Tubal Rupture* This may have fatal consequences, for the tube, gradually distending beyond its

capacity, cannot house the growing embryo beyond six or eight weeks. In some cases the embryo is extruded by retrograde action through the open end of the Fallopian tube into the peritoneal cavity and is absorbed there, in the rare cases, when surgical care is neglected. More commonly, the wall of the tube bursts, resulting in a so-called *tubal rupture* that may endanger the life of the woman. If a woman, who has skipped her last period and believes she may be pregnant, feels a sudden pain in one or the other side of the lower abdomen, followed by more or less vaginal bleeding, or by symptoms pointing to an internal hemorrhage (such as dizziness or fainting), a doctor should be called at once. It may be a case of an extrauterine pregnancy with rupture as described.

375. *Formation of the Germinal Disk* If normal development is taking place, the zygote (cell colony) generally consists of so many cells that, upon reaching the uterus, in size and appearance it somewhat resembles microscopically a mulberry. On its external surface a nutrition-absorbing layer—the so-called *trophoblast*—is formed which "eats its way" into the uterine membrane thus making a kind of *nest* for the zygote. This process is called the nidation of the egg (from the Latin *nidus*, a nest). At the same time the interior of the zygote changes into two blisters that together resemble a figure eight. One blister, which is empty, is called the yolk sac. During the second pregnancy month it is separated from the embryo by constriction. The other blister, filled with a fluid is the *amnion sac*, commonly called the "bag of waters." Where the two blisters touch they form—together with an intermediate layer of cells—a concave disk. *This germinal disk* soon flattens and pushes into the amnion sac. Henceforth it is this germinal disk that develops into the true embryo which is completely surrounded by the amnion sac and thus, throughout the pregnancy period, is floating in a bag of waters which acts as a buffer or shock absorber protecting the fetus from pushing, pressure, jarring, and other disturbances from the outside.

376. *The Whole New Human Being Is Developed from the Germinal Disk* It is thus a rather limited number of cells that

are charged with the formation of the new living being. One can't help experiencing a feeling of awe when considering that this little bunch of cells can grow into a real human being, with a head, neck, and body; arms and legs; eyes to see with and ears to hear with; with heartbeats that may race for joy or slow in grief; with a brain that through confused'and twisted thinking can never stop trying to find out the purpose of life, of birth, and death.

377. *The Cells of the Germinal Disk May Substitute for Each Other*   A huge force is contained in these few cells, a primitive force of which one may gather a faint idea when one learns that during the first month of gestation the embryo grows to fifty times its original size, and to no less than about 8,000 times its original weight! Some of the cells, which by cleavage soon become *groups* of cells, form blood cells. Other cells form brain cells, while still others by cleavage form liver cells, yet others form epidermic cells, etc.

At this early phase there hardly seems to be any hard and fast rule as to whether a certain cell will participate in building up this or that structure. The cells may substitute for each other. Consequently, many cells that were inherently capable of developing into something independent are not being exploited to their full capacity and have to content themselves with functioning as a sort of a reserve for the first team.

378. *When Reserve Cells Start Out on Their Own; Teratoma Formation*   It is possible that a reserve cell, which was excluded from participation in the building up of the fetus, nevertheless slips into the new human being and hides there, often in the part just above the coccyx (the caudal end of the spine). There it stays with all its latent force, all its untamed energy, remaining for years, through the youth and maturity of its host, who may be growing quite old. A growth or a tumor may finally be discovered down there: it is the reserve cell starting out on its own at last and working like fury. When the growth is removed and the surgeon cuts it open to investigate it more closely he may find a whole part of the body *in miniature*, such as a piece of skin with hair glands; or even a tiny set of teeth.

This is evidence of what this specialized cell may have accomplished in its green youth; it was inherent in it, and finally it could wait no longer! Such an abnormal growth is generally called a *teratoma*.

379. *Further Development of the Embryo* It is not essential in this book to describe all the minute details connected with the growth of the embryo. The three cell groups of the germinal disk develop in such a way that one pushes into the other, while the cells continue to divide and increase in size. It does not take long before some cells show some of the characteristics they will bear in the future.

First, about seventeen days after fertilization, the blood cells are formed in groups called blood islands; they rapidly merge and form the great artery, the aorta, which immediately begins to pulse and becomes the foundation for the heart. Almost simultaneously the so-called spinal cord disk is formed on the back of the embryo. It is folded so as to form a tube, the top part of which later develops into the brain, and the lower part into the spinal cord. Similarly, in front, a tube is formed which becomes the alimentary canal. It opens up near the rectal parts and develops into the so-called cloaca, the common cavity for evacuation of urine and feces. With this tube as a basis not only the stomach and the liver are formed, but also the lungs.

When the embryo is thirty days old and a little more than one third of an inch long, it not only is equipped with the organs just mentioned but has traces of arms, legs, eyes, ears, and nostrils. In other words: from the time the blood cells can be distinguished—about seventeen days after fertilization—until the embryo is one month old, practically all of the organs of the human body are distinctly traced and some of them have even begun to function. This major development takes only about fourteen days!

380. *How the Embryo Feeds* At first the embryo gets its nourishment through matter that seeps directly from the uterine membrane into it. As soon as the egg has been fertilized the uterine membranes change in a manner similar to what happens at menstruation, only to an accentuated degree. There is quite a congested blood condition, as the capillary system extends and the glands increase in length, twist and dilate to form a thick soft membrane rich in blood vessels.

The deeper layer of this membrane is loose, providing for the twisting of the glands. The trophoblast digs into the uterine membrane which closes around the zygote. And in its tiny nest it has available all that is necessary to absorb nourishment from the uterine membrane.

381. *The Umbilical Cord* From the third until the sixth week of its life the distribution of nutrient matter in the embryo takes place through circulation in the yolk sac. Later, the embryo gets its nourishment through the blood by way of the *umbilical cord*. This cord stems from the embryo's abdomen in front, in the place which later, when the umbilical cord is severed, remains an indented scar, called the *navel*.

The umbilical cord contains embryonic blood vessels and passes through the embryonic fluid and the so-called *embryonic membranes* of which the *amnion sac* (the "bag of waters") is one. This amnion sac is very close to the uterine wall in which it ends in some extremely delicate ramifications of blood vessels, villi, mainly formed by another embryonic membrane, the so-called *chorion* or *vein membrane*. The umbilical cord is about twenty inches long and a little over one third of an inch thick. It is generally twisted in the opposite way of a corkscrew, which is the way the blood vessels run. When at first removed from the embryo they can easily be distinguished through the mixture of jellylike and filamentlike connecting tissue in which they are encased.

382. *The Placenta* The fine ramifications of the blood vessels in the umbilical cord end blindly in the wall of the uterus, and the fetal blood that fills them, therefore, cannot get further afield. But simultaneously with the development of the ramifications of the umbilical cord, the uterine membrane, on its part, develops into what midwives sometimes call the *mother membrane*. On a more or less large area of the uterus some large cavities develop, through which numerous blood vessels from its

veins are constantly supplied with blood from the mother organism.

It is precisely in these cavities that the ramifications of the umbilical cord end in a blind alley. With their extremely thin walls the portions of the umbilical cord billow back and forth in the blood of the cavities, somewhat in the manner of seaweed at the bottom of the sea following the slow rhythm of the waves.

These structures taken altogether are called the *placenta,* and the ramifications of the fetal blood vessels make up the greater part of it. The mother's blood now carries nourishment to the cavities of the placenta. From the placenta the blood of the mother diffuses through the thin walls into the fetal blood and is absorbed, thus benefiting the fetus. There is no mingling of the mother's blood with the fetal blood as some people are inclined to believe. Mother and fetus both have an independent circulation.

Similarly with nutritious substances diffusing from the blood of the mother organism into that of the fetus, an opposite movement also takes place. Through the metabolism of the fetus a good deal of wastage is formed which it has to rid itself of, for otherwise a poisonous condition may prevail in the fetus. Such waste matter seeps from the umbilical blood vessels into the blood system of the mother and is carried to her lungs, kidneys, etc., and finally evacuated in the same way as waste from the mother's own metabolism.

Chapter 45: SYMPTOMS OF PREGNANCY

383. *The First Miss*   Absence of menses is generally an early sign of pregnancy. It is not, however, a certain sign. A few women menstruate once or more times after pregnancy has actually set in, and on the other hand, menses may stop temporarily for many other reasons. Failure to menstruate as one symptom alone cannot at all be depended upon in determining whether a woman is pregnant or not.

384. *Morning Sickness*   Another early evidence of pregnancy is the so-called *morning sickness,* nausea and vomiting,

generally occurring during the early part of the day. It appears in a rather mild form in about 45 per cent of pregnant women, and in a higher degree—when it is called *hyperemesis gravidae* —in about 5 per cent of all pregnant women, for a shorter or longer period, within the first three months after conception. It is generally considered by physicians that this condition is a symptom of an internal toxic condition, in relation to the toxic condition that may appear in the last three months of the pregnancy period and may be the forerunner of puerperal convulsions, termed eclampsia. The underlying causation is not known. As mentioned earlier, wastage from the fetal blood seeps through the placenta into the blood of the mother and, in conjunction with the higher rate of metabolism in her own body, it results in an increase of toxic products in her blood stream. Some scientists think this may cause the vomiting, possibly in connection with some injury to the liver cells. Hormonal disturbances have also been suggested as a cause—a lack of progesterone, deficient absorption of the gonadtropins, or deficient functioning of the cortex of the suprarenals.

Since pregnancy nausea is closely linked to the presence of the placenta (more than to that of the zygote) scientists are now inclined to believe that the placenta is chiefly responsible for that nervous hypersensitivity whereby a number of influences, internal as well as external that would otherwise pass unnoticed, produce nausea and vomiting in the organism of the pregnant woman now tuned in another key. In case of severe nervous hypersensitivity the vomiting may be extremely violent. If this is accompanied by nausea at the sight of food, a rather common reaction in pregnant women, the mother-to-be may lose a great deal in weight from lack of a proper diet. At the same time the deficiency in important nutrients in the organism, which may entail vitamin deficiency in connection with upsets of the internal metabolism, may injure the liver, the kidneys, and the nervous system. And all this may occur at a time when greater demands are made on the woman's stamina than ever before, during a period when, in fact, she really is eating and drinking for two.

385. *Duration of Pregnancy Vomiting* Usually the vomiting abates about the second or third month and then ceases

altogether. Some women, however, through their entire pregnancy may retain—like a memory—a disinclination, or a direct aversion, to certain foods. About half of all women, however, do not suffer at all and experience neither nausea nor vomiting, as mentioned above in the preceding section.

386. *Treatment of Pregnancy Vomiting* This ailment is often very hard to reduce or curtail entirely. In the most severe cases it may be necessary to interrupt the pregnancy on this basis alone, as otherwise the mother's health might be seriously impaired. Such extreme action is, however, taken only in very rare cases. All sorts of medicines, laxatives, and other remedies have been prescribed, with varying success, in the treatment of pregnancy vomiting. Recently various hormone preparations, particularly progesterone, have been preferred. The use of estrogen seems to improve some cases, but makes others worse. However, experimentation with the various remedies often extends over so long a period that the vomiting has taken place during the usual period and stops naturally. It is, therefore, hard to assess the relative values of the various remedies. The psychological considerations are often predominant ones. Experience serves to prove that an ordinary sedative cure, eventually rational psychotherapy, together with measures to improve the pregnant woman's general health is the very best treatment for nausea and vomiting during pregnancy. The main measure for the improvement of the woman's general health is by giving her the carbohydrate called glucose, the essential vitamins, and—what may prove to be the most important—*lots of water.*

387. *Changes in the Breasts* Changes in the breasts are noticeable rather soon after conception. During the first few months the breasts become tense and sensitive and slight stabbing pains are often felt. The nipples are more erect, and about the beginning of the third month, the coloration of the areola grows darker, its epidermal glands enlarge and appear like small protrusions as big as a hemp seed.

During the latter half of the pregnancy term the lacteal ducts activated by hormonal influences—the exact nature of which is not quite clear as yet—begin to fill, first with a watery, later with a yellowish, milky fluid which may trickle from the delicate aperture of the papillary point and cause them to stick. The mammary gland in its entirety grows and while it distends the deep underlying layers of skin often appear like reddish stripes on the surface of the breasts.

All these signs are uncertain, however, and derive their significance only by being considered in conjunction with other symptoms. The condition just mentioned is particularly noticeable in women who have previously given birth to a child, which she nursed, for the changes then brought about in the breasts are retained later in life. Not even the presence of a milky fluid in the breasts may be taken as irrefutable proof of pregnancy, for in certain illnesses the breasts may contain such a milky fluid, even in little girls and old women.

388. *Changes in the Abdomen* As the pregnancy progresses the abdomen changes more and more, although in the first two or three months there is hardly any alteration. In the fourth month it is possible to feel the uterine fundus above the pubic bone; in the fifth month it extends to about halfway between the pubic bone and the navel. About the sixth month it reaches almost to the navel; in the seventh or eighth month it comes to midway between the navel and the edge of the ribs; and in the beginning of the ninth month it almost reaches the rib.

However, during the last weeks of pregnancy the fetus is somewhat lower. At the same time, on the skin of the abdomen stripes often appear showing that the deep-lying derm is breaking, and finally the navel depression is smoothed out. After parturition a brownish, vertical line generally remains down the center of the abdomen, the so-called *linea fusca* (fusca means dark).

389. *Changes in the Genital Organs* During pregnancy the vulva and the vagina often take on a bluish-red tint somewhat like the dregs of wine; they swell and secrete more mucus than usual. Already at an early stage the neck of the uterus becomes softer which is considered a very important sign of pregnancy. The uterine os changes, occurring differently in women

who are having their first child than in women who have experienced childbirth before. These changes in the cervix and the uterine os are regarded as rather certain symptoms of pregnancy, a particular proof being the very noticeable softening of the uterine neck.

390. *Movements of the Fetus* The fetus is not very old when it begins to move. However, the woman has to be pregnant four and a half months, or "half-term" as the saying goes, before she feels life by more or less noticeable kicking and pushing against the interior of the uterus. The movements may be noticed by a third person too, by putting a hand on the abdomen of the pregnant woman. That is an indisputable sign of pregnancy and, as we mentioned before many primitive peoples calculate the beginning of gestation from the moment life is felt.

391. *Sound of the Fetus* Shortly after "half-term" the heartbeat of the fetus may be heard through the mother's abdomen, and that, of course, makes it absolutely certain that pregnancy exists and that the fetus is alive. The heartbeat is audible as a rapid and muffled tic-*tic*, tic-*tic*, tic-*tic*, noticeable when putting one's ear close to the abdomen, a little below and beside the navel, on the side to which the back of the fetus is turned. The frequency of the sound is from 120 to 140 beats a minute. For convenience one can listen for a quarter of a minute (15 seconds) during which time thirty to thirty-five heartbeats may be counted.

392. *Structure and Position of the Fetus* Feeling the structure of the fetus through the abdominal wall is also a certain sign of pregnancy. The reason this is of special significance is that the examiner can find out then how the fetus is lying. During the early part of pregnancy it often changes position, but toward the end it settles into a definite position which will determine the course of the delivery, as will be described later.

393. *X-ray Examination of the Pregnant Woman* If, on account of obesity or because the fetus may be dead, none of the above-mentioned irrefutable signs of pregnancy can be detected. Nevertheless, if there is a strong belief that the woman is pregnant, she may be examined by X-rays. From the fourth month it is generally possible to obtain quite distinct picture indications. The X-ray photos are the more valuable in that they also show the position of the fetus, eventually whether there are twins and, in certain cases, also whether there is any malformation.

394. *Special Pregnancy Tests* From the very earliest times a definite pregnancy test has been sought. There has been a great desire for a method to determine beyond a doubt—preferably as early as possible—whether a woman is pregnant or not. At the present time several tests are widely employed and are described in the following sections.

395. *The Principles of the Rabbit Test* Very long ago it was observed that mother animals usually eat their own placenta immediately after delivery. This behavior gave rise to the idea that the placenta probably contained some substance important to the nursing of her young. Not until our own day has it been found out that the placenta, in addition to its function as exchange center of matter between the mother organism and the fetus, also functions as a ductless gland by producing hormones. As a matter of fact, the placenta is one of the organs from which the female sex hormone was first prepared for use in therapy. This does not mean, however, that this substance is also *produced* in the placenta. Moreover, it has been observed that considerable quantities of gonadotropine are secreted into the urine of pregnant women. By investigating the placenta the scientists established that it contains great quantities of the so-called chorion-gonadotropine, a substance that has also been found to be produced in the placenta. Moreover, investigations revealed that its effects are similar to those of pituitary gonadotropine.

The ancient Egyptians were already going in the direction toward finding a pregnancy test when they investigated the seed germinating capacity of woman's urine. If the capacity was great, it indicated pregnancy in the woman. However, the first modern scientific pregnancy test was not developed until 1928.

It is the so-called *Aschheim-Zondek* test, in which urine also is tested. A quantity of the woman's fresh morning urine is injected under the skin of five young sexually immature female mice. This injection is repeated six times in the course of twenty-eight hours. One hundred hours following the first injection the mice are killed; if, in only *one* of them, a distinct characteristic showing a ripening of the genital organs is observed by certain changes it may be assumed that the injected urine contained such a quantity of chorion-gonadotropine, the woman from which the urine is taken is, therefore, sure to be pregnant.

This method is very sure, only failing in about two or three per cent of cases, or even less—greater exactitude than that cannot be expected from a biological method of investigation as complicated as that. The only drawback of the test is the lengthy time involved, for it takes about four days to run and get the indicating result.

The principle of the *Friedman-Schneider* test—the so-called rabbit test—is very similar to the Aschheim-Zondek test. Using rabbits, it has the advantage of providing a result in less than thirty-six hours.

396. *The Frog Test (or Xenopus) and the Toad Test* This recently developed pregnancy test is based on the indicative reaction of a South African frog, the species *Xenopus laevis*. A sexually mature frog of this type lays a great number of eggs after being injected with human gonadotropine.

If urine of the woman who is given this pregnancy test contains some gonadotropine the remarkable egg-laying reaction of the injected frog is regarded as positive evidence that the woman is pregnant.

It takes only a very short time to run the test as the frog begins laying its eggs only four hours after being injected with urine containing gonadotropine. The frog may continue to lay eggs for fourteen hours. The test is quite reliable, offering valid results in about ninety-eight to one hundred cases.

It is anticipated that for these reasons this test will become more popular in the future. For the physicians or technicians giving the test there is an advantage in the fact that the same frog can later be used several times on other women.

Recently the common toad has been used for pregnancy

reactions. The urine to be examined is injected beneath the skin of the back of a male toad, and if pregnancy exists in the woman some sperms will be excreted in the course of a few hours. The reaction derived has proved to be just as valid and at least as quick as the Xenopus reaction. This form of pregnancy test has an added practical advantage in that the toads are relatively easy to be found.

397. *Other Pregnancy Tests* In addition to the tests previously mentioned many other methods for determining pregnancy are used. One of these is the Mazer-Hoffman test in which mice are used. In contrast to the above-mentioned tests it does not serve to indicate the presence of gonadotropine but to test the changes in the quantity of estrin. Some additional methods which provide rapid results inexpensively have not yet been thoroughly tested, while other tests have not proved to be sufficiently trustworthy. For this reason physicians at the present usually have confidence only in the previously mentioned methods.

398. *How Soon After Impregnation May Conception Be Determined?* Cessation of menses and onset of vomiting are generally the earliest symptoms of pregnancy. But, as we have said they are uncertain, and if one wants to make quite sure, it is common to supplement them with a pregnancy test. During a normal pregnancy the test becomes positive in the course of one week following the first day of the missed menstruation period. In other words, as soon as one week after the woman *usually* should have had her menses—often meaning three weeks after conception—this test may be undertaken. It is then generally possible to get an answer to the question as to whether she is pregnant or not.

399. *Duration of Pregnancy* In the animal world the period of pregnancy is called the gestation period and its duration seems to have some relation to the size of the animal.

In mice, for example, the gestation period is about 22 days; in rabbits, 30; in pigs, 113; in sheep and goats, 153; in cows, 281; in mares, 336, and in elephants pregnancy lasts no less than 665 days. The pregnancy period in human beings generally covers about 280 days from the impregnation of the egg until the birth of the baby may be expected, and it takes about half that time for the fetus to show "life."

Chapter 46: HYGIENE DURING PREGNANCY

400. *Pregnancy Is a Normal Condition* Among many peoples it is considered a great honor to be pregnant and homage is paid to the pregnant woman, in many different ways. The time is largely past when a pregnant woman felt too embarrassed to appear in public. The pregnant woman is, after all, the fundamental asset of the family as well as of the nation. Her pregnancy is not an abnormal but an entirely normal condition although it makes great demands on her organism.

401. *General Hygiene During Pregnancy* A woman accustomed to living a regular life, using proper hygiene, and with a healthy natural schedule of her day in work, exercise, rest, and relaxation should change her existence as little as possible when she becomes pregnant. Others, who may lead a strenuous life perhaps involving a constant round of parties and entertainment, should adopt a somewhat more tranquil mode of life and see to it that they get enough sleep and rest to feel fit in the morning.

The pregnant woman should not deny herself some quiet relaxation, and she should keep away from crowded, stuffy places and avoid exciting or upsetting influences. All these things may have a harmful influence on her mental state and thus may cause a miscarriage or premature delivery. However, it is absolutely out of the question that any harm may possibly come to the child, physically or psychically from such influences. Any belief to the contrary is superstition and nothing but old wives' tales.

402. *Eating During Pregnancy* A proper diet is of the greatest importance to the pregnant woman as well as to the child she is about to bear. The prospective mother's family doctor or pediatrician will supply her with the proper diet as her pregnancy progresses. Medicine should not be taken except on doctor's orders.

403. Keeping Regular During Pregnancy Regular evacuation of the bowels is most important during pregnancy. It is of primary necessity to a pregnant woman, and is best maintained by eating sensibly. Sufficient exercise should be taken at all times. If difficulties in keeping regular still persist it may become necessary to adopt a special diet, or special laxatives may be employed, but only on consultation with a doctor.

404. Need of Calcium During Pregnancy All the materials that go to build up the fetus are provided by the mother. That is true of calcium, essentially needed for the bone structure and teeth. So when the time comes for the fetus to begin to build up its bones the need of calcium is greatly felt by the mother and she must supply it. If she does not take care to obtain the necessary quantity from outside sources the fetus will exhaust the supply present in the mother's body. That is one of the reasons why some women have their teeth ruined by pregnancy. A lack of calcium may also cause a special form of convulsions (maternal tetany).

Therefore, the mother must be sure that she gets a good supply of calcium in her food. Cheese has very high calcium contents. Other sources of calcium I recommend are cow's milk, yolk of egg, celery, lettuce, kale, cauliflower, cucumber, and oatmeal. In addition, most women, *on the advice of the physician*, take calcium during the later part of the pregnancy, either in tablets or in a solution, possibly with some D-vitamins added which is important for the assimilaton of calcium by the organism. All women should have their teeth examined when they are about halfway through their pregnancy.

405. Need of Iron During Pregnancy In the blood the oxygen-binding coloring matter, hemoglobin, is of the same vital importance for human beings as the substance chlorophyll—which makes leaves green—is to the oxygenation of green plants. Iron is needed to create hemoglobin in the red blood corpuscles of the fetus and the mother has to supply this too. If she does not get a sufficient quantity of iron from the outside to cover her own need and that of the fetus, the unborn child fills its needs from the mother's stock, and this may result in anemia in the mother. Here are some foods that are particularly high in iron contents: blood sausage, spinach, liver, beef, beans, veal, and kidneys. C-vitamins are of importance in facilitating the assimilation of iron in the blood.

406. *How to Dress During Pregnancy* The pregnant woman's clothing must be comfortable and suited to the time of year. Constricting garters should not be worn. Shoes should be sturdy with thick soles and low heels. For women whose abdomen is flaccid a pregnancy corset for the later part of the period may be used on the advice of her doctor. It should support the abdomen from below upwards, and must never fit so tightly as to be uncomfortable. A corset that does not fit well is harmful, not helpful.

407. *Exercise During Pregnancy* Outdoor exercise is generally considered to be good for everyone, including the pregnant woman; however, she must not overdo it as she must avoid getting too tired. Very strenuous physical work (such as spring cleaning, carrying heavy burdens) and stretching her body when putting up curtains, etc., should be avoided. This should apply particularly during the first half of her pregnancy, for it it during these months that the danger of miscarrying is especially great. In respect to sports, long journeys, etc., the pregnant woman should always consult her doctor. Complete rest for an hour or an hour and a half in the middle of the day, or when the pregnant woman comes home from work, is often strongly recommended.

408. *Bathing, Sponging, and Douching During Pregnancy* Frequent bathing is advised, but neither very cold nor very hot, since extremes of heat and cold may provoke contractions of the uterus. Shower baths may be taken all through pregnancy, whereas tub baths or swimming should not, as a rule, be indulged in during the last month of pregnancy, due to the risk of impurities finding their way into the birth tract. If the pregnant woman is swimming she should not swim beyond the point where she can touch bottom, because pregnant women are particularly subject to fainting and to cramps in the calves of the legs. She should never swim alone, nor should she overexert herself in the water. On top of all this, she should thoroughly cleanse her genital organs daily, and after careful drying, perhaps using a little talcum powder to avoid becoming chafed.

In certain conditions douching during pregnancy may entail a risk to the fetus and sometimes also to the health of the pregnant woman herself. Douching should only be done in consultation with a doctor and as a rule not during the last month of pregnancy.

409. *Care of Nipples and Breasts During Pregnancy* Proper care of the nipples during pregnancy is of the utmost importance. During the last half of the pregnancy they should be washed every day with ordinary soft soap and tepid water after which they should be rubbed well with a towel. The purpose of that is to harden them for their strenuous task in nursing the baby. For the same purpose, after having cleansed them, it is advisable to coat the nipples with a mixture of glycerine and alcohol or similar preparations. If the breasts are heavy they ought to be supported by a brassière that holds them up but does not press them in and together.

410. *Sexual Intercourse During Pregnancy* Intercourse may take place during pregnancy but with great care and caution and not during the last month, as impurities may contaminate the birth tract and thus contribute to bringing about puerperal fever. If the pregnant woman has shown any tendency toward having a miscarriage or premature delivery, intercourse should be avoided entirely. However, a decisive factor in determining the *frequency* of sexual intercourse should be the wife's desire for it. Her sex urge may remain unaltered, or it may also grow or diminish, during pregnancy. Her diminished sex urge may frequently be due to the aversion or loathing she feels at certain odors, including the odor of her husband. As a result, it

will often be the *wife's* sexual desire which—perhaps to a greater extent than usual—determines the frequency of intercourse.

411. *Tuberculosis and Pregnancy* It may sometimes be observed in a pregnancy that a disease latent in the woman's organism—which her healthy resistance combated successfully before she became pregnant—now gets the upper hand and is able with marked rapidity to develop. This potentiality is considered to apply especially to a disease like tuberculosis. Recent investigations and research have established, however, that this view is most probably not a true one. But if the physician has the slightest suspicion that tuberculosis is present, or that the woman is at all susceptible to it, he will observe her extra closely during her entire term of pregnancy. Such a precaution thus makes it possible to take immediate steps if there are any signs that the disease is about to break out.

412. *Syphilis and Pregnancy* If the pregnant woman suffers from a case of syphilis it is essential that her condition should be watched with particular care. There is a possibility that the syphilis microbes may penetrate the delicate membrane of the placenta which separates the maternal blood from the fetal blood. If such penetration takes place the child in the womb may become infected. What this may mean to the child before birth and after delivery will be explained in greater detail in the chapter about venereal disease. At this point we only call attention to the fact that a pregnant woman who is infected with syphilis should be given antisyphilitic treatment during her pregnancy, not only for her own sake but also for the sake of her unborn child.

413. *Diabetes and Pregnancy* Diabetics will, as a rule, be able to carry their pregnancy to its full term, if they receive proper care which includes treatment with estrogen as well as progesterone. It is a peculiar fact that when the mother suffers from diabetes the fetus is inclined to grow unusually big. For this reason, as well as the fact that the life of the unborn child will be in danger during the latter part of the pregnancy, and for a short time after birth, such cases should be referred to special medical treatment. If the illness is particularly difficult to treat during pregnancy, or if a marked hereditary charge weighs on the mother, in *rare* instances interruption of the pregnancy may be recommended by physicians.

414. *German Measles and Pregnancy* When German measles, generally regarded as a childhood disease, is mentioned in relation to pregnancy, it is not because the disease attacks the pregnant woman more severely than others. It is because women afflicted with this disease early in pregnancy often bear children with some defects, as a rule in the central nervous system. Therefore, it is a matter for consideration whether it should be possible to give permission for interruption of the pregnancy in such cases on legal grounds. At any rate, a woman attacked by German measles early in pregnancy should certainly consult her doctor about the disease.

415. *Varicose Veins and Hemorrhoids During Pregnancy* As the unborn child comes to occupy more and more room in the abdomen it may press against the veins that carry the blood from the legs and the lowest part of the body back to the heart. Therefore, pregnant women may often suffer from varicose veins in the legs and hemorrhoids (*piles*) around the anus. If the pregnant woman does not keep her bowels in order, hemorrhoids may result.

416. *Albumen in the Urine* Albumen is found in the urine of about 10 per cent of all pregnancy cases. It is important that this is ascertained, for its presence may be the first symptom of conditions that may endanger the lives of both mother and child. Medical opinions differ widely as to the reasons why the presence of albumen can be found in some pregnant women's urine. However, one can say, in general, that it probably has something to do with the accumulation of waste matter in the blood of the pregnant woman resulting in a toxic condition or injury to the kidneys.

417. *Risk of Puerperal Convulsions or Pre-eclampsia* In many cases albumen in the urine is not accompanied by other conditions indicating the presence of a disease. However, there *may* be other simultaneous symptoms. These may include high blood pressure, dropsylike swellings of the tissues, so-called edemas, for instance in the face and hands, and very often in the legs or the feet. It may also be accompanied by deficient urination, pains around the heart, headaches, dizziness, troubled eyesight, etc., etc. This condition is called pre-eclampsia or impending puerperal convulsions. The deeper causes are unknown, but the condition may possibly be brought about by disturbances in the functioning of some glands involved. These glands are the posterior lobe of the pituitary; the thyroid gland, the cortex of the suprarenals. There is the possibility also that the placenta may be functioning improperly.

418. *Puerperal Convulsions (Eclampsia)* If the pre-eclampsia is not properly treated the condition may develop into real eclampsia, i.e. puerperal convulsions. The symptoms are genuine convulsions with immediate loss of consciousness, very similar to those characteristic of an epilepsy state.

If these convulsions occur during pregnancy, childbirth will generally start, as the eclamptic fit may bring on labor. Puerperal convulsions may also occur during the woman's delivery or in her lying-in period. The condition may be very serious for the mother, and the child may face an even greater hazard.

The presence of albumen is often the first warning of this danger and this can be discovered in no other way than by examination of the urine. Thus it should be understood that it is an absolutely essential and unavoidable duty for every pregnant woman to have her urine examined for albumen at stated intervals. It is terrible to reflect that puerperal convulsions may cause the loss of the child's, and sometimes also of the mother's, life when we know that it could have been avoided if only the pregnant woman had taken care to have her urine examined for albumen in time. It is no excuse for the patient to say that she lives far from a doctor or a pharmacy, and that therefore she cannot have her urine examined. It is always possible to send a small specimen of urine by mail or in some other way. It is an absolute *must* for the pregnant woman to have her urine examined regularly throughout the pregnancy period.

419. *If Symptoms of a Disease Occur During Pregnancy* ... As soon as a pregnant woman displays any symptom pointing to a disease the doctor should be called immediately. It is imperative in each of the following cases:
a. If there is any *bleeding*—be it ever so slight.
b. If she feels a rather severe pain, particularly in the abdomen.
c. If there are swellings like dropsy of hands and face (local edema).
d. If she has eye troubles.
e. If she has a constant headache.
f. If vomiting gets beyond control and leaves the pregnant woman in a state of exhaustion with ensuing loss of weight.
g. In the case of skin eruptions which may be the measles.

420. *Arrangements with a Hospital or a Private Nursing Home Should Be Made in Ample Time* It is very important that a number of arrangements be made with a physician in ample time. For example, the woman should undergo the examinations which determine whether the measurements of the pelvis permit normal birth or not. In this respect many women are scandalously negligent. I have often been called to a woman in the throes of labor, or having already been delivered of the child, without her having made the slightest attempt to get in touch with a doctor in advance. In practically every case it was pure negligence on the part of the pregnant woman, often coupled with lack of ordinary intelligence. It seems to me that in such cases the husband ought to be held responsible.

421. *The Last Days of Pregnancy* This section is specifically addressed to the husbands. The days immediately preceding delivery are almost always long, terribly long, for the women. A woman who expects a baby at any moment cannot as naturally as before dispose of her time, because she may feel she ought to be ready for the first pains. If it is her first delivery she will never be able to rid herself of fear, although she may know for an absolute fact that she will get an anesthetic.

Her condition is very much in evidence: she walks with difficulty, loses her breath easily, the skin on her face, limbs, and body is pallid, sometimes quite mottled. She can't do anything with her hair. These are the days when more than ever it is up to the husband to show her his love, to "spoil" her and give her tender care, be near her, serve her, tell her how happy she makes him, show her that he wishes to share in it all, as well as he knows how. He should let her know that this is not only her affair, but his too, and that during these last days he feels a most urgent desire to support her and aid her. This attitude is appreciated a thousand times more than the red roses he may bring her when the whole thing is over.

Chapter 47: CHILDBIRTH

422. Position of Fetus at Delivery During the greater part of the pregnancy the fetus may float about freely in the embryonic fluid, the bag of waters. However, about one month before birth it settles into a definite position that remains essentially unchanged until delivery. In various ways the course of the delivery will depend upon the position the fetus occupies in the uterus and it should be emphasized that as late as about one month before full-term pregnancy, the doctor can change the fetal position and thus help to make the birth easier. The normal position immediately prior to delivery is the head or *vertex* presentation, so called because the top of the head appears first. That is the position in which 87 or 88 per cent of all babies are born.

423. Size of Baby's Head in Relation to Birth Tract There seems to be a wrong proportion between the size of the baby's head and the narrow birth tract. But this difficulty is partly remedied by the fact that the soft parts of the birth tract are capable of very great expansion, and partly by the fetal head being able to yield a little, as the bony parts have not yet hardened completely to form a firm skull.

424. The Birth Force Adapting the baby's head to the birth tract and expelling the fetus from the womb requires a certain force called the birth force. It is supplied by the contractions of the uterus that cause the labor and pains attendant upon childbirth.

425. Onset of Labor The hormones of the pituitary gland —pituitrin or oxytocin—constantly activate the uterus, trying to make it contract. Their action, however, is hindered by the hormone, progesterone, produced in the yellow body or *corpus luteum*—mainly during the first months of pregnancy. Later it is mainly produced in the placenta and exercises its influence throughout the pregnancy term. When childbirth is at hand production of the progesterone diminishes, and the pituitary hormone, oxytocin, which also seems to be produced in the placenta during pregnancy, has the opportunity to bring its full influence to bear on the uterus that consequently contracts. The woman's labor thus starts in this manner. Quinine is sometimes administered to bring about premature birth. Such treatment makes the womb more sensitive to the pituitary hormone.

426. Labor Is Independent of the Childbearing Mother's Will The muscles in the body are either striated or smooth. The difference between them, largely speaking, is that the striated muscles—to which all voluntary muscles belong, with a few exceptions—can be flexed or unflexed at will. The nonstriated muscles—found in the intestines or in the walls of the arteries and veins—are involuntary ones, independent of a person's will. The uterine muscles are nonsmooth muscles, and consequently the uterine contractions producing the labor pains are independent of the will of the childbearing woman.

427. Frequency of Labor Pains At the onset of labor the pains come at intervals of twenty minutes or half an hour or more; as a rule they are rather slight and are called "plucking pains." The woman feels them like a pinching or a small pain in the abdomen radiating to the small of the back. By and by they grow more frequent and at last occur at intervals of only half a minute up to a few minutes. At this time the pains are usually very strong.

428. Duration of Labor How long the labor lasts differs in different women. If it is her first childbirth, it may last for about twenty hours from the onset of the first pain until delivery is over. For the woman bearing her second or third child the labor pains are generally much more brief. In some instances a woman has been known to bear her child at the second pain, not even realizing that she was about to give birth.

429. *Pains at Regular Intervals*   The pains come regularly, alternating with intermissions free of pains. These intervals of quiet are absolutely necessary to the fetus and are nature's help to the mother. While the pain is felt and the uterus contracts the uterine blood vessels are so strongly constricted that only a small quantity of blood can get to the fetus. If the pains were not interrupted the fetus would finally suffocate from lack of oxygen. But thanks to the intermissions the fetus at intervals gets the necessary blood for circulation and at the same time gets its oxygen supply. For the mother too, the intermission is very important. She may lie back and relax completely, gathering strength so she may be ready to follow the directions of the obstetrician who exhorts her to apply all her forces to further the delivery, at the onset of the next pains.

430. *Anesthetics in Childbirth*   Labor pains are extremely painful and have always been so. Primitive peoples also know birth pains. One should not believe that labor pains, as was once maintained by some, are a phenomenon exclusively connected with civilization. There *are* a few women even nowadays, who experience almost no pain at childbearing, although they certainly are the exceptions. The pains are so directly linked with the uterine contractions that if they were made to cease immediately the first small pains started, the uterus would stop working with the result that the childbirth would be arrested. So it will be amply clear that it is quite impossible to suppress birth pains entirely, and the broad claims in the advertising of new remedies are not wholly true. It is, however, possible to alleviate the pains considerably, partly by initially employing laughing gas and eventually following up with anesthesia during the latter part of the delivery. At the end of the delivery, when the pains are at their height, eventually so strong a dose may be applied that the mother is put to sleep. Anesthetics harm neither mother nor child, and the endeavor to give to every childbearing woman who so desires this pain-relieving admin-

istration must be considered among the finest humanitarian achievements. Not only physicians, but every person should give strong support to every woman's inalienable right of access to anesthetics during childbirth. Obstetrically, too, administration of an anesthetic is an advantage as under such circumstances the expulsion of the fetus does not occur so violently or suddenly. The outer birth tract is given time to distend and the risk of tears and splits, particularly of the perineum, is greatly reduced.

431. *Period of Dilatation* The initial, and longest, period of a birth is the period of dilatation or expansion. In the pregnant woman the fetus lies in the upper part of the uterus while the cervical canal more or less maintains its usual dimensions, with a slight difference in mothers who are bearing their first child and women who previously have had other children. It is, therefore, necessary to dilate the cervical canal to prepare it for the passage of the fetus. This happens after the onset of labor, when the embryonic membranes with their contents are pushed into the uterine neck. Every pain helps to distend the canal as the "bag of waters" descends, further preparing the way for the fetus.

432. *Breaking of the Bag of Waters* When the cervical neck is completely distended the "bag of waters" generally bursts; the water passes. It often happens, however, that only part of the water flows out, the so-called "fore-water" preceding the head of the fetus. In some cases, however, the "fore-water" may pass at a still earlier moment which makes the fetal head participate more actively in the process of dilatation.

433. *The Period of Expulsion* When the membranes have burst and the fore-water or the entire bag of waters has passed, the pains generally increase; each pain then is usually divided into three to four "turns." This means that the actual expulsion of the fetus has begun. The vagina and introitus, the vulva and the perineum have by then become so limp and adequate in size that splits and tears occur only very rarely. When the pain grips her the mother bends over as much as possible, chin on chest, exerting her will power on the abdominal muscles (striated or voluntary muscles) to make them do their share in extruding the fetus. When the fetal head has performed the last of the screw movements necessary to make it pass through the birth tract, and shows in the vulva the doctor takes hold of the back of the baby's neck (which generally shows first) to help it through, at the same time supporting the perineum. After that comes the face and the chin and then, all that is needed, is a couple of quick twists of the baby's shoulders to bring forth the rest of the little human being—a finishing touch, taking only a few seconds.

434. *Care of the Navel* However, the birth is not entirely over, since the baby is still connected with the placenta in the uterus by the umbilical cord. Now it is no longer essential to the child; as soon as it is out in the open a number of changes take place in its lungs, heart, and circulation. For the first time the child sucks in air and expels it as its very first cry. Then the umbilical cord is severed and the stump is cared for, whereupon the child is fully removed from the mother for the time being.

435. *Apparently Stillborn* However, sometimes the baby's first breath does not come at once, and this is largely due to an accumulation of embryonic water and mucus in the infant's windpipe. Then the obstetrician must suck out this matter by using a small tube and thus procure a free passage for the air. If the child still does not breathe it may be because it is apparently stillborn. Then it is necessary to bathe it, alternately in cold and hot water, give it artificial respiration by using a pulmotor or give it a couple of smart smacks on its little posterior, which often has a most amazing effect on the respiratory functions. In rare cases it is necessary to give the baby an injection of *lobeline,* an oily fluid prepared from a North American plant which has a strongly stimulating effect on the respiration center.

436. *The Afterbirth—Closing Phase of Childbirth* A quarter of an hour or twenty minutes generally elapse before the placenta or *afterbirth* comes loose from where it was imbedded

in the womb. It happens like this: After the fetus has been expelled the uterus continues its contractions and the placenta not being particularly tensile or yielding cannot follow the uterine movements, with the result that it is gradually pried loose from the uterine wall. Together with the tissue of broken embryonic membranes it is then pushed and pressed out through the dilated birth tract where the fetus had preceded it. The placenta is a round or oval disk about six to eight inches in diameter and more than an inch thick weighing about one pound. The placenta, the embryonic membranes, and what is left of the umbilical cord make up what is described as the *afterbirth*. When this is expelled the birth is completely over; the uterus contracts violently until it is hard as a hand ball, whereby the bleeding from the large open wound left by the departure of the placenta usually stops. Some medication is often necessary, particularly if the uterus gives evidence of once more getting limp and lax.

437. *Treatment of the Baby's Eyes* In some cases great parts of the baby's body are covered with a rather thick layer of fat. This has to be removed, usually with oil, after which the child must be washed. Finally its eyes must be treated with drops of a nitrate of silver solution. Before this treatment was generally introduced there was an unfortunate number of cases in which a childbearing woman suffering from gonorrhea would infect her newborn baby. The infected child would thus get a terrible ophthalmo-blennorrhea.

438. *The Newborn Baby* A newborn, full-term baby generally is about twenty inches in length, weighing on an average seven pounds. For boys to be full-term babies the testes must have descended into the scrotum, and a sign that baby girls are full-term is that the labia majora cover the labia minora; and, in both sexes, that the end of the nails protrude beyond the fingertips. The proportions of the various parts of a newborn baby in relation to each other are entirely different from those in adults. The baby's navel is the center of its body. The size of the head is one quarter of the length of the entire body, the limbs are relatively short, the trunk plump, and

the liver represents one twentieth of the baby's total weight. In adults the center of the body is the upper edge of the pubic bone; the head is only one-eighth of the person's height and the weight of the liver represents only one-fortieth part of the entire weight of the body.

439. *Mal Position of the Fetus* Sometimes the fetus may be so situated in the uterus that the abdomen appears first at birth, which is called abdominal presentation. Most common among such positions is the *breech presentation,* meaning that after one or both legs have come down the birth tract the buttocks, trunk, and arms emerge with comparative ease. However, the head sometimes has a hard time passing through, because it has had no chance to participate in the gradual dilating of the birth tract and adapting itself to it, thereby permitting relatively quick passage. As a result, the umbilical cord, whose one end is fixed to the future navel on the fetal abdomen and extends to the placenta in the uterine wall, may get stuck between the baby's head and the birth tract. If this pressure continues for any length of time (over fifteen to twenty minutes) the fetus risks suffocation. If it proves impossible to wriggle the head out by special manipulations it may become necessary to use a forceps (rarely, though), an instrument employed in various forms of complicated births. Like the palms of two hands the forceps is brought up around the head compressing it very gingerly and extracting it with the greatest care.

If the face shows first and emerges first the fetus is said to be born in *face presentation.* If the forehead or brow comes first, it is a *brow presentation.* However, such mal positions which complicate delivery are very rare.

440. *Difficult Birth (Dystochia).* The term *dystochia* is a term which refers to a birth that is particularly lengthy, or painful, or difficult in some other way. Since, as we know, the real magnitude of a difficulty depends upon how well prepared one is to meet it, it is evident that the chances of dystochia may be considerably reduced by careful health control throughout pregnancy.

Let us, for instance, mention the *Caesarean section*, which consists in surgically opening the woman's womb and removing the unborn child through this opening rather than through the natural manner of birth. Among the few forms of dystochia that necessitate a Caesarean operation, the most compulsory form is the one in which the woman's pelvis is so narrow that the full-term baby cannot possibly pass through the natural birth tract. Such a contraction of the pelvis may be a result of the woman having had rickets of the pelvis as a child. However, if a contraction of the pelvis is ascertained during the pregnancy it is possible to bring about a premature birth, i.e. before the child has become too large to pass through the natural birth tract. A Caesarean section may thus be avoided.

In the same way the so-called *maternal tetany*, a special form of painful paroxysms, which is more likely to occur during pregnancy and nursing than during actual birth—as differing from puerperal convulsions (eclampsia)—has become very rare indeed. The fortunate reduction in incidence comes as a result of the public's increased awareness that it is essential to provide a proper diet and a sufficient supply of calcium and phosphorus for the pregnant woman's organism. The preventive treatment of puerperal convulsions has been described earlier, and if the obstetrician fears that a certain *fetal position* may cause dystochia, he will always take proper steps to circumvent the difficulty in time. If, for some reason or other, the fetus grows *disproportionately* during pregnancy the future mother's diet may be regulated, or childbirth my be prematurely brought about. *Insufficient labor pains* during delivery in most cases require only patience and some exercise; if the deficiency occurs in the last stages of delivery it may be remedied by injecting *oxytocin* or in some other way, whichever seems most practical in each case. As a matter of fact, dystochia is a rare occurrence nowadays, found only in less than 2 per cent of all deliveries, and this figure might be still further reduced if *all* pregnant women would adopt a really sensible hygiene during pregnancy as described in the preceding chapter. Thereby they would also be creating the best possible conditions for making the birth of the child a completely normal termination of a completely normal pregnancy.

Chapter 48: THE LYING-IN PERIOD

441. *Importance of Lying-in Period* The period of lying-in, confinement, is sometimes understood to be the six weeks or so following the baby's birth. But in a narrow sense it covers only the first ten days or two weeks, and it is in this sense that the term is used in this section. During the lying-in period the woman must recover after the upheavals of childbirth, which have particularly affected her abdominal organs. In some cases, she must also start nursing the baby. In connection with these two things—the return of the abdominal organs to their normal state, and nursing—a number of matters come up that are also of great importance to the woman's sexual well-being and sexual bloom in the future.

442. *What Happens to the Abdominal Organs After Childbirth?* At every childbirth some degree of injury is done to the abdominal organs through tearing of tissue. These tears must be given an adequate time to heal. Moreover, during pregnancy the uterus has been so distended that it requires some time until it returns to normal by contractions. This process is called the *involution* of the uterus. The *lochia,* the so-called *birth discharge,* a sero-bloody emission from the large wound-surface of the uterus and genital passage, continues for five or six weeks after childbirth.

443. *Risk of Prolapsus of the Uterus* During pregnancy all the muscles of the uterus have been very much enlarged. In addition, for a short time after childbirth the uterus is heavier than usual. If the mother gets up too soon, perhaps overexerting herself, the result may be retroversion, descent or sometimes, prolapsus of the uterus. The longer the woman rests in bed the less risk there will be of prolapsus of the womb.

444. *Risk of Puerperal Fever* Puerperal fever is an abdominal infection that may be contracted by women soon after childbirth, caused by bacteria making their way into the still highly susceptible internal genital organs. It was the Hungarian doctor Semmelweis who, in 1847, as an assistant at the Obstetrical Institute in Vienna, made the great and beneficent discovery that puerperal fever was due to infection, and that it could be prevented by strict cleanliness. The concept of bacteria at that time was unknown.

Before his discovery up to 30 per cent of women in certain hospital wards died of puerperal fever after childbirth. At the present time the disease is almost unknown and the few cases that still occur are almost entirely due to self-inflicted infection, so-called self-infection.

445. *Risk of Blood Clot (Embolism)* At every childbirth the blood coagulates and small blood clots normally form in the uterine blood vessels. This clotting is absolutely necessary in stopping the bleeding when the afterbirth is loosened from the uterine wall. Normally, these blood clots do not give rise to any symptoms, but in rare cases they may also occur in other places besides the uterus. Only little is known about the reason for this. Many people believe that remaining in bed too long after the delivery is a contributing cause to blood clots forming. This view has no basis whatsoever in fact, and the danger of blood-clot formation will not, therefore, influence our considerations as to what may be regarded as the proper length of confinement.

446. *Duration of the Lying-in Period* Opinions on this point have changed considerably over a long period of years. In former days the mother remained in bed for two or three weeks, or even longer as for several months, and during all that time she was regarded as a patient. Later on, in the generation of our parents, the general practice was for the mother to get up a couple of days or so after having given birth, and this, in many circles was regarded as a real act of courage. The basis for this conception, as indicated above, was mainly that a long confinement was believed to increase the risk of blood clots, a viewpoint that we now know to be false.

The reply to the question of how long the mother should remain in bed after delivery would be something like this: The longer the mother remains in bed after having given birth, the greater the guarantee that her abdominal organs will be restored to normal and especially that there will be no risk of prolapsus of the uterus or the vagina. For this, ten or twelve days would be a suitable period, rather more than less. In America some doctors have recently permitted mothers to get up after only three or four days—and without regrettable consequences—but on condition that they were given energetic medical and other treatment almost immediately following delivery in connection with keeping up regular exercises.

447. *Exercises for Women After Childbirth*   In our own day and age there is a widespread and probably correct prevailing opinion supporting carefully planned and faithfully executed exercises already at an early stage of the confinement and in the period thereafter. It is considered that such exercises can play a great prophylactic role, in the prevention of flaccidity of the vaginal walls, descent of the uterus, phlebitis and limp, or pendulous abdominal muscles, and also may contribute importantly in restoring the mother to a normal condition, carried on in conjunction with other measures to that effect.

Many physicians make a pamphlet of comprehensive postnatal exercises available to mothers, recommending specific ones more than others, as depending upon specific cases.

448. *The After-pains*   On top of the regular questions as to whether her child is healthy and not deformed, many mothers immediately after delivery make this remark: "Now, I hope I am not going to have too many after-pains!" One may reply negatively to this, for simply through the administering of some hormone preparation (progesterone or androgen) or some quite harmless anesthetic or sedative it will be possible to make the after-pains practically nonexistent. A special teamwork gets under way between the breasts and the womb: sucking at the nipple will cause the womb to contract. These contractions are the essential cause of the after-pains. They occur mainly in women who have had more than one child. The after-pains are very important, inasmuch as they contribute to the uterus' return to normal proportions, which comes about more quickly and effectively in women who nurse their babies than in women who do not.

449. Nursing the Baby During pregnancy the breasts have already increased in size, and toward the end of pregnancy they begin to secrete an amber-colored fluid called *raw milk* or *colostrum*. This milky secretion is brought about by a so-called *lactogene hormone* from the anterior lobe of the pituitary gland, possibly simultaneously or later supplemented by a lactogene hormone from the suprarenals. During the very first day after childbirth—the time for the milk to commence flowing—this raw milk or colostrum continues to be secreted. This raw milk is particularly important to the baby because it acts as a laxative on the contents of the baby's bowels which have accumulated while in the fetal state. This bowel content is called *meconium*.

How soon after birth the child should begin to nurse depends entirely on the mother. During the first twenty-four hours the baby really does not require any nutrition, and is inclined to sleep. Therefore, it is principally the mother's need for rest which must determine at what moment the child should be laid to her breast for the first time. Before and after each of the baby's meals the nipples should be bathed in boiled water or in a boracic solution (in the interim they should be protected as carefully as possible against dirt and any kind of impurity).

How long the mother should continue to nurse the baby, and the proper time for weaning it is rather outside our subject here. However, it might serve a practical purpose to mention a number of undesirable disturbances in nursing that may occur as early as the lying-in period.

450. Disturbances in Nursing As was rather evident from the preceding remarks secretion of milk is a complicated process. For its initial start as well as for its continued flow, the milk depends upon a delicate teamwork between a number of factors, more than have been mentioned here. It is not surprising, therefore, that lactation may easily encounter difficulties.

A mother with an insufficient supply of milk is said to have *hypogalactia*. If the condition is in evidence immediately after childbirth it is termed *primary hypogalactia*. If the secretion of milk was normal to start with, but stopped after a shorter or longer period before the normal time for weaning the baby is at hand, the mother is said to have *secondary hypogalactia*.

The breasts may possibly be at fault and this may be due to abnormal hormone conditions or the mother's improper diet, or some unfortunate way of living.

The treatment must be adapted to the underlying cause or causes. It is yet impossible to make a hard and fast statement regarding the value of treatment with lactogenous hormone, which can now be obtained by extracting it from the anterior lobe of the pituitary glands of oxen. A so-called *pseudo-hypogalactia* is a condition in which a normal quantity of milk is produced, but that for some reason or other there is difficulty in getting it through the nipple. In case of complete absence of milk production the term sometimes used in describing it is *agalactia*.

A flow of milk so ample and persistent that the baby, even if it is entirely healthy, cannot possibly exhaust the supply, is a condition called *hypergalactia*. This condition is rare, but where it does exist it may cause much discomfort. In some large cities facilities for distribution of mothers' milk are proving to have great value.

Hypergalactia is often accompanied by a discharge of milk, which is also called *galactorrhea* and may also occur outside the normal period of nursing, according to some scientists. The causes are numerous and may be connected with widely varying diseases in organs far removed from the breasts, and that is why a woman with symptoms of galactorrhea should consult a doctor for examination and possible treatment.

Because of her general health or that of the child, sunken nipples, or the infant's death, or possibly unfortunate social conditions, the mother may be unable to nurse her baby. Her flow of milk may be stopped by administering estrogen or androgen immediately after delivery and the following days. Under these circumstances it is also necessary to bind the breasts.

If the nipples are sunken or inverted, and if they cannot be pulled out by hand or by applying a cupping glass, it is usually impossible to suck out the milk, and in that case the mother has to give up nursing her baby.

If very painful cracks or sores appear in the nipples, so-called "fissures," the child may sometimes suckle through a nipple shield, a glass funnel with a broad collar placed over the nipple equipped with a teat at the other end. If that method is unsuccessful the milk must be milked or sucked out. Sensible care of the nipples during pregnancy greatly aids in avoiding such conditions.

Should bacteria gain entrance to a fissure, inflammation of the breast, *mastitis,* may result, a condition that may require surgical treatment. If, however, the bacteria penetrate through the mammary ducts—and this cannot always be avoided despite very special care of the nipples after and between nursing—inflammation of the mammary glands may arise. The scientific name for this is *galactophoritis.* This disease generally comes on very suddenly and is accompanied by a high temperature. However, if it is treated as early as possible it is not otherwise dangerous. The infant must suckle as usual (strange to say the child is not affected adversely by the presence of bacteria in the milk) whereupon the breast must be sucked or milked empty every time; in the intervals between nursing the baby, hot compresses should be applied. The condition generally clears up in the course of from two to four days.

451. *Composition of Mother's Milk*   Woman's milk contains all the great variety of substances essential for the nutrition of a baby: proteins, carbohydrates, fats, vitamins, mineral salts, etc. In a little over two pints of human milk the sugar content is about five and a half ounces. Another substance is vitamin A which helps to protect the baby against infectious diseases. In spite of the fact that mother's milk is considered the best possible and most appropriate food that exists, babies should not live exclusively on breast milk for more than their first six months. If nursing at the breast extends over a longer period, the baby may become anemic because there is an inadequate amount of iron in the milk and a complete absence of copper which is also required to provide the red blood corpuscles with the oxygen-binding coloring matter, hemoglobin. If, nevertheless, anemia is not generally in evidence in the infant, it is because at birth it has a surplus of iron available, mostly accumulated during the latter part of the pregnancy.

452. *Return of Menstruation After Childbirth*   Many women menstruate regularly during their entire nursing period, while the menses of others may be completely absent until nursing is terminated. It is rather common to find women who think that by protracting the nursing period they will be shielded from a new pregnancy. This opinion is erroneous. Not only do women frequently get pregnant during the nursing period, but there are also many cases of their becoming pregnant before menses has returned at all.

453. *Sexual Intercourse After Childbirth* Having been stretched and dilated so considerably during labor the vagina must be left undisturbed for a time so as to permit it to return properly to its normal proportions. If a small tear or split came about during the delivery that also, of course, must be given time to heal. As a general rule intercourse should not take place within the first four weeks following childbirth. Thus it is best not to have intercourse for one month before and one month after childbirth.

454. *How Long an Interval Should Elapse Between Two Pregnancies?* It is depressing to see a woman already exhausted and dispirited from too frequent childbirths and, with her last baby still at the breast, pregnant again. A woman should be given enough time and quiet to regain those feminine qualities that are so essential to her ability to fulfill her task as a wife and mother. She should be permitted to have the time and strength to give care and tenderness to her small baby. When a new pregnancy is started she must be able to devote a great part of her energy and concern to it. Therefore, two pregnancies should not follow immediately upon one another. It is, of course, difficult to establish completely valid rules. However, one that certainly comes nearest to meeting the biological requirements advocates at least one and a half or preferably two years, should elapse between babies. Thus the means to prevent pregnancy by various forms of contraceptive devices, which we shall describe later, have their distinct mission, particularly during the first year after childbirth.

455. *The Cycle Is Completed* For both the child and the mother, the cycle of pregnancy is completed upon delivery.

Motherhood is the greatest task in a woman's life. Conception, pregnancy, childbirth, and confinement are merely episodes, regarded as links in the woman's sex life, which is our subject here. If they have passed normally, she is now ready to take up her life as a sexual being the same way as before she became pregnant.

11

INTERRUPTION OF PREGNANCY

Chapter 49: ABORTIONS AND MISCARRIAGES

456. *What Is Meant by Interruption of Pregnancy?* Pregnancy that stops or is arrested at a time, or in such a way, that full-term childbirth does not occur, is termed interruption of pregnancy. On that point interruption of pregnancy differs in principle from the prematurely induced miscarriage. This type of birth may sometimes be imperative as a precautionary measure, for example, cases in which the pregnant woman risks eclampsia or in order to avoid certain other forms of dystochia.

457. *What Are Miscarriages and Abortions?* The terms abortion and miscarriage refer to pregnancy which is interrupted or terminated before the twenty-eighth week—i.e. before the fetus would be capable of living if it were born.

458. *How Frequently Do Abortions or Miscarriages Occur?* Much more frequently than people generally imagine. The figures —especially the actual number of abortions—are difficult to obtain and usually unreliable. But according to most available statistics nearly every fourth pregnancy ends in an abortion or miscarriage. Hence there is really nothing surprising in that a woman who has borne five or six children may also have had a miscarriage either before she had her first child or after she has borne one or more children.

459. What Are the Forms of Interruptions of Pregnancy? A distinction is usually made between *spontaneous interruptions* or *miscarriages*, which occur unintentionally, and abortions. We shall consider each of these categories separately.

Chapter 50: MISCARRIAGES

460. The Two Forms of Miscarriage or Spontaneous Interruption a. If a miscarriage—apparently by accident and quite unexpected—occurs in a woman who otherwise has been able to complete her pregnancies normally and bear her children, it is called an *accidental miscarriage*. b. If, however, a woman has a miscarriage *every* time she gets pregnant the proper term to be used is *habitual miscarriage*. The majority of miscarriages occur in the second or third month of pregnancy.

461. Accidental Miscarriage Sometimes the cause of accidental miscarriage may be traced and sometimes not. It may be due to a disease in the mother or in the father. However, in recent years the results of scientific investigation point to the conclusion that the cause of a miscarriage may quite well be inherent in the egg proper. Likewise it is rather logical to conclude that some deficiency in the sperm that fertilized the egg could be the cause of the zygote's failure to develop normally, resulting in a miscarriage. Some deficiency is often found upon close microscopic examination of a colony of cells evacuated at a miscarriage, distinctly indicating that this group of cells would not have been capable of developing into a normal human baby. To realize that may, after all, be somewhat of a comfort to a married couple when they grieve about a miscarriage. The sooner an embryo like that is evacuated the better it is for the woman.

462. Possible Influence of External Factors A woman who has had a miscarriage generally believes she can remember something she has done that she shouldn't have done, such as having carried a heavy load, cleaned the topmost windows, driven over a rough road, etc. But those are things that many pregnant women constantly do without a resultant miscarriage; and, to tell the truth, nothing is actually known as to whether that sort of ordinary activity may or may not provoke a miscarriage. It is probable that events like that are simply the incidental or final factor that cause an egg, which at any rate would have pried loose sooner or later, to be expelled by the accidental strenuous effort. However, one external cause that—apparently without a shadow of doubt—may hasten the advent of a miscarriage, due sooner or later, is a sudden, violent fright. For such a fright is accompanied by uterine contractions that may lead to a miscarriage.

It is common knowledge that air-raid alarms, fires, and earthquakes may hasten births as wells as miscarriages.

463. *Habitual Miscarriage* What causes habitual miscarriage is not known either. Tests using doses of progesterone in cases of treated miscarriage might point to the fact that hormonal conditions may be of importance in certain cases of habitual miscarriage. Some believe it is due to a deficiency of C-, E-, and K-vitamins in the pregnant woman; and the E-vitamin is considered particularly necessary to help carry a pregnancy to its full and normal term. Another treatment, therefore, consists in feeding the pregnant woman E-vitamin, extracted from alfalfa.

In recent years, particularly in America, a campaign has been going on for introduction of a treatment, now generally adopted, to give all pregnant women E-vitamin although it is maintained that in the United States such treatment is not essential inasmuch as the average diet in the country is well balanced in respect to vitamins.

464. *The Importance of the Rh-factor* In 1940 it was discovered that a special substance present in the red blood corpuscles of a monkey species called *rhesus macacus* is also present in the red blood corpuscles of most human beings. Therefore the substance has been called the *rhesus factor*, or, short, the *Rh-factor*. If a pregnant woman lacks this substance, in which case she is said to be *Rh-negative*, whereas it is present in the father, who is said to be *Rh-positive*, the fetus in most cases will be Rh-positive. In certain circumstances such a fetus will be able to

cause production of antisubstances in the blood plasma of the Rh-negative mother.

By way of the placenta these substances pass into the fetus and through their reaction to the Rh-factor present in the fetus may cause various diseases, often causing the death of the fetus. This condition has proved to be at the bottom of many cases of miscarriage; but whether they have any close connection with the repeated occurrence of "habitual miscarriages" is not yet known.

465. *Bleeding at Miscarriage* When the fetus and the placenta abnormally break away from the uterus some blood vessels always burst. Consequently, a miscarriage is always accompanied by *bleeding*. It may be a large flow of blood, or it may be only slight. In some cases it stops quickly, while in other cases the blood keeps gushing forth for quite a long time, and women who have started a miscarriage often feel they will bleed to death. Let me say right away, to still the fears of these women, that it is among the rarest of rare occurrences for a woman to bleed to death from a miscarriage. As soon as the pressure abates somewhat, the blood vessels in the uterus quickly close up, so the bleeding is apt to stop spontaneously. Moreover, the female organism seems to be so constituted that loss of blood in a woman apparently is replaced much quicker than in a man.

466. *Pains Accompanying Miscarriage* The uterine contractions connected with a miscarriage often give rise to violent *pains*, often as painful as real labor pains. This may be due to the fact that the tissues in the uterine neck are not as soft and tensile as those involved in a full-term birth to permit even a small premature fetus to pass.

467. *What Is Delivered in a Miscarriage?* What is entailed in a miscarriage is dependent upon how early in the pregnancy period it occurs. If it takes place within the first six to eight weeks after conception it may emerge as an unbroken little bag composed of the embryonic membranes, including the embryo, the bag of waters, and a small placenta. If the abortion

or miscarriage occurs later in the pregnancy, both the fetus and the afterbirth are evacuated.

468. *Treatment of Miscarriage*   The first thing to do if bleeding occurs during pregnancy is to go to bed and call your doctor who will prescribe proper treatment. It is entirely possible that with proper medical care the pregnancy may be saved. The details involved are too medical in nature for discussion here.

469. *The Fetus and the Afterbirth Must Be Completely Removed*   If the fetus is dead and the hemorrhage keeps on, it is an essential rule that no trace of the fetus or the afterbirth should be left in the uterus. First, as long as there is anything left at all, it may cause bleeding and prevent the uterus from contracting to its normal proportions. Secondly, there is (as mentioned before) a possibility that very strong cells that were part of the little fetus and its afterbirth may develop into growths or tumors, settling in the uterus and perhaps twenty or thirty years later cause some grave disease.

If the miscarriage is well under way when the doctor comes, it is, therefore, important that everything that has been evacuated be kept until he can examine it. If he has not personally observed that the afterbirth too has been expelled, he will probably order a *curettement* of the womb.

470. *Confinement in Bed After a Miscarriage*   What happens in the uterus is in many respects exactly the same in a miscarriage as what occurs at a birth. The uterus contracts violently, a hemorrhage follows, and in the place where the placenta has pried loose a lot of tiny blood vessels have burst that now have to be closed with coagulated blood—small blood clots. What I said about staying in bed after childbirth remains an essentially valid recommendation as a postlude to miscarriage also. The uterus should be given time to contract to its normal proportions and size and heal, and this requires rest and quiet. At any rate, the woman should remain in bed about a week.

471. *Consequences of a Miscarriage*   If a miscarriage has been properly cared for there need be no unfortunate conse-

quences for the woman's future health. It is another matter that many women suffer real injury by undergoing a miscarriage. But it should be noted that this is not because of the miscarriage as such but because the women were not given proper care.

Chapter 51: INDUCED ABORTIONS

472. *Two Forms of Induced Abortions* As long as the concept of an undesired pregnancy has existed, artificial or induced abortions have been significant problems. In former days interrupting a pregnancy before it had reached half-term was not considered illegal. However, interrupting a pregnancy during the latter half of its term was regarded as murder of the fetus, because it was considered that by that time the fetus had gained its "soul." In modern times we are concerned more with the fact that all of the future physical qualities of the human being are already present in the genes from the very moment of conception and that interrupting a pregnancy at any stage of fetal growth will always be identical with destruction of a potential life. The only legal abortions, therefore, are those which are performed on the basis of valid medical indications. All other abortions are considered illegal or criminal, while the legal ones are called therapeutic abortions. For such an abortion to be legal, certain medical indications must be met. When the woman's life or health is not in serious danger, a pregnancy must not normally be interrupted after the end of the third month of pregnancy.

473. *Diseases Endangering the Pregnant Woman's Life or Health* It would lead too far to list those diseases that spontaneously and unconditionally justify interruption of pregnancy; or to note all the diseases that justify it in certain circumstances; and to list all those diseases that do not justify it, for that would require classification in separate groups of each and every known disease.

The fact that a pregnant woman may be suffering from some ailment is considered by many women as justifying her in having a therapeutic abortion performed. This widespread viewpoint is quite a wrong one. The following diseases are regarded as justifying a therapeutic abortion. a. aggravation of certain mental diseases or states of insanity, if former pregnancies have proved that they are apt to reappear or to be aggravated during pregnancy; b. certain forms of epilepsy that were rapidly aggravated by preceding pregnancies; c. certain acute and chronic nervous complaints; d. certain potentially dangerous diseases of the blood; e. certain eye complaints; certain malignant tumors; f. certain cases of chronic rheumatoid arthritis that had proved to become worse during a former pregnancy; g. cancer of the uterine cervix, as a rule; h. and the same for tuberculosis of the larynx. There are no other *absolute, unconditional indications*.

To these indications may be added a number of diseases that —provided certain very definite circumstances are present— also indisputably entitle a woman to have her pregnancy interrupted. For example, that may be the case in respect to syphilis if the patient cannot tolerate the necessary antisyphilitic treatment requisite for the mother and child during pregnancy. But the concerned pregnant woman can obtain more detailed information about all these matters from her physician. Tuberculosis of the lungs was formerly considered a medical indication permitting interruption of pregnancy, and it used to be one of the most frequently cited legitimate bases for therapeutic abortions. However, in recent years it has been established that tuberculosis of the lungs in its active phase follows almost the same course in pregnant as in nonpregnant young women, and as a result, there is no longer any logical reason to believe that the disease is aggravated to any considerable extent by pregnancy. From a medical viewpoint, therefore, tuberculosis of the lungs will not always be considered a justifiable reason for recommending an abortion.

12

REGULATION OF FERTILIZATION

Chapter 52: PROBLEMS OF FERTILITY

474. *What Is the Crux of the Problem?* From the point of view of the community the problems associated with fertility and sterility present themselves like this: It is desirable to bring about a certain balance between the number of births and deaths in order that there may always be as many people as possible at their productive, active age to take care not only of themselves, but also of those in the nonproductive age-groups: children and old people.

The individual couples are confronted with these alternatives: "How are we, who have not hitherto been able to have any children, to find a remedy that will enable us to have them?" There also is this question: "How are we, who do not, for the time being, wish to have children, able to avoid it?" It is such conditions as these that each category separately tries to remedy.

475. *The Great Population Surplus of the Past* If the population of the nineteenth century continued to increase at its previous rate, in one hundred years there would be ten million inhabitants in Denmark (today about four million) and in another 500 years there would be more inhabitants than the entire population of Europe as of today. If the population increased by 1 per cent yearly for 638 years Denmark's population would equal that of the whole world now. In one thousand years there would be seventy billion, which would correspond to two persons per square meter throughout the country.

476. *But Sterility Is on the Increase* If we estimate how many women are born who later attain the age of childbearing, we arrive at the amazing result that 1,000 women born in 1946 will become the mothers of only about 900 girls, who will live long enough to become mothers in their turn. They will bear only about 810 girls who will live to become mothers. One may deduct from this that as early as 1970 births and deaths will already balance each other in Denmark, and by then there should be a little more than four million; from 1970 on the population would diminish. That is a warning and a symptom; it means that fertility is on the wane, or that sterility is increasing.

477. *The Law of Gradual Sterility* Fertility may decrease gradually because of hereditary causes. The downfall of the Babylonian and Greek civilizations may have occurred principally because of such causes. In the present era certain statistics seem to point to a regular law of probability with respect to the possibility of having offspring, that may be surprising to most people. A few years ago a poll was taken among a great number of married couples whose greatest wish was to have children, as many as possible. It disclosed that 15 per cent of these couples, despite their great desire for children and efforts toward having them, were absolutely incapable of having offspring! Twelve per cent of the couples had succeeded in having one child, but no more, although they ardently desired more children. Eleven per cent had proved themselves capable of having two children, and that was their limit. Ten per cent of the group polled would have three children. In Denmark, statistics from an investigation of 14,121 marriages show that 44 per cent of modern marriages still remained childless after five years of marriage, and that fertility is 55 per cent lower than thirty-five years ago.

478. *The Practical Approach of Individual Problems* The main lines have already been stated: Certain people consider their fertility is greater than they desire it to be; others find it less than they should wish for. The members of the first group specifically desire to avoid having children as a result of sexual

intercourse. In actual experience this can be accomplished by contraception or induced abortion. From these two alternatives the latter and its narrowly conditioned legitimacy has already been mentioned in Part XI. Contraception will be mentioned below. The members of the second group want concretely to beget children but are frustrated. The practical tasks are to cure a definite sterility or a pseudo sterility and to prevent miscarriages. The latter has been mentioned in Part XI.

Thus, in the following, first psuedo sterility, then sterility, and finally contraception will be considered.

Chapter 53: PSEUDO STERILITY

479. *What Is Pseudo Sterility?* A very frequent cause of lengthy childlessness is that the couple quite accidentally may have had no sexual intercourse during the fertilization periods. A second possibility is that intercourse in some other way has been improperly or inadequately performed. In such cases there is no genuine sterility. Under proper circumstances the parties may be fertile. The condition is named *pseudo sterility*.

Impotence during intercourse, however, is not the same as being sterile should artificial insemination prove successful. Perhaps, in such a case, the state of the man might be described as *pseudo sterility*.

Nor is it correct to call a woman who habitually miscarries sterile. On the contrary, she is not sterile, for the basis of her repeated miscarriages may lie in her capacity for being fertilized, without, however, the ability to carry her pregnancy to its full term and to deliver her child. This state too—which some scientists classify under sterility—is more correctly characterized as *pseudo sterility*.

Physiological sterility means the sterility (pseudo sterility in my opinion) that normally exists before puberty, during pregnancy and lactation, during and after the menopause, and during certain periods of the menstrual cycle.

480. *Guidance in Intercourse* In case of pseudo sterility the physician must determine whether intercourse is carried out in such a way that the seminal fluid is actually being deposited as far back in the vagina as is necessary.

However incredible it may sound, physicians are sometimes consulted by couples who, on direct questioning, are not able to say for certain—even after several years of marriage—whether they have ever achieved normal intercourse, whether the introduction of the penis into the vagina has really taken place. In such cases of pseudo sterility it may be necessary to give the husband some guidance about the proper way of carrying out intercourse. If the obstacle to a complete intercourse is due to deficient erection in the husband, or to vaginism (genital spasm) in the wife, these complaints must be treated separately. It may also be advisable to enlighten the wife about certain positions in intercourse that will permit the seminal fluid to pass as far back into the vagina as possible, and eventually prevent it from flowing out.

481. *Fertilization Terms* There has been much speculation as to whether one or more periods between two menses might offer exceptionally great possibilities of fertilization. In the deliberations of the possible and practical importance of such fertilization terms the question of the fate of the egg cell and the sperm cells in the female organism is most essential.

According to experiments and calculations made about twenty-five years ago by the Japanese, Ogino, ovulation must occur twelve to fourteen days prior to an expected menstrual period. More recent investigations, by Knaus, revealed that the ovulation always takes place fifteen days before menstruation.

In 1948, Farris, the American gynecologist, found through a special examination method that the ovulation in forty-six examined women took place between the sixth and twentieth day of the menstrual cycle. In the case of 64 per cent of these women between the eleventh and thirteenth day. The time was very constant as the variations were less than three days in 93 per cent of the women examined while the menstruations only in 77 per cent showed a similar degree of regularity.

Furthermore, it will have been observed that the unfertilized (but eventually mitotically-divided) egg during its passage through the tube is surrounded by an albuminous membrane secreted by the tube which the sperms are not able to penetrate. If the egg cell is not fertilized it dies rather quickly. This means that the egg is only capable of being fertilized for a couple of hours or, possibly, for a couple of days after ovulation has occurred.

As previously mentioned, opinions are much divided as to the fate of the spermatozoa after coition. However, according to observations made their activity is not particularly pronounced when exposed to a temperature which is, as in the scrotum, two to seven degrees below the body temperature, but they become even very active when entering the vagina which has the ordinary body temperature. However, the activity ceases presumably because the substance energy of the spermatozoa carried along is quickly used up owing to the intense activity. Thus attempts have been made to remove oviducts with active semen cells. After the lapse of twenty-four hours all the cells had ceased to move about, and it is therefore thought that semen cells, under normal conditions, can remain alive only three or four days in the female sex organs.

482. *Determining the Time of Fertilization* Taking it for granted that the fertilization is most likely to take place around the days of the ovulation, our task will be to determine when the ovulation occurs during the menstrual cycle.

The method employed by Farris, which is of great value in scientific research, is much too troublesome and costly for ordinary purposes.

On the other hand, the rise in temperature that occurs simultaneously with the ovulation in a healthy woman may be of great practical importance for the determination of the moment of ovulation. It has been found (Diddle) that this rise in temperature in most women fails to occur once or several times a year from which fact the conclusion is drawn that no ovulation has taken place in such cases.

483. *Knaus' Tables* On the basis of the consideration that the ovulation always occurs fifteen days before the menstruation, Knaus has worked out his well-known *menstruation table*. The date on which the menses begins is noted down on the left. The

duration of it is marked by a waving line extending over as many spaces as the number of days it lasts, and the succeeding menstruation is marked in the space that indicates the number of days between the onset of two successive menses. By counting backwards fourteen to fifteen days from this space one may determine the day in the menstrual interval on which the ovulation that provoked the menses marked in that space must have occurred. The days just around ovulation are the so-called fertile days, or the fertilization term proper. The days close to them are, in practice, where the lifetime of the semen cells also must be taken into consideration, the questionable days. The remaining days constitute the sterile period, sometimes called the "safe" period.

The register should preferably be kept over a couple of years before one dares to rely upon it. And even then one may hardly dismiss the possibility that irregular ovulations may take place outside the calculated moments of ovulation. This, of course, makes the calculation somewhat unreliable. In respect to the practical application of the method as a contraceptive measure, a study among 379 women indicated that in 15,924 cases of completely natural intercourse on days outside the fertilization term fertilization did not occur in a single instance.

484. *Important Information for Childless Marriages* In some cases of lengthy childlessness the fertilization term is very short, perhaps only a single day a month. To obtain fertilization in such cases, the point is to determine the date of ovulation as exactly as possible. Knaus' table may offer some help in this connection. However, it is of greater value in that it is often possible to fix the individual moment of the ovulation with great accuracy through regular measurings of temperature. One should primarily choose such days for intercourse.

Chapter 54: STERILITY

485. *What Is Sterility?* Sterility in man mean the inability to fertilize and in woman the term indicates incapacity to be fertilized. The word sterility as such gives no indication as to

its origin or what causes it. Sterility is the same as *impotency at begetting and conceiving,* impotency at reproduction.

486. *Whose "Fault" Is It?* If, after several years of marriage, a couple has had no children there might be justification for examining them for possible sterility.

It is almost invariably the wife, not the husband, who consults the doctor in such cases, for it is a common belief that when a couple doesn't have any children it is always the woman's fault.

This widespread opinion is quite wrong. Recent tests have disclosed that the man is the inadequate party as often as the woman. It is impossible, however, to offer a valid estimate as to the normal relationship of men to women among the general population. In some cases both husband and wife are more or less sterile, with one partner's partial sterility, in effect, supplementing the other's.

487. *Examination and Treatment of the Husband* · As a rule the doctor will ask for the husband to be tested first, because it is easier to check male sterility. His genital organs are examined for: infantilism and a blocked passage for the sperms, double cryptorchism, and double epididymitis—all of which may be the cause of sterility.

If the organs are in a normal condition, his seminal fluid is examined. The doctor will instruct him how to get a specimen of his seminal fluid for examination. It is very important that the sperm cells are exposed to a suitable temperature which means suitably low and to a proper degree of humidity during the transportation to the laboratory. Such care must be taken, for the test is to provide a means for showing not only the quantity of sperm cells present in the seminal fluid, but also the number of *motile* and otherwise normal sperms. The sperms, for example, may not be properly developed, possibly by reason of double cryptorchism, or mumps. Another cause for male sterility may be when the secretions from the prostate gland and the seminal vesicles—with which they are to be mixed—are not present in sufficient quantity, or they may be so composed that the sperm cells get only an inadequate impetus for spontaneous movement although a greater propulsion is essential if they shall reach the egg and fertilize it.

A complete absence of sperm cells in the seminal fluid is called *azoospermia*. Complete absence of mobility in all sperm cells is called *nekrospermia*. In case of aspermia (deficiency of seminal secretion) there may be good reason to try a treatment with gonadotropine. In the case of cryptorchism this is always effective. Such a treatment may therefore always be recommended as a preventive measure for all boys suffering from double cryptorchism which may cause sterility.

Furthermore, the test comprises some other physical and chemical examinations of the seminal fluid as, for example, a consideration of the contents of *hyaluronidase* which plays a special part. Extensive scientific examinations have provided evidence that the amount of hyaluronidase in the seminal fluid is usually correspondingly larger the more sperm cells the seminal fluid contains per cubic centimeter. Furthermore, in the case of a number of childless marriages the scientists have found that the man's seminal fluid—which was normal in every other respect—did not contain any hyaluronidase at all. These examinations seem to indicate that the absence of hyaluronidase in the seminal fluid is a cause of sterility—and not a rare cause—in man. Before intercourse an adequate amount of hyaluronidase is placed in the woman's vagina; thus the otherwise sterile man will then be capable of begetting children.

488. *An Evaluation of Sterility Tests for the Husband* If the husband's sperm cells prove to be capable of fertilization the question may arise, as to whether his sperm cells and the woman's egg cells possibly do not harmonize chemically, for if they don't there is little hope of remedying the sterility. Chemical incompatibility is, however, considered rare, and the doctor would then investigate whether the cause of the couple's childless state might be associated with the wife, as that would seem to be the logical conclusion. If, on the contrary, the husband's sperms prove to be too few in number or to lack proper mobility, or possibly be entirely absent, or lacking *hyaluronidase*, one will naturally be inclined to consider *that* to be the cause of the sterility. However, the result must be judged with the greatest

tact and circumspection. It must be remembered that the husband's general capacity to fertilize has not been tested, only an incidental specimen of his seminal fluid. Therefore, the physician will insist on several tests, and even if these should continue to prove "negative" he must still be very cautious about establishing with certainty that the man is incapable of begetting children. There are a good many examples of married couples having had a child five or ten years after it had been "established" that they couldn't have any children. And it is easy to imagine what the husband would feel justified in accusing his wife of, just because they were told too definitely that he was sterile. In paternity cases many "negative" sperm tests are necessary before ruling out a particular man who is under accusation.

489. *Investigation of the Penetration of Sperm Cells into the Mucous Clot* An absolutely necessary condition for fertilization is that the sperm cells be able to make their way through the clot of mucus at the cervical canal. This may be tested by the so-called Miller-Kurzrok test in which a little sperm and some mucus from the cervical canal are placed side by side, quite close, on a glass plate, and covered with another very thin disk, whereupon it may be seen through the microscope how the sperms penetrate. The so-called Huhner test consists in examining shortly after intercourse a specimen of the seminal fluid deposited in the posterior vaginal vault and a specimen of the mucus from the cervical canal.

This latter method is of special value if the husband refuses to permit a test, as it gives information as to whether any ejaculation of seminal fluid occurs during intercourse at all, and, if so, more detailed information about the composition of the seminal fluid ejaculated under normal conditions, as well as its capacity to penetrate the mucous clot in the cervical canal.

490. *Examination of the Woman* The causes of sterility in woman are more numerous than those in man. In the same manner that deficiencies in the male sperm may cause sterility, so some deficiency in the egg may bring about the similar result in woman. More detailed examination, however, could hardly

bear upon the egg, at least not with the methods at present available.

The examination must therefore consist of an investigation of the passageway the sperms must use from the moment they are ejaculated into the interior of the vagina until they meet the egg in the Fallopian tube. Every obstacle the sperms meet on their way through the vagina, uterus, and tubes may become a cause of sterility. Such an examination at the same time affords an opportunity to investigate the woman's birth tract. The result of the examination shows that by far the most frequent cause of sterility in woman is inflammation of the Fallopian tubes (salpingitis). The second most frequent cause is infantilism.

491. *Infantilism as a Cause of Female Sterility* The female genital organs may often be so stunted in growth that either the ovulation or the passage of the egg does not take place normally, or it may be that the sperm cells are not given the chance to get as far as the egg. In all of these circumstances infantilism will be the cause of the woman's sterility.

This condition requires hormone treatment with estrogen preparations, or a local operation in order to facilitate the passage of the sperm cells, or a combination of both.

492. *Changes in the Vagina as Causes of Sterility* It was formerly believed that sperm cells can withstand only a certain degree of acidity. Very recent investigations of sperm cells have revealed that an abnormal amount of acidity did not impair the motility of the sperms. There is, therefore, little validity in the suggestion that an acid secretion of the vagina such as is found in vaginal inflammation (*vaginitis*), could have any decisive influence on the life or motility of the sperm cells, or that *that* could cause sterility as was formerly maintained. However, there is no doubt that inflammation of the vagina of a *grave nature* may cause sterility. In each case the treatment must be adapted to the exact nature of the complaint.

493. *Long and Narrow Cervical Canal as Cause of Sterility* Particularly in narrow, comparatively long, cervical canals the mucous plug may (cf. secs. 58 and 364) form an impenetrable barrier to even normal sperms, thus causing sterility, whereas the narrowness of the canal as such does not prevent their passage. Dilation of the canal by a small operation does away with the sterility in 50 per cent of cases, probably because a wider outlet is thus provided for the mucus, which no longer is so likely to form a firm clot or stopper. Perhaps the favorable result may also have something to do with the operation influencing the tubes indirectly so that the sperms are afforded better chances of passage to the egg.

494. Sterility Caused by Retroversion of the Womb Abnormal positions of the womb, particularly retroversion, may, in relatively rare cases, be a cause of sterility. The uterine os may thereby be turned at such an angle in relation to the vagina that it practically touches the front of the vaginal vault. This makes the penetration of the sperms through the uterine os difficult, if not impossible. The passage from the uterus to the tube may, as a second possibility, form an "elbow" obstructing partly or completely the passage of sperms at that point.

The uterus may be brought back to a normal position by using a ring, or by a surgical operation; such treatment will eliminate the sterility.

495. Changes in the Uterine Mucous Membranes as a Cause of Sterility Occasionally sterility may be caused by modifications in the uterine mucous membranes. If the secretions of the glands within the mucous membranes are insufficient the zygote cannot imbed itself in the uterine wall. On the other hand, if the mucous secretions are too ample, the result may be a discharge that will also prevent the zygote from digging in.

In the first case the mucous membranes are said to *atrophy*, in the second, to *hypertrophy*. *Inflammation of the uterus* (*endometritis*) is an inflammation of the uterine mucous membrane which, as long as it lasts, may be considered to some extent a cause of sterility. Endometritis may be due to many causes, such as exposure to humid cold and draughts; use of dangerous contraceptives, untrained interference, and introduction of impurities in the uterine cavity. It may also occur as a result of pregnancy, inflammation of the Fallopian tubes, cystitis, etc.

The treatment is often a very lengthy process. In some cases it will consist in a curettement; in others by applying heat, as in diathermy. If the uterine inflammation is caused by some special disease, that, of course, must be treated simultaneously. If the deficiency is a resultant of the uterine mucous membrane's inability to prepare for nestlike function—the nidation—of the egg the treatment calls for the use of the hormone progesteron.

496. Blocking of Passage by Uterine Tumors Sometimes a woman's sterility may be due to unfortunately located uterine tumors. They may not be dangerous, but small nonmalignant polyps or *fibromes* (a form of growths of connecting tissue) or muscular formations (*myomes*) may have settled in places where they block the passage of the sperms into the cervical canal or into the Fallopian tubes. Surgical treatment may be necessary.

497. *Inflammation of the Fallopian Tubes as a Direct Cause of Sterility* Tubal inflammation (*salpingitis*) is undoubtedly the most common disease of the female organs, and may be the direct cause of sterility. There are many causes for this great incidence: a. exposure of the abdomen to cold and draughts, for instance, by the woman being too scantily clad, or by having to stay constantly in cold, humid places; b. appendicitis; c. various contagious infections, of which by far the most frequent is the venereal disease gonorrhea that will be described later; moreover, tuberculosis, influenza, etc., may cause salpingitis; d. use of dangerous contraceptives; e. faulty care at confinement.

498. *Examination of Fallopian Tubes by Blowing Air Through Them* Many of the more modern gynecologists test whether the passage through the uterus and the tubes is open by blowing air through the cervical canal (the so-called persufflation method). Antispastic medication may be administered before the test, if the physician believes that the tubes are contracting convulsively. If the air passes through the tubes and into the abdominal cavity a characteristic, crackling, bubbling sound is heard. Some doctors consider this method dangerous on the grounds that bacteria may be blown from the uterus and the tube into the abdominal cavity and give rise to inflammation there. Actually, however, this testing method has proved to be not only harmless but, in most cases, painless as well.

499. *Testing by Injection of a Tracer into the Tubes* A method similar to that just described (and which may also be preceded by administering antispastic medication) but permitting a more accurate appreciation of the condition of the Fallopian tubes, consists in introducing into the uterus and the tubes an opaque substance that will show on an X-ray plate. Such a substance acts as a tracer, and on the X-ray picture the uterus will show up as a column between the two tubes extending to the left and to the right, like two threads, widening where they approach and meet the ovaries.

500. *Treatment of Changes in the Fallopian Tubes* The best treatment for salpingitis under a doctor's care (inflammation of the tubes) is rest in bed, together with the employment of hot douches, hot compresses or some other hot application on the abdomen, sometimes supplemented by diathermic treatment. Diathermic methods involve placing electric heating tubes, electrodes, in the vagina from where the heat radiates to the Fallopian tubes.

If the salpingitis is due to *gonorrhea, tuberculosis*, or to some other grave disease, these more deep-seated ailments must of course receive appropriate treatment too. Experience has proved that examining the condition of the tubes by blowing air through them sufficed to do away with the sterility in twenty per cent of cases. The conclusions drawn from these figures is that the sterility was simply due to some purely mechanical obstruction of the passageway through the tubes, and therefore needed no further treatment. However, if the examination reveals *adhesions* of one or both of the tubes to adjacent organs the question of using some surgery may arise.

501. *Adhesions as Causes of Sterility* Adhesions may sometimes result from salpingitis, i.e. the Fallopian tube, for instance, adheres to the peritoneum, the appendix, the intestine, etc. Salpingitis has a tendency to spread to the ovary and cause *inflation of the ovary*. Such a condition may bring about shrink-

ing and constriction by scars and adhesions with other abdominal organs obstructing or completely blocking the passage of the egg from the ovary into the tube. Salpingitis in conjunction with oöphoritis is called *salpingo-oöphoritis* or *annexitis*. If both tubes are affected, the physician will, as a rule, recommend a surgical operation.

502. Deficiency of Ovarian Function In rare instances the ovaries are not developed at all, not because the woman suffers from infantilism but probably because of some disturbance in the hormonal balance of the organism. For that reason the woman has no menstruation. However, the woman's missed menses do not necessarily point to her ovulation being abnormal. She may have normal ovulation and may also become pregnant. The physician may try hormone treatments.

A special fault in the eggs may be their *barrenness*, that is, they ripen, but cannot be fertilized and develop further. If this is the case nothing can be done, at least not within the knowledge we currently have available.

503. Sterility Without Any Discoverable Cause In many cases it is impossible to point to a definite cause of a person's sterility. Some scientists have advanced the hypotheses that there might be some chemical disharmony, so-called negative *chemotaxis*, between the egg and the sperm, so that instead of being attracted to each other, they repel each other. The attraction is called positive chemotaxis. No method is known of changing the possible chemical attraction between the spermatozoa and the eggs.

A great deal of sexual intercourse with the same man might also make a woman immune to that man's sperms. It is very likely that a hyaluronidase-restrictive substance may be present in some sterile women, the substance having been perhaps produced through too frequent sexual intercourse, which renders the passage of the sperm cells to the egg impossible.

There is still no general medical agreement about these theories. However, it is a fact that when a childless couple divorce they sometimes prove capable of having offspring in a new marriage, the husband with another woman, and the wife with another man.

A great deal of resignation is often required in such childless marriages. If the desire for a child of their own is very strong the couple in many cases agree to divorce. In other instances, they may adopt one or more children so as to gratify their parental urge in that way. There are frequent cases in which women who were considered barren became pregnant shortly after having adopted a child. This may probably be due to the fact that they no longer are under the nervous tension developed from believing that they are incapable of having children of their own.

In effect, fertilization and conception seem to depend greatly upon a number of physical as well as emotional factors not yet sufficiently investigated.

Many married couples will resign themselves to their childless fate if they love each other very much.

504. *Artificial Fertilization (Insemination)* This means that, under observation of the most thorough aseptic precautions, seminal fluid is gathered and injected directly into the uterus or into the cervical canal. We mentioned earlier that impotence at intercourse may raise the question of artificial insemination. However, it is of still greater practical importance that, by having recourse to artificial insemination, the sperm cells—normally too few in number or too weak to survive the passage through the vagina—are helped to penetrate directly into the cervical canal. Finally, artificial insemination is increasingly applied with sperm of a—usually anonymous—third person, a so-called *sperm donor,* in marriages where the husband is sterile but where the husband and wife all the same wish to have a child, with the wife as its actual mother.

Chapter 55: CONTRACEPTION

505. *Contraception or Not* Contraception is one of the subjects in recent times that has been capable of stirring up the greatest commotion in the discussion of sex. Discussion of it has

been stamped to a great extent by purely personal opinion. A large percentage of the general public quite seriously maintains that sexual intercourse should not be indulged in except for the definite purpose of bringing a baby into the world. Another large percentage of the public insists just as earnestly that such an idea is completely erroneous. The latter group considers that most married couples, on the basis of economic reasons alone, are excluded from rearing more than three or four children, and that it would be unreasonable to believe that an individual's sexual need should be permitted an outlet only during three or four brief periods in a whole lifetime.

The United States Government, as well as more than half of the states themselves, has enacted various laws regulating the distribution of contraceptives and of information concerning their use.

Couples contemplating use of contraceptive devices (chemical or mechanical) must seek the advice of their physicians.

506. *Practical Remarks about Sexual Abstinence* The terms prevention of pregnancy and contraception denote not only that the object is to avoid impregnation but also that something has to be done with this end in view. Sexual abstinence leads *automatically* to the fulfillment of this object, and the method, therefore, cannot really be called a method to prevent but, rather, a means to avoid pregnancy.

In this connection a few practical remarks would be rather expedient. The term *sexual abstinence* is generally understood to be abstinence from sexual intercourse. However, it has been found that it cannot be left out of consideration with any degree of certainty that impregnation may take place if sperm cells and a sufficient quantity of hyaluronidase are introduced in another way than through intercourse. For example, with the fingers, they are introduced into vagina or the entrance to vagina. On the one hand, sexual abstinence is, therefore, one of the methods that ensures avoidance of impregnation. But, on the other hand, the method is only safe if the abstinence is sufficiently comprehensive. This should not be forgotten whenever the point is to give an exhaustive explanation of the methods that aim at the avoidance of impregnation.

507. Two Positive Methods for the Prevention of Pregnancy Among the methods for the prevention of pregnancy some are safe, although the majority are unsafe. There are two safe methods: sterilization of the woman or of the man, and castration of the woman or the man.

508. Sterilization of the Female This either means closing of the Fallopian tubes, or, by a surgical operation called *salpingectomy* or *resection tubarum*, which involves removing part of each tube, whereby the passage of the eggs is cut off. Moreover, many women, perhaps unwittingly, become involuntarily sterile when local disturbances occlude their Fallopian tubes; in this respect gonorrhea is the most common offender.

509. Sterilization of the Male This is obtained by removing part of each *vas deferens* or by blocking (tying) them to prevent the passage of the seminal fluid. From ancient times man has possessed the knowledge that such cutting (*vasectomy*) or tying (*vasoligatur*) could cause a pronounced improvement in the general health of the patient. After such an operation old, senile animals have been seen to become quite youthful, also sexually speaking. One explanation offered is that following the operation, the production of spermotozoa in the testes ceases; these glands, to make up for it, produce more sex hormones. On this basis it was held that by undergoing a similar operation senile males might regain their youthfulness, be "rejuvenated" (Steinach). The results of such *re-erotization* have fallen short of general expectations, as they have proved to be only temporary.

510. Castration of the Female This consists in removal of both ovaries, or destroying them some other way. Such an operation frequently proves necessary if a disease in the ovaries endangers the permanent health of the woman, which would be the case if there were a possibility of cancer. In such cases the ovaries may be destroyed by X-ray or radium treatments, or may be removed by a surgical operation.

511. Castration of the Male In order to castrate a male both testicles must be removed. We shall later see how this radical method is applied in certain parts of the East to procure eunuchs to guard the harems. For the sole purpose of preventing a man from begetting children this operation is, of course, far too radical and should hardly be considered in that connection. If the object is sterility, that can be achieved, as we have seen, by simply cutting the *vas deferens* whereby the important production of sex hormones which is part of the task performed by the testes, is kept intact.

512. *Evaluation of the Five Completely Effective Methods for the Avoidance of Pregnancy* They naturally fall into two widely differing groups, relative to a consideration of principle. Continence or abstinence is in a group by itself, inasmuch, as a method of preventing pregnancy, it is not irrevocable. That a man and a woman are completely abstaining from intercourse does not make them less capable of begetting and conceiving a child should they decide to abandon their self-restraint. Sterilization and castration, on the other hand, are *irrevocable* methods. Once a person has been sterilized he is at the point of no return. He or she will never be able to have offspring; and neither will castrated persons. And that is precisely why the laws in the different states usually establish very severe rules governing the cases in which these operations are permissible.

513. *Uncertain Methods of Preventing Pregnancy* With the exception of the methods mentioned above, all other methods are uncertain. They are based on the following two principles:

a. By taking glandular hormones the object is to curtail the ripening of follicles or to induce a condition in the uterine mucous membranes that makes a normal, full-term pregnancy difficult or impossible.

b. By using various mechanical appliances or devices or chemical compositions the couple seek to prevent fertilizing sperm cells, deposited in, or close to, the vagina, from reaching an egg cell capable of being fertilized. These methods do not aim at permanent, but only at temporary sterility. It is, therefore, important to call attention to the fact that the possibility cannot be entirely excluded that the use of contraceptives may reduce the reproductive capacity for a longer period than may be intended by the couple.

514. Sterilization by Hormone Treatment For a long time it has been a matter of common knowledge that by administering various glandular sex hormones to animals temporary or permanent sterility may be induced. This form of prevention of pregnancy is called *hormone sterilization*. It is, however, rather difficult to evaluate the significance of these experiments, because *pure* hormone extracts were not always used, and the sterilizing effect *may* have been due to accessory poisonous matter in the drug. Whether sterilization by hormone treatment has any future as a preventive method *in human sex life* and, if so, whether it will prove to induce temporary or permanent sterility, are several points on which it is yet too early to make a definite statement.

515. Coitus Ante Portas This expression refers to intercourse in which the seminal fluid is deposited outside the *introitus*, i.e. at the entrance to the vagina. By this procedure the seminal fluid may either be placed on the labia majora or between them. But the method is a very unsafe one, since the sperms move spontaneously and thus are able to work their way further up through the female genital tract.

516. Carezza (Coitus Reservatus) This is a form of intercourse which was used in India. Neither partner seeks to reach an orgasm; the sexual pleasure consists solely in the intimate proximity of their genital organs. As a contraceptive measure this procedure is hardly to be recommended.

First of all, it requires such an inordinate measure of self-control on the part of the man that there is absolutely no guarantee that he can avoid ejaculation. Moreover, as a rule, there will be secretions from the large mucous glands of the urethra which, as it will be remembered, are located deep within the innermost curve of the urethra and whose task it is to act as lubricants.

If the man has just had an ejaculation, sperm cells may remain in the tiny ducts that lead from these glands into the *vas deferens* and when the glands begin to function in response to the stimulation of a later "carezza," the sperms may join the lubricating fluid which means that this fluid may contain sperms capable of fertilizing an ovum. This contingency makes the method still more hazardous.

517. *Coitus Interruptus* This birth control method consists of the man's withdrawal of his penis just before he feels his oncoming ejaculation, so that he empties it directly outside the female genitals. The uncertainty of this method is the same as that of *coitus ante portas*. There is the definite possibility that the sperm cells if they get to the vulva may be able to work their way into the vagina and, as mentioned in connection with *coitus reservatus* (*carezza*), that the clear lubricating drop already contains living spermatozoa so that these may be present in the vagina, be it in ever so small quantities, before the regular ejaculation. Moreover, if the woman attains her orgasm easily, and if the man is considerate and has control of the moment of his ejaculation, then she will suffer no emotional harm from the interrupted intercourse. *But* if she reaches her climax later than the man, and he disregards this fact, she will with this method, as a rule, not obtain any orgasm at all. In effect, this actually means that as the method is employed over a number of years, she risks getting a sexual neurosis.

518. *Douching* We have repeatedly stated that inserting a syringe into the uterus rather than the vagina constitutes a hazard to a woman's life. The contraceptive method is in reality not an effective method at all. When many women nevertheless maintain that they have used it for years with success, it should not be forgotten that 15 per cent of all women cannot conceive at all. Twelve per cent can conceive only one child, 11 per cent only two children, and there is no guarantee that the women who advocate this method may not belong in one of these groups.

Moreover, this method, like *coitus interruptus*, definitely conflicts with the central idea inherent in intercourse. It is certainly not the object of intercourse that the wife, as soon as she has had her orgasm, get out of bed and prepare her douche. That deprives her of the complete satisfaction, which she should and must derive from intercourse.

519. Sperm-blocking Means It is not unusual to employ certain chemicals intended to block or stop the spermatozoa, and which, prior to intercourse, are placed in the vagina on a moistened sponge or in the form of creams or tablets or otherwise. It should be emphasized that there is no real basis for the assumption that if a semen cell, damaged by such substances, should nevertheless fertilize an egg cell, it would cause the child to become in any way defective. Frequently a fully blocking chemical substance called oxycinolin-sulphate is employed, for instance in the form of so-called *oxycin tablets*. The tablets develop a foam which completely or partly fills the innermost part of the vagina. The uncertainty as to applying sperm-blocking substances is, *inter alia*, due to the fact that there is no real guarantee that each and every one of the sex cells comes into contact with substance particles which can block their forward movement or kill them, just as it is not possible to check whether the substance has developed in a spot in vagina where it really closes off the uterine orifice.

520. Vagitoria Contracept By a *vagitorium* (plural: *vagitoria*) is understood a pill suppository intended for introduction into the vagina. The so-called *vagitoria contracept* contain the strongly sperm-blocking material *fenylmerkuriacetat*. The vagitorium is introduced into the vagina immediately prior to intercourse, and six to eight hours later douching is carried out with physiological salt water. This method is considered to be very safe, but the active material, which is also to be had in the state of a solution or cream, has not yet (1950) been sufficiently tried out so that it is not possible to have any definite opinion of the value of its method.

13

MASTURBATION

Chapter 56: MASTURBATION, SELF-GRATIFICATION

521. *What Is Masturbation?* Masturbation means fingering, touching, or rubbing the genital organs for the purpose of provoking voluptuous sensations tending to sexual gratification; in men, as a rule, it is accompanied by ejaculation.

522. *Practice of Masturbation* That *small children* masturbate is not a rare occurrence. It has been estimated that up to one fifth of all children have masturbated before they are six years old. As a matter of fact the practice is so widespread that it is also estimated that almost all men at one period or another in their lives have been given to it. Kinsey states 92 per cent of all American men have masturbated. It is not considered to be so common among women. However, certain other authors claim that about 80 per cent of all women at some period or other have in some way or another touched their genitals—particularly the clitoris—for sensuous effects.

523. *How the Practice of Masturbation Was Formerly Regarded* Our grandparents' generation—often including many members of the medical profession—preferred to avoid mentioning the matter at all. But should some bewildered young person finally succeed in getting some information from his elders concerning the problem, he was generally told that masturbation was a bad disease, or a sin, which would bring about dire and terrible consequences, physically and mentally.

In many countries masturbation was called by the dreadful word of self-pollution, a word which, used for propaganda purpose, has harassed and tormented many boys and young men and several women. The young people came really to believe they had infected themselves or committed a crime for which sooner or later they would be called to account and be punished for. They were told that the lunatic asylums were filled with people who had lost their minds through the practice of masturbation. Some people even believed, quite seriously, that the gray matter of the brain ran down through the spinal cord and was spilled with the seminal fluid at ejaculation, and even today one may encounter people who are absolutely convinced that those who have masturbated will have feeble-minded offspring, or have even lost the capacity of begetting or conceiving any children at all.

524. *Fear of the Consequences of Masturbation* We are happy to say that the dire consequences of masturbation are pure invention and miserable phantasies. Let us look more closely at the question which is generally put to the physician when a patient consults him on that score. Is masturbation harmful? Is it harmful to the brain? Does it influence a person's capacity for having offspring? May masturbation mean that one will beget children not sound in body or mind? How about the loss of matter at masturbation?

525. *About Masturbation Affecting the Brain* In respect to the brain, and in what possible way masturbation may affect it, it is true that the person who masturbates induces in himself a condition of excitement which is often very violent and which eventually—but I say *only* eventually—may have a certain effect on the blood pressure over a long period of years. However, the excitement in that respect is probably no more dangerous in the person who masturbates and is scolded for it, than in the other person who becomes very excited himself by giving the scolding.

526. *The Influence of Masturbation on Begetting and Conceiving* As to the possibility of begetting and conceiving children the spermatozoa in the man and the ovae in the woman who have masturbated have exactly the same value as the reproductive cells of those who have not practiced masturbation. The habit, therefore, does not affect the potency, nor does it affect the possible offspring.

Yet in this connection there is just one particular circumstance which we must mention. The degree of excitation necessary for satisfaction at masturbation is generally considerably more violent and quite different from the excitation of intercourse. Therefore a person who has practiced masturbation to an exaggerated extent, may find it difficult to obtain release during ordinary intercourse. This potentiality is something every young man, and every young woman too, who contemplates marriage should remember. However, this effect is not permanent. It is only a question of a habitual disposition in the *sex organs* and the *excitatory fields* on the whole, and by stopping masturbation completely for some months the person regains his or her capacity for obtaining normal release. It would seem most embarrassing for the person in question, and extremely unpleasant for the marriage partner, if it should materialize that this quarantine would have to be instituted *after* the wedding.

527. *About the Loss of Matter at Masturbation* Concerning the loss of sperms, the following may be established as fact: The boy or man who masturbates loses a certain amount of sperm cells, but not any more than is ejaculated at nocturnal emissions or by intercourse.

The frequency of a man's natural need for intercourse may, as previously mentioned, vary very much. Nocturnal emissions, or "wet dreams," may also occur with varying frequency. They may occur on several nights in succession or at intervals of weeks, months, and even years. Thus every man has a natural need for ejaculation with a certain frequency, and if masturbation is not performed very often, it cannot be said to involve any real *loss* of sperms.

528. *Masturbation and Sex Hormones* But—for there is a very big and important BUT—among those who practice masturbation there are hardly any who do it only once a week and not more often, at any rate not among men. There is that strange thing about masturbation that the tendency, the more it is being indulged in, becomes more and more insistent, and the person who starts masturbating once a *month* will soon do it twice or more times a *week*, or every *day*, sometimes several times a day. And that will deprive the organism of bigger quantities of sperm cells than intended by Nature. A terrible feeling of exhaustion follows upon the act if too frequently repeated. And, as we know that if ejaculation of seminal fluid is hindered by tying or cutting the vas deferens, the testes manufacture an exceptional amount of sex hormones, so one might similarly imagine that the testes, when they have to be busy constantly producing sperm cells to make up for the loss caused by repeated ejaculation, do not have a chance to produce the necessary quantity of sex hormones required to make a man a really *masculine* man, as their task is. However, there is no scientific proof as to whether this is correct or not.

529. *The Solitary Person*   Moreover, there is this decisive point on which masturbation differs from normal sexual intercourse. At the normal sex union there is a principle: there must be two, a couple. And it is a fact that intercourse, more than anything else, satisfies that deep urge in man of feeling a common bond, a sense of community, which to the very great majority of persons (since the human being has been called a social animal) is a necessary condition for peace and happiness. There lies a deeper truth in the words, "It is not good for man to be alone," than meets the eye.

In complete contrast to this, masturbation generally is a solitary act. Just as normal sexual intercourse is rich in strengthening the ordinary feeling of a common bond with humanity, the most characteristic emotional result of masturbation is a very pronounced sense of loneliness, which increases as the act grows more frequent.

530. *Masturbation in Adolescence*   This feeling of loneliness is particularly sharp in the very young person who is plunged in the sensitive period of adolescence. It is true that

the deep feeling of isolation may last only for a very brief period —maybe only a couple of hours; then he is restituted after having masturbated, and once again feels like himself, but to an older adolescent even a couple of hours may seem like an eternity. He has entered the realm of loneliness and to him it seems like a loneliness effectively lasting an eternity.

The bright light and laughter of the summer day does not reach him or penetrate his isolation in all eternity; the pure air and high clear sky on an autumn day, the cold of winter, and the finest pale green beech leaves newly unfolded in May do not exist for him. He is dead; dead and removed from everything for all eternity. From that feeling springs the *depth* of his despair, that bottomless, deep despair the very young may keenly experience.

531. *It Is the Character That Is Threatened by Masturbation* And yet it is not the feeling of being isolated which finally drives so many people to seek a physician with the express resolve that now they *must* rid themselves of their bad habit. No, the explanation is rather like this: That feeling of fatigue and dullness which is the result of frequently repeated self-gratification sooner or later makes the masturbator resolve that next time the urge crops up he or she will not succumb to it. But when the desire next time comes, they do it just the same. *That* is the crucial point. In that case they do something which they did not intend to do, and the bad habit is, in their estimation, becoming a *vice*. The consequences of a vice do not long remain absent. Not the direct consequences of masturbation, but the consequences of being the victim of a dominating habit. He feels like a slave. He begins to have contempt for himself, and this contempt in return may affect his other psychical and emotional life. Perhaps he grows despondent, ashamed, a victim of inferiority complexes. He may feel loathing for himself, become vacillating and insecure, lose his mental and emotional health—*not*, mark it well, because he masturbates, but because he has discovered that he has no will power, no character, that he is not in harmony with his own self. And this is of catastrophic importance, particularly for a young person who is at that period of life where generally it is determined whether he will grow into

an integrated personality or the contrary, whether he will lead his own life, or he will be at the beck and call of his urges.

It should be especially noted that masturbation cannot be considered according to the ordinary conception of a good or a bad action, a moral or an immoral one. Here, a part of the body is used at cross-purposes to that for which Nature—one might say, *biologically*—intended it. To draw what may be a strained analogy: A smoker may be up against the same problem. The smoker may become such a victim to his need that smoking eventually develops into a dominating habit. To a young person, smoking may become the touchstone of his strength of character, of the logic and integration of his personality. Viewed objectively, one thing cannot be said to be "worse" than the other. *But*, what is essential in this connection is that he who permits himself to be mastered by an inclination which he *does not want* to let himself be mastered by, is a house divided against itself. And he who is divided in that way, *sins*, at any rate from the point of view of character.

532. *Treatment of Masturbation* The remedy for masturbation is, therefore, first and foremost psychological and mental therapy. To every person who really feels himself possessed by an urge to masturbate so intense, that he feels it as a habitual, weakening burden, a vice, there is a very clear way out.

Do not fight a desperate battle; such a battle cannot be carried through without constantly having one's gaze fixed on the adversary, and that is no good in this case. One must realize that one is in the midst of a battle to find one's own self, to become an integrated personality, acquire self-possession. It should be realized that masturbation is only *one* of several obstacles to this goal, and not the one that one must conquer first, even if it is the obstacle which at the moment is considered the most embarrassing. Masturbation is only a symptom of what is wrong at bottom: lack of character, or the real risk of losing one's character. Therefore the only means of treating masturbation lies in adequate training in general character building.

14

SEXUAL ABNORMALITIES

Chapter 57: HORMONE-CONDITIONED ABNORMALITIES

533. *Influence of Hormones* As our knowledge of hormones was gradually extended it was only natural that attempts were made to explain deviations from normal sex life (and that included sexual abnormalities that have always been known to exist) as due to irregularities in the hormone production of the pituitary gland and of sex hormones. In some cases it proved possible to find a hormonal explanation; in others not.

534. *Adiposogenital Dystrophy* It is self-evident that disturbances in the hormone production of the pituitary gland, particularly if it occurs just about the age of puberty, must influence the organism powerfully.

The disease *adiposogenital dystrophy* is a result of failure by the pituitary gland to produce its gonadotropic hormones. If this happens before the age of puberty, there will be no puberty. The sex organs will fail to develop. No sex cells are secreted and no sex hormones produced. Growth of pubic hair will fail to appear on and around the external sex organs, a girl's breasts will not develop, a boy's voice will not change, and neither boy nor girl will feel erotically attracted to the opposite sex.

On the other hand, a special kind of obesity always appears, particularly about the breast, abdomen, mons veneris, buttocks, and that part of the arms and legs which is closest to the body, i.e. at the shoulders and thighs. If such persons get the proper doses of gonadotropic hormones in time, that will "start" the testes and the ovaries (the gonads) which, once started will continue to function and these persons will have a chance to develop normally.

535. *Early and Precocious Sexual Maturity* If puberty occurs as early as at the age of eight or nine, it is called an *early puberty*. If it occurs even earlier, the condition is called a *precocious puberty* (*pubertas praecox* or *macrogenitosomia praecox*).

One may, for example, see boys no more than six years old with a large penis and marked pubic growth around the sex organs. And girls of about the same age may become pregnant. The illness which occurs about three times as often in girls as in boys, is extremely rare; up to 1938, only 565 cases had been described in the entire medical literature of the world.

The cause of the disease was thought to originate from the pituitary gland's premature production of gonadotropic hormones. However, this opinion has not been able to withstand criticism. The direct cause of the disease is held to be due to disorders in the sex center of the central nervous system which in turn may be due to various influences such as hormone-producing sex glands, tumors, inflammations, lesions, congenital deformities, and a diseased condition in or near the interbrain, or some peculiarity in the chromosome contents of the body cells, etc. Moreover, certain forms of tumors in the cortex of the suprarenal glands may produce a so-called pseudo precocity, whereby, as a rule, only the external sex organs develop too early, whereas the internal genitals remain undeveloped and fail to function.

536. *Castration of Men and Boys* History offers many sad examples of what happens if the sex glands proper do not function. In the Orient emasculated men were formerly much in demand as guardians of the harems. What was usually done was this: before puberty boys had both testes removed. In other words, they were castrated. When the gonadotropic hormones of the pituitary gland began to circulate with the blood stream at puberty there were no gonads and no testes for them to activate. So there could be no question either of producing sperms or sex hormones, and almost all the characteristics otherwise indicating the boy's change into man remained absent. A castrated person is called a eunuch or castrate. Since a castrate's pituitary gland is not needed for producing certain quantities of gonadotropic hormones it sometimes, in compensation, secretes a larger quantity of other hormones, one of which activates unusual growth of the arms and legs. In other cases it may be a hormone that causes a peculiar distribution of fatty tissue, half male, half female. A eunuch, therefore, often has ample deposits of fat on his body, insignificant external sex organs without pubic hair, a shrill, thin voice like a child's and frequently is devoid of emotions in regard to the opposite sex; in other words, he feels no sex urge.

In modern times the problem of castration has unfortunately gained renewed actuality. For during the wars of the first half of the twentieth century, it not infrequently happened that the men's testes were destroyed by bullets, shell splinters, or land mines. It is, therefore, a most welcome progress in medicine that some cases of eunuchism now yield to treatment with androgenic substances.

537. *Influence of Castration on Sex Needs* The question as to whether the removal of the sex glands also meant the disappearance of the sex urge has always aroused special interest. The nature of the matter makes it inherently impossible to carry out any systematic experimental research on it. Steinach, the Austrian professor who deserves great praise for his studies of the biology of sex life, found that fully grown white castrated male mice remained accessible to sexual influences and were ready for mating, but gradually became impotent at intercourse. It was also found that animals castrated before puberty showed considerable sexual sensitivity. They made attempts at initiating intercourse, sniffed at, and licked the female mice. At intercourse, erection was generally very imperfect and there was no ejaculation of sperm. This sensitive condition lasted for a year, whereupon sexual desire began to diminish and signs of premature senility made their appearance. Similarly, it is not un-

usual to observe steers and geldings simulate attempts at mating with cows and mares in heat. Geldings are often capable of mounting a mare, and are even especially fiery, but, of course, without being able to procreate.

In the human species, too, castrates have proved in most cases to retain their sexual emotions for a certain length of time. Pelikan writes about Russians, that individuals castrated in puberty are capable of having intercourse for a long time after the operation, and that even in maturity their potency and sex desire hardly abate.

A French physician at Peiping at one time reported that Chinese eunuchs have sex feelings. He stated these men seek the society of women and satisfy their sex urge as best they may, having no external genitals. From the Negro eunuchs at Istanbul, from Egypt and other parts of the Orient similar reports have come pointing to the fact that in the male sexual desire, or sex need, is to some extent independent of the presence or absence of testes.

538. *Artificial Menopause* Conditions may be observed in castrated women corresponding to those found in the behavior of the male castrate. If a malignant disease occurs, such as cancer of the ovaries, the growth must either be removed by surgery or eradicated by X-ray or radium treatment. In both cases the ovaries can no longer function which is tantamount to female castration.

The consequences rather closely resemble those accompanying menopause and the term used to describe the operation is, in fact, *artificial menopause*. Ovulation and menstrual flow cease, a great many special symptoms characteristic of the menopause appear and are treated in the same way as they would have been if the menopause had been natural. Both sex need and enjoyment of sexual intercourse may remain unchanged after the artificial menopause as may also be the case after the natural menopause, or else these conditions may undergo certain changes. In some women sexual desire, as well as sexual pleasure, diminish. This, however, may in part be due to autosuggestion, the women imagining that they are now different from other "normal" women. In others, on the contrary, sexual desire becomes very insistent, and this is sometimes taken to be due to the certainty of no longer risking pregnancy. However, we quite realize that a great many other conditions must also be considered in this connection. But even before treatment by hormones was introduced the great majority of scientists, through close study of the artificial menopause and its consequences, had reached the same conclusion: namely, that in somewhat more than 50 per cent of the women examined the artificial menopause had in no way curtailed their sex urge nor their capacity for sexual enjoyment. After the introduction of hormone treatment it is usually considered that removing or destroying the ovaries need not have any influence on a woman's sex life, except in so far as she will no longer be able to conceive.

539. *True and False Hermaphroditism* The presence of both male and female sexual characteristics in the same individual is termed hermaphroditism. This is a condition that has been known from ancient times. In *true hermaphroditism* female and male sex gland tissue appears in the same individual, but this is extremely rare in human beings, and the presence of sperm cells capable of fertilizing, and ripe egg cells capable of being fertilized, has never been observed at the same time in one individual. In contrast, the condition, that is called *false hermaphroditism* occurs much more frequently among men and women. Among them the question is of persons with a definite disproportion between their exterior genitals and their sex glands proper. Frequently the external sex organs already at birth rather resemble female genitals, although often with an unusually large clitoris, in which case the child is generally considered to be a girl. At puberty, however, it becomes evident that not the ovaries but the testes have developed, bringing about male hormonal sex characteristics. The individual is then called a *false male hermaphrodite*. In some cases a successful surgical operation creates the possibility of transforming such a person—who, after all, feels like a man—into one capable of also performing a man's sex functions. In other cases the operation did not succeed and this makes for a very unfortunate condition indeed. *False female hermaphroditism* characterized by external masculine sex organs and feminine sex glands is extremely rare.

In the entire scientific literature on the subject only two cases have been described.

The term hermaphroditism which is still used in everyday language has been discarded by science as a result of the research findings on heredity in relation to the mechanism of sex determination. The new concept of *intersexualism* has been introduced.

540. *Intersexualism and Gynandromorphism* According to the modern conception, there is a type of transition from the normal masculine to the normal feminine organism, and the normal forms are the result of a certain balance between the sex-determining genes. There may be, however, cases of individuals who are properly termed feminine intersexual. In such persons the original genetic sex destination begins to develop predominantly female, at a certain moment in the embryonic state—the so-called *turning point*, but due to some influence, perhaps hormonal, changes into a male direction. Scientists are of the opinion that masculine intersexuality does not exist.

While in the intersexual, *all* of the sex cells in accordance with their genetic tendency, are of the *same* sex and all change together to the opposite sex, a person of doubtful sex (a *gynandromorph*) may develop, for example, if two sperm cells, one of them X-chromosome-bearing, and the other y-chromosome-bearing, both fertilize an egg cell with pronuclei that contain *both* masculine and feminine sex cells with the result that part of the individual develops into a male, and part into a female direction. Gynandromorphs are extremely rare among human beings; up to the present only a single case has been described that might point to gynandromorphism.

Some scientists have also held the opinion that certain forms of intersexualism might originate in this way: During pregnancy a feminizing substance from the mother organism might change a fetus, genetically male, into a female direction. This explanation, however, is only a theory, as yet unproven.

541. *Gynecomastia and Hirsutism* *Gynecomastia* is a rare condition. It refers to the enlargement of male breasts and their development as female breasts. This is probably due to hormonal disturbances. *Hirsutism,* a condition in which most of the body is covered by hair, depends to a certain extent on hormone conditions. It is frequently seen in men in which case it must be considered physiological, even if it is present to an excessive extent. In women it is observed in connection with certain diseases.

Chapter 58: ABNORMAL SEX LIFE

542. *Homosexuality and Analogous Conditions* A person who is homosexual is sexually attracted only to persons of his own sex and seeks a sort of sexual intercourse with them, for instance in the form of pederasty. Kinsey has determined that at least 37 per cent of all adult men—more than every third man one meets in the street—have had homosexual experiences. No exact figures—either for men or women—are known from any other country. There are probably at least as many homosexual women as men. However, what frequently occurs is that an individual *fears* he or she is a homosexual and so gradually comes to *believe* it, and for that reason does not dare seriously to contemplate becoming engaged or married. This condition which can be relieved or remedied by psychotherapy might properly be termed *imaginary homosexualism.*

The causes of homosexuality are the subject of much discussion. However, there is rather general agreement on the question of a special disposition beyond the control of the individual and consequently that it is not due to any form of sexual debauchery or moral laxity as the vast majority of people formerly believed.

The origin of homosexuality may be a glandular influence from within or a psychological influence from without. Quite valid reasons may be cited in favor of both conceptions. As is known, the sexual differentiation occurs at a rather late stage in the development of the fetus, and hormonal disturbances might easily arise at this stage. In many cases—but by far not in all—conspicuous signs of the appearance and behavior of the opposite sex are also found in homosexual persons—particularly feminine men and particularly masculine women.

On the other hand, many cases of homosexuality are apparently based on sexual experiences in previous life, perhaps as far back as the earliest childhood. Otherwise the borderlines of homosexuality are particularly vague and may change all through an individual's life, even with periods of heterosexual tendencies, i.e. with the sexual urge directed against the opposite sex.

Among homosexual persons there seems to be a quite obvious division of "sexes"—of individuals with a "male" ("positive" tendency) and individuals with a "female" ("negative" tendency). Connections occur which have the character of "marriages" where only both partners, according to the general conception, in actual fact are of the same sex. Connections between two women are called *tribadism* or Lesbian love, after the island of Lesbos, where in antiquity a circle of young homosexual women lived under the direction of the poetess Sappho. Such women are called *tribades*.

As a matter of fact, homosexuality was generally accepted in ancient Greece and in many other countries too, which should serve to remind us that all moral codes are based on generally accepted custom. Such accepted customs may last for longer or shorter periods whereupon other customs take their place. Then a new moral code comes up and that, in turn, is considered the one and only proper code as long as it prevails. And in regard to homosexualism the accepted moral code seems to differ considerably in its application to the two sexes.

A special form of homosexuality is the so-called bisexuality. The bisexual persons feels erotically attracted to both sexes, sometimes at the same time.

A person who, for erotic reasons, dresses in the manner of the opposite sex is called a *transvestite;* such persons are, as a rule, homosexual.

Men with typically feminine looks or women with typically masculine looks are called *metatropes;* it appears from the foregoing that this need not be a sign of homosexuality.

543. *Pederasty* Pederasty, or pedicatio, really means sexual intercourse with children. Its present meaning, lawfully, has gradually changed in the United States to denote: a. sexual intercourse between members of the same sex; b. sexual contact with animals; c. so-called "unnatural" sex between a man

and woman. Pederasty is not considered synonymous with sodomy though at times confused with it.

544. *Autoeroticism* The term autoeroticism or self-eroticism comprises the following three forms of eroticism:

a. *Automonosexuality or Narcissism.* Like Narcissus in the Greek mythology who fell in love with his own picture which he saw mirrored in a pool of water, and longed for it, so the sex urge of the automonosexual person is directed toward himself or herself. He or she may dress up and perhaps admire his or her own person in a mirror, eventually masturbating while looking at it.

b. *Erotic daydreams.* A constant flow of sexually exciting phantasies in which the person imagines himself or herself to be an active partner in intimate erotic situations constitutes erotic daydreaming. Such dreaming may end with an orgasm with or without masturbation. In the latter case it is called *psychical coitus.*

c. *Masturbation.*

545. *Erotomania* This term denotes an abnormal heightening of the sex urge. In women it is called *nymphomania, metromania,* or *huror uterinus.* In men it is called *satyriasis* or *salacitas.*

546. *Nymphomania (Abnormally Strong Sex Urge in Women)* This disorder requires the greatest watchfulness from a social point of view, because many women thus afflicted walk the streets promiscuously selecting one man after another for the purpose of having intercourse with them. These women are potentially very dangerous as carriers of venereal disease. They are often mentally deranged. Only in very rare cases does nymphomania prove to be due to hormone conditions, and most cases, therefore, do not respond to hormonal therapy.

547. *Satyriasis (Abnormally Strong Sex Urge in Men)* Men with abnormally developed sexual desires also frequently present a great social danger; still, not as potential carriers of contagious disease in the same degree as women, since the male capacity for intercourse is quantitatively more limited than that of the female.

They are, however, dangerous as sex fiends, offenders against sexual morality, as it is called, for instance, by committing rape. Only the very infrequent cases that are due to hormone disturbance respond to therapy.

548. *Algolagnosis (Sensuous Pleasure through Pain)* Sexual pleasure, algolagnosis, obtained through pain, includes *sadism* and *masochism*.

Sadism is named after the French Marquis de Sade, who described this form of abnormal sex life in several books. The sadist may bring on his orgasm by humiliating, torturing, beating, kicking, tearing, and in other ways physically maltreating his victim. A special form of sadism is killing for lust, sadistic murder. In that case the sadist does not confine himself to maltreating his victim; he kills it. Such killers are, of course, extremely dangerous and must be taken into custody by the public authorities. They are rarely wicked, but mentally abnormal and there is not much chance of their being improved by punishment.

History abounds in examples of sadists. Several of the old Roman emperors were sadists as also many Nazis in Hitler's time.

Masochism, term derived from the name of Sacher-Masoch who has described this disease. In extreme forms of masochism the masochist only feels sexual pleasure if he is maltreated in some way, as by being beaten or whipped, etc.

549. *Fetichism* This is an abnormal condition in which a person experiences sexual gratification by looking at or touching an object which belongs to a person of the opposite sex, for instance, a shoe or an article of dress. *Pygmalionism,* a special form of fetichism, is a term denoting that a person obtains sexual release by looking at statues and pictures. The name is taken from the Greek sculptor Pygmalion who fell in love with the statue he himself had sculptured.

Also the *cisvestite* who obtains sexual gratification by wearing children's clothes, dressing up in clothing from former days, or similar things, may be said to be among those who practice Pygmalionism.

550. Exhibitionism   The person who suffers from exhibitionism feels an abnormal urge to show his naked body. In men the compulsion centers particularly on the genitals which they want to show; in women it is mostly the breasts.

Old men are often exhibitionists and so commit what is called *senile immorality*. Their act generally consists in taking a stand in a gateway or in a passage showing their sex organs to casual passers-by, or they may suddenly uncover themselves in front of young girls and women.

Apart from the shock such persons give their "victim" they are comparatively harmless, but as a rule they are taken into custody on an accusation of moral turpitude.

551. *Scoptophilism*   This term, the exact opposite of exhibitionism, refers to an abnormal urge to see the naked bodies of *other* persons, in particular their genital organs. A scoptophile may become sexually excited by looking at nude children (in which case the abnormality is called *paedophilism*) or by witnessing erotic situations, such as seeing intercourse between human beings (*voyeurism*) or between animals (*erotical zoophilism*).

552. *Sodomy, Bestiality*   *Sodomy, bestiality* refers to a man's or a woman's sexual intercourse with animals, as a rule, dogs, pigs, cows, or mares. Such sexual contacts can never result in progeny. According to Kinsey, not less than 17 per cent of young men in the country are said to have taken part in this at one time in their lives. Sodomy is not considered synonymous with pederasty though at times confused with it.

553. *Necrophilism*   *Necrophilism* or *Vampyrism* denotes sexual intercourse with dead bodies.

554. *Urolagnosis and Coprolagnosis*   The literal translation of *urolagnosis* is "urine voluptuousness." One of the partners lets his or her urine on the body, into the mouth or into the vagina of the other in whom it produces voluptuous sensations. The same term refers to *coprolagnosis*, feeling of lust at emptying of bowels, feces and intestinal air.

555. *Cleptolagnosis and Pyrolagnosis* These terms are mentioned here—like the preceding ones in the main to round out the enumeration of sexual abnormalities. They indicate sexual sensations abnormally brought about by filching, thieving (*cleptolagnosis*) or on seeing fire (*pyrolagnosis*).

556. *Where Is the Borderline between Normal and Abnormal Sex Life?* In reality it is actually impossible to draw a sharp or completely accurate dividing line between normal and abnormal sex life. In every human being there is a trace of incipient hermaphroditism or intersexualism, inasmuch as every single cell in the organism is created by a merging of a male and a female sex cell. Moreover, at an early stage in the fetus there were incipient female and male sex organs and sex glands. Such vestiges remain in the body of the opposite sex all through life, as mentioned in an earlier section of this book. In the normal pendulum motion—oscillation between periodical comparative lack of interest to the highest sexual tension and urge for release—there are traces of *dyspareunia* (lack of sex interest) on the one hand, and nymphomania and satyriasis on the other hand.

In respect to normal sex life, what really significant conclusions may be drawn from Kinsey's documentary evidence that sexual behavior differs widely in the various social groups, and from his information that every third man has homosexual experiences? There is probably something of a sadist in every normal male and something of a masochist in every normal woman. He wants to show that he is the master, the strong cave man, and she loves being the vanquished, the weak woman. Where is the "normal" borderline? And what about fetishism? What about pressed flowers and old love letters from him or her, and what young man in love has not caressed his loved one's shoes or a dress of hers that she had left in his closet? And to the beloved every person is certainly an exhibitionist and a scoptophile.

It is, therefore, very difficult to draw a line dividing normal sex life from abnormal sex life. In no other human field is the lofty and the base; the fine and the ugly so terribly close, as in sex.

The all-important thing is that the *two partners* should be in harmony, suited to each other. This they can only determine through exchanging of confidences and if they are really trusting and honest with one another. That is the vital core of the whole relationship. Trust, moreover, is a necessary condition for mutual adaptation. Therefore, the wife, from a sense of *false* modesty, must not refrain from letting her husband know all her longings and desires, for we now know that as a woman she possesses a sweeping sex urge capable of spanning the whole gamut of feeling and sensations. The same is true of the husband. What the two, husband and wife, mutually regard as normal is normal for them.

15

DISEASES OF SEX LIFE

Chapter 59: VENEREAL DISEASES

557. *What Is Understood by Venereal Diseases?* Venereal diseases are those illnesses that most frequently, partly or entirely, are connected with the sexual organs and which are subject to various types of legal control.

These diseases are principally transmitted through sexual intercourse, but they may also be transmitted in other ways. Conversely, every disease transmitted by intercourse may not be a venereal disease in the sense the law ascribes to this term.

558. *How Are Venereal Diseases Transmitted?* Contagious diseases in which category the venereal diseases belong, have this one thing in common: they are due to germs or other contagious substances. Germs cannot penetrate into completely healthy skin or mucous membrane. Only where tiny tears and scratches are present is it possible for germs to gain access. Inasmuch as such microscopic tears and scratches will almost always be present to some degree in the sexual organs there is a definite chance for germs to penetrate there.

It is, therefore, characteristic of venereal diseases that they are mainly transmitted during intercourse. However, they *may* also be passed on from one person to another in some other way, for instance by kissing or by touch.

559. Contagion Through Objects A question that occupies the minds of many persons is whether they may become infected with a venereal disease through various commonly used objects.

As we shall see in the following, there is a possibility that a disease like syphilis (if at the stage where it is accompanied by festering sores in the mouth or by contagious spit) may be transmitted through the patient's pipes, cigar butts, drinking glasses, etc. However, note that contagion can only be transmitted if the pipe, the glass, or whatever the object may be passes directly from the lips of the diseased person to the lips of the healthy person. It will also be described further on, how gonorrhea germs may be transmitted by the hands from the sex organs to the eyes. In any case, touching another person's genital organs always may involve the risk of venereal infection. Cases of venereal diseases being transmitted by contagion through objects are, however, comparatively rare, largely due to the extreme sensitivity of venereal germs. For example, in order to survive they require a suitably warm temperature and a suitable degree of humidity. The germs simply perish if they are exposed to too much dryness, and the same thing happens if they are exposed to a sufficient degree of cold. A humid, but cold towel in a public lavatory will therefore hardly present any great danger as a carrier of disease unless it has just been used by a person suffering from an infectious venereal disease. The same is true of a completely dry towel. A drop on the toilet seat, if it is cold, will rarely contain contagious bacteria. However, since there is always the risk that the drop may have come there so shortly beforehand that the germs have not yet perished, but may possibly have gained in vitality as they again found a conveniently favorable and suitably humid place, such a drop must of course be wiped off or covered up.

Such measures can be taken by everyone, and should be taken. Reports from various countries often mention cases of syphilis transmitted by way of washing utensils, sponges, etc., just as gonorrhea is passed on from one woman to another through using the same douche.

In order to prevent contagion by objects the following rules should be observed:

Whoever suffers from a venereal disease must not share a

bed with another person, nor use another person's items of personal hygiene, as his sponge, douche, wash rag, or towel. After every contact with the sex organs hands must be washed carefully with soap and water. Touching of toilet seats with the genital organs must be avoided. If the disease is syphilis, such caution should apply with respect to other parts of the body too, with contagious eruptions or sores. Moreover, the sharing of handkerchiefs, toothbrush, bedclothes, etc., should be absolutely avoided with others, and eating utensils must be thoroughly cleansed after use.

560. *Prevention of Venereal Disease* Although good remedies exist in the treatment of the various venereal diseases it goes without saying that, as in every illness, prevention is better than cure. This is particularly true of gonorrhea and syphilis, the two prevailing venereal diseases.

For the woman there is nothing to do. That is a fact she must know and realize. She can do nothing at all effective to protect herself against the disease; the precautions to be taken are entirely up to the man she is with. Diaphragms *do not* protect a woman against contagion. Many women do not even know that they have acquired a venereal disease, but find it out incidentally. This may be most unfortunate, for as a result of a woman's ignorance treatment is delayed, other persons may become infected, and resultant diseases may have time to develop.

As far as the man is concerned we must stress that we do not know of any completely effective method for the prevention of infection. However, the risk may be inconsiderably curtailed if the man will use a condom. If it should break he should take the following precautions: immediately after intercourse the genital organs should be carefully cleansed with soap and water; a swab of absorbent cotton should then be dipped in a two per cent solution of nitrate of silver, and following urination this swab is introduced less than half an inch into the urethra. It must stay in for half a minute. The entire penis, but particularly the glans, the furrow behind it, and the foreskin must be rubbed for a few minutes with a calomel ointment. The salve must be left on and not be touched for at least four hours.

It should be pointed out to the public, and in as urgent a

manner as possible, that a person infected with a venereal disease is a great risk to others, even before visible symptoms of the disease appear. The disease is frequently transmitted by persons who themselves are recent victims and believe they are all right because the disease has not yet manifested itself by any symptoms. Sexual relations, particularly promiscuous relations, always represent a risk; so the danger may be there every time a person has had sexual intercourse with a casual acquaintance, notwithstanding the prophylactic measures that may have been taken. At this juncture it is very important to remember what we have stated previously, that a very high percentage of the patients seeking treatment for venereal diseases disclose that they were under the influence of liquor when they caught the infection.

561. *New Methods of Treatment of Venereal Diseases* As is widely known, recent medical discoveries have made it almost miraculously possible for human beings to master a number of diseases that formerly were almost, if not entirely, impossible to cure. Some of these remedies have proved extraordinarily effective in the treatment of various venereal diseases, and we shall, therefore, give a description of them here.

The so-called *chemotherapy* was introduced as far back as 1909 by Ehrlich in the preparation called *salvarsan*, a preparation that contained arsenic, formerly the most effective medication in the case of syphilis. But chemotherapy was not applied on a wide scale until in 1935 when the first preparations of sulfa drugs were experimentally produced, which proved extremely effective for use as remedies for certain diseases due to germ infection. In 1938 a sulfa drug was manufactured that gave fine results in pneumonia and at the present the number of different sulfa drugs on the market exceeds 2,000. Of these sulfa drugs *sulfanilamid, sulfapyridin,* and *sulfathiazol* have proved to have a curative effect, for instance, in case of gonorrhea.

However, as early as in 1928 the English scientist Fleming discovered a substance produced by the mold fungus *penicillium notatum*, which proved to be a specific germicide. Widely known now as penicillin the product was not thoroughly tested until 1938 though (Florey and others), but since the preparation in

1940 and 1941 proved to be extremely efficacious in various grave diseases medical periodicals continuously print new reports on it. Penicillin is now used as a link in the general treatment of syphilis, as well as a prophylactic in congenital syphilis. In treating gonorrhea penicillin has proved to be far superior to the hitherto so popular sulfa drugs. Future sections of this book include more detailed discussions of each of these diseases. Scientists all over the world continue their search for new remedies. Thus, in 1943, *streptomycin* was extracted from a germ in the soil. Still more recently developed remedies are drugs such as *chloromycetin, aureomycin,* and *neomycin,* the last as yet untested in humans. And it is permissible to anticipate future remedies being found that will be still more effective in the battle against venereal diseases.

Chapter 60: GONORRHEA

562. *What Causes Gonorrhea?* Gonorrhea is an inflammation caused by a small germ, called a gonococcus, which is shaped like a coffee bean. One single pus drop of gonorrheal discharge contains millions of gonococci. The time that elapses from the moment a person is infected until the disease manifests itself, the so-called *incubation period,* is generally from two to six days, but it *may* be several weeks longer.

563. *How Can Gonorrhea Be Traced?* It is often possible to discover the germs, the *gonococci,* in pus or scrapings from the infected spots. Such a test is the basic method for proving whether or not a person has gonorrhea. The germs may be cultivated on particularly suitable extracts of nutrients and stained by special methods whereupon it is possible to observe them in a microscope. In other cases the presence of the infection may be proven and demonstrated by the so-called *gono-reaction* (*gonococci complement-fixing-reaction*). This is made possible because the presence of the disease brings about certain changes in the blood serum of the patient, which may be established by a rather complicated process.

To perform such a test, the doctor takes a specimen of the

patient's blood. It takes two or three weeks after the infection has been transmitted for the reaction to become positive, and if it is only slight, the positive reaction may not show up. The changes in the blood serum probably keep on for rather a long time; at any rate for months after the infection has cleared up. So it is sometimes possible to find a positive gono-reaction in a patient otherwise well, which then only shows that he *has* suffered from gonorrhea.

564. *Dissemination of Gonorrhea* Of all venereal diseases gonorrhea was for a great many years undoubtedly the infection that brought about the greatest social consequences, as it was, also, by far the most widespread venereal disease. When the sulfa drugs were introduced shortly before the Second World War, there was a great reduction in the incidence, but it flared up again during the war.

565. *Genital Gonorrhea in the Male* Genital gonorrhea refers to gonorrhea located in the sex organs. In men the following forms of genital gonorrhea may occur: a. inflammation of the urethra (*urethritis gonorrhoica*); b. in the ducts about the urethral orifice, the para-urethral ducts; c. in the urethral mucous gland ducts (peri-urethral infiltrations); d. in the lymphatic glands and lymphatic vessels (lymphangitis and lymphadenitis); e. in the prostate gland (prostatitis); f. in the bladder glands (spermatocystitis); and g. in the epididymis (epididymitis).

We shall now examine these forms of genital gonorrhea separately.

566. *Urethral Gonorrhea (Urethritis Gonorrhoica) in the Male* This is the most common form of gonorrhea in the male. Incipient symptoms are a sort of itching at the tip of the urethra, increased mucous secretion, and smarting and cutting sensations at urination. For the first two days the mucous discharge is almost clear, but later on (two to five days after contagion) it is filled with gonorrheal pus and the discharge is more ample, and yellowish in color. Sometimes a whole week or more may elapse after the actual contagion took place, before the first symptoms are felt.

567. Urethritis Anterior If the inflammation is confined to the foremost part of the urethra it is called *urethritis anterior*. In many cases the disease does not spread further. However, after some weeks it may change into a phase likely to be more permanent, with a thicker, yet smaller, mucous discharge.

568. Urethritis Posterior If the infectious germs penetrate deep into the posterior part of the urethra, the disease is called *urethritis posterior*. Symptoms accompanying this form of gonorrhea will often be an urge to very frequent urination, and sometimes the last drops of urine may be mingled with a little blood. In order to find out whether a gonorrhea has spread to the posterior end of the urethra the doctor usually makes a so-called *two-glass test*. The patient urinates into two glasses and by comparing the appearance of the two specimens the physician will generally be able to determine whether the infection has spread to the posterior part of the urethra. It is very important to establish this distinction, for a *urethritis posterior* represents a complication as compared to the simple, so-called uncomplicated gonorrhea in the anterior part of the urethra. Such a complication may indicate that the disease is on the point of penetrating into, and perhaps lodge itself, in other organs.

569. Gonorrhea of the Para-urethral Ducts Around the urethral orifice (meatus) particularly near the foreskin band there may be some tiny ducts ending blindly (without any issue). These ducts are called the *para-urethral* ducts. They may become infected by gonococci and may show up as tiny, fiery red points. When pressed, a little drop of pus may be forced out. Before a gonorrhea patient can be declared completely well, it is of the utmost importance to make sure that no such tiny foci—potential sites for a generalized disease—remain hidden in the para-urethral ducts which would permit the infection to flare up again.

570. Gonorrhea of the Urethral Mucous Gland Ducts (Peri-urethral Infiltrations) The mucous membrane of the urethra is not entirely smooth. It contains some tiny saclike protrusions and also a lot of small mucous glands. Inflammation in these or in the big mucous glands of the urethra may give rise to the so-called *peri-urethral infiltrations* on a gonorrheal basis. These infiltrations are rather hard spots as big as a pea or even bigger, and they may develop into regular abcesses filled with gonorrheal pus.

571. Gonorrhea of the Lymphatic Vessels and the Lymphatic Glands (*Lymphadenitis Gonorrhoica*) In relatively rare cases the lymphatic vessels, those tiny vessels that carry the tissue fluid to the lymphatic glands, become the seat of a gonorrheal inflammation that may spread to the lymphatic glands. As a result, various parts of the penis and of the lymphatic vessels located in the groin may become very sensitive and cause pain.

572. Gonorrhea in the Prostate Gland (*Prostatitis Gonorrhoica*) This complication of gonorrhea in men requires constant and undeviating attention, as it occurs very frequently. As determined from experience, it is very difficult to effect a complete cure. Very often a *prostatitis gonorrhoica* develops in the wake of a urethritis posterior and in its *acute stages* it shows the same symptoms. This complaint is accompanied by pains at evacuation of feces, by painful erections and pollutions, and by a peculiar sensation of tension and heaviness in the direction of the anus. In those cases the prostate gland is generally swollen and sensitive to the touch, as the doctor can find out by feeling it with his finger through the anus.

A gonorrheal prostatitis has a definite tendency to become *chronic*. If this is the case the gonococci will stay in the inflamed prostate gland for months, perhaps for years, and become the starting point for extragenital gonorrhea, that is, a gonorrhea that spreads to other parts of the body besides the genital organs. The chronic *prostatitis gonorrhoica* is often followed by changes in a person's general health. The patient tires easily, feels depressed, and may suffer from headaches. The sex need may be influenced so that it either disappears or increases. Impotence at intercourse may occur, and also nocturnal emissions and erections without any apparent cause. The disease may be accompanied by different sensations of itching or pins and needles right out in the glans. The examining physician by pressing the swollen prostate gland (that is filled with gonococci) through the anus may cause the puslike discharge to be evacuated through the urethra.

573. Gonorrhea in the Vesical Glands (*Spermatocystitis Gonorrhoica*) This means a gonorrheal inflammation of the cystite. The disease is similar to prostatitis in several ways, and both localizations may gradually become a focal point for the spreading of infection both in the patient's own organism and as a carrier of infection.

574. Gonorrhea of the Epididymis (*Epididymitis Gonorrhoica*) *Epididymitis gonorrhoica* is a very frequent complication in gonorrhea. The gonococci either penetrate through the vas deferens or the lymphatic channels to the epididymis where they give rise to an acute inflammation, almost invariably accompanied by high temperature and swelling of the epididymis. They may swell to the size of a hen's or goose's egg, at the same time becoming tense and very sensitive to the touch. The inflammation generally reaches a climax in the course of four or five days, and then gradually goes down. A peculiar thing to note is that patients who get an *epididymitis gonorrhoica* are often cured unusually quickly of their general gonorrhea. This *may* be due perhaps to the very high temperature that generally goes with epididymitis since gonococci get along badly at temperatures of 103 and 104 degrees. Sterility generally is one of the consequences of double epididymitis.

575. Extragenital Gonorrhea in Men This term refers to gonorrhea that is not located in the sex organs. These cases originate either by direct contagion of gonorrhea pus, or the gonococci are carried to the various organs by the blood stream.

576. Gonorrhea of the Anus (*Proctitis Gonorrhoica*) in Men This is a rare complaint. In the few cases that appear the prevailing cause is unnatural sexual intercourse like pederasty.

577. Ophthalmo-blennorrhea This means a gonorrheal inflammation of the conjunctiva of the eye. Formerly many babies were infected during birth because the mother suffered from genital gonorrhea. To a great extent this is now a thing of the past; it happens rarely, since the eyes of newborn babies are required by law to be treated with a ⅔ per cent solution of nitrate of silver.

578. The Quartermaster on SS Ignota Ophthalmo-blennorrhea may occasionally be found in both adults and children. In former days I sometimes had occasion to be on duty in a medical station which the Danish government had established at one of its radio stations. Danish ships at sea could radio the symptoms of patients onboard to the radio station in question and the physician on duty replied by radio, instructing the captain what to do, as he had always before him a list of the contents of the medical kit available on each ship.

One day the captain of the SS *Ignota* radioed that during a shore leave the quartermaster had caught gonorrhea and now showed symptoms that might point to ophthalmo-blennorrhea. "Please send instructions for treatment!" My response consisted of directions for preparing a 2 per cent solution of nitrate of silver with which the patient's eyes had to be treated at definite intervals, and for making a solution of kitchen salt to bathe them with every quarter of an hour, and in conclusion I said: "The treatment must be kept up without stop day and night; if not, there is danger that he may lose his sight."

Three hours later another radio message was received from the skipper: "Have effected ten treatments. Patient requires constant attendance. Must the treatment really be kept up day and night and the patient not allowed to go to sleep?" My reply was the briefest radiogram I have ever sent. It consisted of one brief word: "Yes!"

579. Gonorrhea in the Joints In this and in the following forms of extragenital gonorrhea the gonococci are carried by the blood stream to various parts of the organism. Gonorrhea in the joints is by far the most common of these complications. It generally does not appear until at least three weeks have elapsed after the original infection. It is characterized by fever and pains. Sometimes the pain shifts from one joint to another, but finally it concentrates in one of them. The joint swells and a tumor appears, very sensitive to the touch, and if the patient attempts to move the joint he suffers very great pain. The joint most frequently attacked is the knee joint. Smaller joints may also be infected, but it is mostly the big joints that are attacked. The correct diagnosis may sometimes be obtained by sucking out a little of the fluid that causes the swelling of the joint, and test it for gonococci.

580. Other Localizations of Gonorrhea The *eyes* may be affected by gonococci. The lung membrane, *pleura*, and the *heart membrane* may also be affected. On the skin and in the glans penis symptoms may appear as a result of the spreading infection through the blood stream, and in rare cases real *blood poisoning* may occur.

581. Genital Gonorrhea in Women Women can become infected with gonorrhea, the same as men. In them it most frequently settles in a. the urethra. (In adults the vagina rarely becomes the seat of the disease probably because the mucous membranes in the vagina of the adult woman form a defense against the penetration of the gonococci. There is also the possibility that the vaginal secretions offer an unfavorable soil for the development of the germs.) On the other hand, gonorrheal inflammations often occur in: b. the greater vestibular glands (bartholinitis); c. the cervical canal (cervicitis); and d. the Fallopian tubes (salpingitis).

582. Gonorrhea in the Urethra (*Urethritis Gonorrhoica*) in Women Here the disease shows in the same way as in male urethritis. The symptoms, however, are much less marked, probably because of the shorter length of the female urethra. Apart from the discharge, the patient as a rule feels nothing, at most a slightly burning or smarting sensation which may be intensified at urination.

583. *Gonorrhea in the Greater Vestibular Glands (Bartholinitis Gonorrhoica)* The greater vestibular glands are very often attacked by gonococci, which sometimes may show only as a slight inflammation with but scant discharge. As a rule, however, the glands swell until they are as big as pigeon eggs and become more and more painful. One of the glands may develop into an abcess. There are also other forms of *bartholinitis*, but as a rule the complaint is of gonococcic origin.

584. *Gonorrhea in the Cervical Canal (Cervititis Gonorrhoica)* This, next to the urethritis gonorrhoica, is the most frequent form of gonorrhea in women. When, during intercourse, the gonococci have been evacuated from the male urethra they are deposited directly in front of the external uterine or at the entrance to the cervical canal, and thus the gonococci are afforded a most favorable opportunity for further penetration into the cervical canal. This disease is difficult to detect because it is rarely accompanied by any spectacular symptoms. Only when the germs have penetrated still deeper into the womb a discharge appears that is ample enough to point to a diseased condition. At the same time there may be abdominal pains, and menstrual irregularities may also occur.

585. *Gonorrhea of the Fallopian Tubes (Salpingitis Gonorrhoica)* Salpingitis is an extremely frequent complication following upon female genital gonorrhea. Like bartholinitis, salpingitis may be caused by bacteria other than gonococci. Its main symptoms are abdominal pains which may radiate into the small of the back, and a discharge that is often of a yellowish-brownish color, sometimes smelly and purulent, and always very dangerous as a carrier of infection. A man who has intercourse with a woman suffering from gonorrhea of the tubes can hardly hope to avoid infection. When the gonococci have been active in the tubes for some time the interior may have been transformed into a gruel-like substance, most of all like Camembert cheese. Sooner or later this cheesy mass will block the whole tube. Such a condition existing will mean the woman will not be able to conceive, thus will not be able to have any children.

586. Extragenital Gonorrhea in Women These forms of gonorrhea in women do not differ from the corresponding forms in men, and so the reader is referred to what has already been said about them. Only gonorrhea of the anus in women requires special mention.

587. Gonorrhea of the Rectum and the Anus (*Proctitis Gonorrhoica*) in Women The discharge from the vulva may sometimes flow by way of the perineum to the anus. This is the most frequent cause of proctitis gonorrhoica in women, a not altogether uncommon form.

588. Genital Gonorrhea in Little Girls Unfortunately, this is not a rare complaint. The infection is transmitted either through some form of sexual immorality, or by the mother or nurse using sponges and other objects that have been in touch with purulent gonorrheal discharge. The seat of the disease is generally in the urethra, more rarely in the vulva and the vagina, and very rarely further back in the internal genital organs. The rectum may be affected too, and that happens not infrequently.

589. Treatment of Gonorrhea Genital gonorrhea in little girls has in the past been treated with estrogen, either applied locally or by injection. Otherwise treatment of gonorrhea may consist in a. *syringe and vaccine treatment;* b. *sulfonamide treatment;* c. *artificial fever eventually combined with sulfonamide treatment;* and d. *penicillin treatment.*

590. Syringe and Vaccine Treatment Injections by syringe was formerly the only known method for combating gonorrhea, but the days of the syringe treatment are almost over. Treatment with vaccine is already old-fashioned. Vaccination is an extremely uncertain method but was formerly much used in special cases, such as in certain chronic, deep-seated forms of gonorrhea.

591. Sulfa Drug Treatment As soon as the sulfa drugs—in which category the much used modern cure for pneumonia belongs—were made available they aroused great expectations in respect to their possible effectiveness in treatment of gonorrhea. These expectations have only been fulfilled to a limited degree, inasmuch as only some forms of gonococci have been able to resist the sulfonamides. As a result of treatment with such tablets one may succeed in killing only the weaker type of germs, which means that by this treatment one, in effect, isolates those germs that are capable of resistance and gives them a chance to spread and multiply, whereas only the feebler germs perish. As a result, most gonorrhea cases that persist now are due to sulfa-resisting germs. Local applications of sulfa powder in the urethra may in such cases sometimes bring about good results.

592. *Artificial Fever Combined with Treatment by Sulfa Drugs* Furthermore, it is also possible to give a combined therapy that has proved to be very effective. At the same time that the patient is given his sulfonamide tablets he gets an injection of a special vaccine intended to bring about artificial fever; a fever up to about 104 degrees is then produced for three days in succession. As a rule, the fever keeps up only for some hours at a time. By this treatment, which requires hospitilization, we have succeeded in curing the great majority of cases recalcitrant to sulfonamide treatment alone.

593. *Penicillin Treatment* At the present time penicillin has proved to be the sovereign cure for gonorrhea. According to comprehensive English, American, and UNNRA statistics penicillin cures almost all cases of gonorrhea, including those that resist sulfa therapy. Recently acquired gonorrhea is generally treated with four or five injections in the course of a day, and, as a rule, no untoward secondary effects are noted. The gonococci disappear from the urethra in from three to twenty-four hours; the discharge stops in about twenty-four or forty-eight hours, and the patient is cured in from three to five days. There are many examples of cases in which a single, very concentrated injection of penicillin has cured a fresh gonorrhea. Older cases, particularly if accompanied by epididymitis, may require more energetic measures. Penicillin treatment of peri-urethral abcesses and of gonorrhea in the joints hitherto, i.e. up to October, 1946, has not produced any satisfactory results.

DISEASES OF SEX LIFE 279

In penicillin treatment of gonorrhea the most important thing to remember is that penicillin may also make syphilis germs disappear from chancrous ulcers and that it may therefore be difficult to establish whether syphilis is or is not present at the same time. And it should be remembered that syphilis is *not* cured by the penicillin treatment used in gonorrhea.

594. *When May a Gonorrhea Patient Be Said to Be Cured?* Such a question is very hard to answer. Gono-reaction, as mentioned earlier, keeps on for months after the infection seems otherwise to have been ousted, and yet there is no certain guarantee that the patient may not still present a danger as a carrier of gonococci germs. On the other hand, as the cure progresses, one expects the reaction to get weaker and weaker. If it does not develop that way rather quickly, there is a possibility that some complication has arisen, such as gonorrhea of the Fallopian tubes or of the prostate gland or something else.

Three weeks is considered to be the very shortest period during which a gonorrhea patient must be watched after the acute symptoms have disappeared. Until then there can be no question whatever of declaring him cured. To establish that a gonorrhea is cured after such a short time is really impossible.

Chapter 61: SYPHILIS

595. *What Causes Syphilis?* Syphilis is an infection caused by a tiny germ the Latin name of which is *spirochaeta pallida*. It is extremely small and twisted in a spiral, generally with six to fifteen twists. It is found in syphilitic ulcers and in recent syphilitic eruptions of a different nature on the skin or in mucous membranes. The period of incubation generally lasts from two to six weeks.

596. *How Is Syphilis Tested?* By scraping lightly on a syphilitic ulcer, with a specially designed instrument, after having moistened the surface of the ulcer with a drop of salt water, it will generally be possible to obtain scrapings in which living syphilis germs will be found through microscopic investigation. Moreover, an extremely valuable diagnostic resource exists in the so-called *Wassermann* test.

597. *What Is a Wassermann Reaction or Test?* While syphilis is developing changes take place in the blood that can easily be traced by a special test. The most frequent test used is the Wassermann and Kahn reactions. When the term a WR is used, it refers to a Wassermann reaction plus a Kahn reaction. If a sufficiently clear answer is not obtained by the WR test an "extended WR" may be undertaken which generally includes an ordinary WR plus several analogous examinations of the blood serum. The value of the Wassermann test resides in the fact that only very few diseases or sickly conditions besides syphilis give a positive reaction. A positive Wassermann reaction may occur in leprosy and malaria, and immediately upon a complete anesthesia, but these conditions are easy to recognize in their own right, and so, as a rule, do not come into consideration at the evaluation of the significance of a positive Wassermann test. A very faint reaction may appear, making it essential then that renewed tests will generally have to be made to find out for sure whether the patient has syphilis or not.

In the so-called *secondary* stage of the disease the Wassermann reaction is nearly always positive. In tertiary syphilis, or when a patient formerly treated for syphilis has a relapse, the reaction is not always positive.

598. *Acquired Syphilis* The most frequent form of syphilis is the acquired syphilis. Its course runs in three, rather unique, phases.

a. Primary syphilis: comprising the first weeks after inoculation, is mainly characterized by the syphilitic ulcer, the so-called *primary affection,* and by changes in the adjacent glands.

b. Secondary syphilis: which may last for one or more years, calculated from the moment the disease "entered the blood" and spread to other parts of the body.

c. Tertiary syphilis: which appears some years—maybe fifteen to twenty—after the original inoculation, and is characterized by a number of changes of a very varied and often deeply disturbing nature.

599. *Primary Syphilis* After the infection has taken hold from two to six weeks may elapse, as mentioned formerly, before the disease is discovered. This happens when the so-called *primary affection, the hard chancre,* appears.

600. *The Hard Chancre* The primary affection, the hard chancre, appears as a little ulcer in the place where the germs have penetrated, most often with a smooth, lacquered-like surface. When the rims of the ulcer are pressed together between two fingers, it feels peculiarly stiff, almost as when one presses a small deck of cards together in the same way.

The most common point of access is the penis in men and in women, the labia majora. However, as mentioned before, the infection may also penetrate into the organism in other ways. It may gain access through the lips by a kiss, through the mucous membrane of the mouth, if sharing eating or smoking utensils, or a toothbrush, with someone who has syphilitic sores on the lips or on the tongue, or through little sores on the fingers. Doctors assisting syphilitic mothers at delivery may, therefore, get it. For the untrained layman it is not easy to establish whether a sore is harmless, or whether it is a syphilitic chancre that can be detected. It must be stressed, therefore, most emphatically that on discovery of a sore on the genital organs, or some other suspicious sore, a doctor should be consulted as soon as possible, for during this phase the disease is very contagious.

601. *Adjacent Lymphatic Glands Swell* Simultaneously with the appearance of the chancre the lymphatic glands in the corresponding parts of the body generally swell, which includes the glands located in the groin. In syphilis they become hard, round, *insensitive* to touch. Such a condition is a rather sure sign and provides the physician with a valuable means of establishing his diagnosis. However, quite a number of persons have glands noticeable in the groin that have nothing whatever to do with syphilis. The lymphatic vessels leading to the glands may also be infected.

602. *Secondary Syphilis* In the hard chancres of the primary phase many nontypical forms occur, and an amazing degree of negligence prevails in the general public. As a result, the early stage of syphilis may frequently not be discovered. The patient may not, therefore, get any treatment, and the infection has the opportunity to progress unchecked in his organism. Very quickly after a person has become infected (often, as a matter of fact, before the chancre appears), the disease has spread throughout the body by way of the lymphatic vessels and the blood vessels. The first symptom indicating this has occurred, is (as mentioned above) that the WR becomes positive. Such a positive reaction occurs about five to six weeks after the inoculation has taken place. Thereupon follows rapid swelling of the lymphatic glands in very different places, as in the neck, in the armpits, at the elbow joints, etc. About eight weeks after the original contagion, symptoms on the skin and the mucous membranes may show up. At this stage, also, the disease is very contagious.

603. *Changes in the Skin*   The onslaught of the disease on the skin may show up as rosy spots, *roseola*, of somewhat varied appearance. In cases that are not treated, the spots, as a rule, change into a darker red and become slightly scaly. Sometimes only small welts appear on the body; in other cases there appear faintly colored calluses in the palms and on the soles of the feet. *Corona venerea* (or *veneria*) is a term used to describe something like a semicircle of raised skin, on the forehead. Nails and hair which, in an evolutionary sense, are part of the skin, may also be affected. Characteristic loss of hair may occur about three or six months after the first infection took place. *Leucoderma* also occurs, likewise three or six months after inoculation, most frequently in women. It appears as white spots about the size of half a pea in a network pattern of grayish brown, most often on both sides of the neck.

604. *Changes in the Mucous Membranes*   These changes are generally localized in the genital organs and their adjacent parts as well as in the mouth. In secondary syphilis the changes often appear in the form of the so-called *papillae*, of rather varied appearance according to where they are located. In the female genital organs the *papillae* may be pink, like protrusions, making the vulva and its surroundings look rather like a moon landscape with mountains, high plateaus, and valleys. These eruptions may become the seat of ulcers. Such cases are more rare in the male sex organs, whereas they are often found around the anus in both sexes. In the mouth similar eruptions, although not quite as marked, may occur, as for instance on the tonsils. The tongue, too, may be infected, and syphilitic germs may be secreted into the saliva.

605. *Tertiary Syphilis* Generally the secondary phase of the disease is limited to two or four years after the infection started, although it *may* extend over a longer period. Tertiary syphilis is an indication that the *spirochaeta pallida* now holds complete sway and has every opportunity of carrying on its ruthless destruction in various organs. This phase of syphilis, consequently, has so many aspects that it would require volumes by specialists to describe them in detail. In a general way, however, it may be said that the disease at that stage is particularly marked by: a. infection of the skin and of the underlying tissue; b. by changes in the circulation organs; c. by changes of the bones; and d. by changes in the nervous system. As mentioned before, tertiary syphilis may not show any of its symptoms until fifteen to twenty years after inoculation.

606. *When the Skin and the Internal Organs Are Affected* A very characteristic development is the formation of chancres. A single or several chancres may form on the skin or in one or more organs, and very often they develop into ulcerating sores. These may grow further and present two aspects: either the sores dry up and become confined by a scab or crust, or the whole chancre may dissolve and real wound hollows may appear. In such a manner the disease may *corrode* entire parts of the body, as, for example, an eye, a cheek, or large parts of the calf. The tongue may corrode in spots and the palate too, which may cause great discomfort at swallowing, and impediment of speech. A syphilitic chancre of that nature is galled a *gumma*.

607. *Changes in the Organs of Circulation* Syphilis may also affect the organs of circulation, which is not too surprising if one considers that the contagious germs are carried all over the organism in the blood stream.

Some of the most marked changes then take place in that part of the circulatory system in which all the blood contained in the body passes once a minute, namely the great artery trunk, the *aorta*. The disease centering upon this artery is called *aortitis syphilitica*. It generally manifests itself by a dilation of the aorta, sometimes accompanied by bulbous protrusions, in the way a bicycle tire, when being blown up, will form balloonlike protrusions at some especially worn spot. If the disease hits the valves (which unfortunately is very often the case) at the spot where the aorta leaves the heart, it may result in their shrinking, or there may be adhesions that in turn may cause a tragic upsetting of the heart's functioning. If the disease attacks the little arteries in the heart proper, through which the muscles of the heart are nourished, constrictions in spots may result.

608. *The Effect on the Bones* It has been mentioned already that the bones may also be affected. A syphilitic who may not have any idea that he had been attacked by the disease may some day break a bone through only a very slight cause. It may be an arm that is broken, merely by uncorking a bottle, or a leg becomes broken only through kicking at a pebble in the road, or by stumbling over some rather small object. This sudden breaking of bones is due to the fact that the *spirochaeta pallida* has burrowed into the bones and so corroded them that only a fragile fretwork remains at the spot that later breaks, or that an adjacent *gumma* has worked its way into the bone. One of those bones on which corrosion has its way most easily is the nasal bone. If the disease is sufficiently progressed a slight blow may break the nasal bone at the root. And since the nasal bone is the foundation of the shape of the nose, it will change completely, cave in and become what is called a "saddle nose."

609. *Changes in the Spinal Cord* The spinal cord consists of numerous nerve threads; some issue *from* the brain and connect with it as, for example, with a muscle. They are, so to speak, telegraphic wires through which the brain sends out messages to various muscles and other organs, telling them how to function.

The spinal cord, on the other hand, contains other large sheafs of nerve threads, charged with taking messages *from* the various organs *to* the brain on how things are going in the place where the nerve threads end. For example, from all joints such nerves connect with the brain and inform it how the knuckles that work in connection with the joints are operating in relation to each other, in such a way that even if one keeps his hands in his pockets one knows whether the finger joints are bent or not, whether the hand is balled up as a fist, or not. One will always be able to say with eyes closed, at least with some degree of exactitude, what position each part of the body is in. It is precisely those nerve paths in the spinal cord that the syphilitic germs attack. The effects of such a destructive attack are tragic. When the syphilitic walks he is not completely aware of which leg is in front and which one is behind. To know for sure he must look at his legs while walking, or else he has to count "one two, one two" all the time to know what leg to put forward first, for he cannot feel it. That gives his walk a unique, jerky appearance, rather like the movements of a mechanical doll. If such a person closes his eyes and with arms half outstretched tries to make the points of his index fingers meet, he will rarely succeed, for he cannot really feel whether his arms are bent or *how* they are bent. Thus, it will, in the same way, be difficult for him to put the heel of one foot on the opposite knee with eyes closed. If he stands erect with eyes closed he will soon fall (*Romberg's symptom*) because he does not, like healthy persons who are about to fall, immediately feel the impending fall, because the weight of the body comes to rest more on one, than on the other foot.

The disease is called consumption of the spinal cord or dorsal tabes (*tabes dorsalis*) and gives rise to *locomotor ataxia* as described. The disease is often first felt as rheumaticlike pains that come in lancinating flashes "as if one were stuck by knives" the patients say. They disappear as quickly as they came. Trouble in urinating is another rather early symptom, but since that is also a symptom of several other more ordinary ailments, it is less decisive an indication for the diagnosing physician. Only later do all the other symptoms appear, such as certain changes in the pupils of the eyes, which do not react to light any more, no longer having their former size and may no longer be circular. There is a failing sense of balance, and failing sensitivity, as to pain, for example, and a reduced capability in coordinating body movements, as shown, for example, by the test with the index fingers, and the heel and knee, mentioned above. Gradually the patient also loses what is called the knee or patellar reflex.

610. *Effect on the Nervous System* Syphilis may affect the peripheral nerve filaments and cause nerve inflammation, and of course a *gumma* may form in the brain or in other parts of the nervous system. However, what particularly characterizes tertiary syphilis, in relation to the nervous system, is the change in the central nervous system, which includes the brain and the spinal cord.

611. *The Patellar Reflex* Healthy persons have a rather unique reflex that can easily be demonstrated. The person who is to be tested sits or lies down, one knee crossed over the other in a relaxed position. Now, if with a small heavy object, or with the side of the hand, one strikes fairly lightly against the sinew just below the kneecap, the big muscle on the front of the thigh contracts spontaneously, making the leg jerk up. The sensation of the light blow made beneath the kneecap was carried via the sensatory nerve paths of the spinal cord to a subsidiary nerve center in the spinal cord from which it was sent directly, without the intermediary of the brain, through the motor nerves of the thigh muscle. This reflex movement does not occur in some persons whose nerve paths—that were to expedite the message of the blow to the spinal cord—have been destroyed, as may be the case in a person suffering from tertiary syphilis.

612. *Test of the Spinal Fluid ("Spinal Cord Test") in Syphilis* Many people falsely believe that a "spinal cord test" is carried out by thrusting a needle into the spinal cord. The test merely involves the tapping of a little of the so-called *spinal fluid surrounding the spinal cord*. The correct description of the test is "spinal fluid test." Even before a Wassermann reaction becomes positive in a blood test, it may be possible to conduct a

WR on the tapped spinal fluid to find possible changes in it that indicate a syphilitic infection. In secondary syphilis such changes are rather frequent. If in tertiary syphilis a Wassermann test of the spinal cord fluid gives positive results, it is taken for granted that the syphilitic germ has infected the central nervous system.

613. *Changes in the Brain* The brain may also become affected, and such a development takes place on the average of twenty years after the patient was first exposed to the disease. It is a peculiar fact that the later in life a person contracts the infection the quicker this form of the disease develops. In a young person who acquires syphilis about the age of sixteen changes in the brain will not show until twenty-five years later, whereas a person infected at the age of forty-three will generally have reached the brain-affection stage before he is fifty. These two examples are based, of course, on the supposition that the disease has not received proper treatment. The brain disease called *dementia paralytica,* or *general paralysis,* manifests itself by the patient's inability to collect and coordinate his thoughts, his power of thinking being affected. It often starts as nervousness, fatigue, failing power of concentration, and depression. This introductory phase may be followed by megalomania. The patient may believe he is a millionaire, the emperor, the Pope, or God himself, and this condition is, in turn, usually followed by a dullness that may lead to complete mental decay.

If the disease affects certain arteries in the brain so-called softening of the brain (*encephalomalacia*) may ensue, with symptoms very similar to those of apoplexy. As a matter of fact encephalomalacia is one of the most frequent, and, therefore, one of the most serious forms of syphilis in the central nervous system.

614. *Syphilis During Pregnancy* The syphilitic germs may penetrate into the placenta and thus be transmitted from the mother to the baby before it is born. If the physician knows that a woman has—or formerly had—syphilis he will always give her particularly severe antisyphilis treatment, as soon as her pregnancy is an established fact. The child thereby generally avoids suffering infection. If the woman does not receive any treatment

the pregnancy may terminate in various ways, all of which are disastrous. What most commonly occurs is the death of the fetus in the womb after five or eight months and its expulsion as a miscarriage (if it is before the twenty-eighth week of pregnancy), or as a still-born baby if the fetus is more than twenty-eight weeks old. A third possibility is that the pregnancy may be carried to its full term, but the baby is dead, and when the cause is investigated it will be discovered that the syphilitic germs have changed the fetal liver into a so-called *brimstone liver* teeming with spirochaetae pallidae.

615. *Congenital Syphilis*   The baby of a syphilitic mother may be alive at birth and apparently not diseased. Nevertheless, the infection may be present, but hidden, and may break out some days, weeks, or months following birth. A special form of syphilis, the so-called late *congenital syphilis*, may remain latent up to fifteen to sixteen years or more, before the disease is recognized. Symptoms may then appear in the teeth, the eyes, and the ears, followed by blindness and deafness. Feeble-mindedness may also be one of the results of congenital syphilis.

616. *Systematic Wassermann Tests*   Efforts aiming at discovering as many cases of syphilis as early as possible are to be greatly encouraged. By systematic blood tests, as required in many states, very good progress is being made. With the effective remedies for syphilis now available the tremendous importance of such tests becomes more obvious.

617. *Therapy of Syphilis*   Some of the old remedies like *mercury iodine-kalium,* are now rarely employed and then only in special forms of syphilis. After the discovery of *salvarsan* a therapy was introduced that is still being employed. The test consists of a series of injections into the blood stream, as a rule with the so-called *neo-salvarsan*. At the same time injections of an entirely different substance, *bismuth,* are administered into the muscles of the buttocks. The treatment is given in series, generally consisting of six to eight neo-salvarsan injections and ten bismuth injections over a period of from six to ten weeks. Moreover, at intervals of about one and a half to three months a few more series are administered, as a rule three to five, the number depending upon how the disease and its symptoms (among others the Wassermann reaction) react.

Secondary syphilis is generally treated for at least two years, even if all symptoms disappear quickly. If it takes very long for the Wassermann reaction to become negative, it may be necessary to prolong the treatment over a still longer period.

If tertiary syphilis has started, the ordinary series of treatments are given for a couple of years, and it is often necessary to treat the accompanying symptoms separately. It has been found, for example, that both attacks on the spinal cord and brain syphilis or softening of the brain may yield to the artificial fever therapy. The sooner these diseases are found out—as by a spinal fluid test—and are treated, the better the results to be expected. Formerly fever cure was used exclusively as a *treatment for malaria*. The patient was vaccinated with malaria germs, and when a suitable number of fevers had occurred, the treatment was interrupted, whereupon the patient was given quinine as a cure for malaria. Then the patient was placed in a sort of sweatbox, a *hyper-therm*. The fever may also be induced by an injection of the *fever vaccine*.

In recent years there have been especially difficult cases of syphilis that resisted eradication by means of the neo-salvarsan and the bismuth treatment. In such cases it has proved beneficial to hospitalize the patient, inducing artificial fever, combined with injections that are best initiated in the first or second phase of the disease.

Concerning penicillin treatment of syphilis, it has been pointed out that penicillin treatment of gonorrhea may bring about a change in the syphilis infection which may be present at the same time in the patient. The dose of penicillin that cures gonorrhea may make the syphilitic germs (on whose presence the *early* diagnosis of syphilis so absolutely depends) disappear from the chancre. However, such a reaction does not mean that the deep-seated syphilis is cured. Very large doses of penicillin are necessary in treating syphilis, requiring, for example, a rather strong injection every three hours throughout seven or eight days and nights. Such a therapy is capable of curing about 85 per cent of freshly acquired syphilis. It is impossible, however, to say anything definite about the permanent effect, until the patients who were treated have been under observation for a number of years. Excellent results have been obtained by a therapy combining salvarsan, penicillin, and bismuth. Penicillin may also be applied in the treatment of infants with congenital syphilis and in the treatment of the mother in the latter stages of her pregnancy, as such treatment keeps the disease temporarily in check.

618. *When May a Syphilitic Be Considered Cured?* It is impossible to produce any positive proof that a patient suffering from syphilis is *definitely* cured, cured forever. However, this must be determined in each separate case, for there is no over-all valid rule. The patient must be kept under observation for a long time.

619. *How Long Should a Syphilitic Be Kept Under Observation?* In order to make certain that symptoms of tertiary syphilis do not crop up unexpectedly (symptoms may remain latent for twenty years, as mentioned earlier), the syphilitic patient, as a general rule, should be observed at intervals all through life. After the completion of the first treatment, the patient should present himself for observation every three months during the first year, twice during the following year and then once yearly. The observation includes a general check-up and a Wassermann test. After three or four years a spinal fluid test should be made, and that is even more important if the WR should happen to be negative at this time. Syphilitics later in life should always be able to give an exact account of the treatment they have undergone, and if a syphilitic is being treated for some other illness, no matter *which* one, he should never refrain from disclosing to his physician the fact that he formerly had syphilis, for such restraint may involve risking his health and life. One should never take offense if the consulting doctor inquires whether you have had syphilis: he only asks as a matter of routine and for your own sake.

Chapter 62: VENEREAL ULCERS

620. Venereal Ulcers Venereal ulcers, or *soft chancre*, is a venereal disease caused by the Ducrey-Krefting germ. It is almost exclusively transmitted by intercourse. The ulcers which appear (as a rule, several of them at one time) two to three days after infection, are mostly irregular and red, the base of which are covered with creamy yellow pus. They vary greatly in size, are very sensitive to the touch, and very contagious. In men they mostly appear under the prepuce and on the rim of the prepuce. In women the ulcers occur particularly on the vulva where the labia meet near the anus. Venereal ulcers generally disappear spontaneously; however, inasmuch as syphilitic infection may be mixed up with the complaint, the patient should have the doctor check on his condition even after the ulcers have healed. The patient should return for checking as long as the physician considers it necessary.

621. What Are Buboes? In case of a venereal ulcer the lymphatic vessels, particularly on the penis ridge, may often be infected. About from eight to twenty days after contact swelling and a little pain not infrequently occur in one or more of the glands in the groin. In that case the lymphatic gland is called a *bubo*. It may grow to the size of a hen's egg or even bigger, and develop into a real abscess that may burst open through the skin.

622. Treatment of Buboes Tablets of the sulfonamide type are used for this complaint together with injections, as for example, with the so-called *Dmelco-vaccine*. This Dmelco-vaccine treatment brings about a rise in temperature, and, therefore, it can be carried out properly only if the patient stays in bed. There is only incomplete statistical material available about the effects of penicillin treatment of this ailment.

Chapter 63: THE FOURTH VENEREAL DISEASE

623. The Fourth Venereal Disease—Lymphogranuloma Inguinale Lymphogranuloma inguinale (or as it is also called, the fourth venereal disease) is caused by an unknown infectious substance, and is almost exclusively transmitted by intercourse. The incubation period is not definitely known; it may have a duration of a few days to fifty days. The disease is rare. Sailors frequently bring it from tropical and subtropical regions or from the Mediterranean or Baltic countries. At its initial stage the illness resembles both the soft and the hard chancre. But these early symptoms generally disappear so quickly that the doctor rarely has an opportunity to see them. In the following stage the infection spreads to the glands in the groin which in the course of some weeks swell terribly, stick together or adhere to the skin which often gets very red. There may be softer parts in the tumors which only rarely perforate the skin. The illness may be accompanied by fever and various types of rash.

624. *The Frei Test* It was extremely difficult formerly to diagnose the fourth venereal disease. Now it can easily be accomplished by means of the so-called *Frei Test*. A little fluid containing some of the infectious substance, in inanimate form, is injected directly under the skin of the upper arm. If the person suffers from the disease, a small, firm protrusion circled with red, at the spot where the needle was inserted, will appear after one or two days. This reaction remains throughout life, even after an acute attack of the disease has been cured. The cure itself generally requires a period of several months.

625. *Treatment of the Fourth Venereal Disease* The treatment consists in applying hot compresses, with rest in bed for rather a long period, eventually combined with X-ray treatment. The diseased glands cannot, as a rule, be removed by surgery as elephantiasis of the legs may ensue. The most recent therapy prescribes sulfa drugs in the same way as used in gonorrhea. Experimentation has proved that penicillin treatment is counterindicated in the fourth venereal disease.

Chapter 64: NONVENEREAL DISEASES OF THE SEXUAL ORGANS

626. *Nonvenereal Diseases of the Sexual Organs* In addition to the venereal diseases proper many different complaints within or upon the genital organs may occur. But all of them differ on some point or other in such a way from the real venereal diseases that they have not been included in the special laws covering venereal diseases. The point is, not every disease affecting the sexual organs is necessarily a venereal one.

627. *The Itch* (*Scabies*)   Scabies is caused by the so-called *itch mite* acarus. The male lives on the surface of the skin where it fertilizes the female. She, thereupon, burrows into the epidermis, making a tunnel. While burrowing the female lays her eggs until she reaches the deepest end of the duct where she dies after a few weeks. The eggs develop into larvae and work their way out to the skin where they develop into itch mites. Scabies may be transmitted in several ways: for instance, by shaking hands or by similar contacts. That, however, occurs only very rarely. The disease is almost always transmitted by a person sharing the bed of another afflicted with "the itch." Among adults there is almost always a strong possibility that it was transmitted by intercourse. However, pure "family endemics" occur. Scabies is treated by a special ointment cure: first a hot tub, and soaping with soft brown or black soap, followed by hard brushing particularly of the hands and feet; then drying and applying the ointment with a brush, or smearing with a special preparation. Then the patient generally puts on the same clothes he wore; on the next day he takes an ordinary bath, just for cleanliness, and not until then should he put on a change of clean underwear. The bedding should be aired for a day and a night, and the bed linen changed. As a rule, it is preferable to treat all the members of a household.

628. *Crab lice or Morpions*   Crab lice (also called *pediculus* [*or phtirius*] *pubis*) are an especially strong kind of lice with extraordinarily large pincers on their two hindmost pair of legs. It may be found in the hair under the armpits and in the hair on the head, but the pubic hair is their preferred hunting ground. They fasten their eggs on the hairs where they may be observed as tiny oblong structures growing out with the hairs. The disease is treated by brushing with *Cuprex* or by sponging or swabbing with special remedies, for instance, with hot vinegar or sublimate vinegar or sabadilla vinegar. At the same time one should attempt to remove the eggs with tweezers, or by using a very fine comb, and similar methods. The treatment should be repeated after a week.

629. *Venereal Warts (Condylomas)* Condylomas are wartlike growths that usually appear on the genital organs, both in men and women. What infection causes them is not known. The disease is generally transmitted directly by intercourse and erupts two or three months after inoculation. Venereal warts may grow to rather large dimensions, particularly on the female sex organs, and they show a marked tendency to grow during pregnancy. Their removal may require surgical treatment.

630. *Bladder Rash (Herpes)* Herpes, or bladder rash, is due to some small infectious matter, the nature of which has only been recently established. An attack of this rash begins by a small part of the skin becoming red and itching. Then, as a rule, subsequently smaller or larger spheric blisters appear, and these contain a transparent fluid. Herpes may occur all over the body, but most frequently it is located on the lips and on the sex organs. In women the rash may occur frequently in connection with menstruation. Whereas the blisters on the skin proper soon dry up and form yellowish brown scabs on the mucous membranes, they easily break and may cause insignificant sores. Treatment should include: powdering, salve, cold compresses, or compresses saturated with a solution of boric acid.

631. *Simple Urethral Inflammation (Urethritis Simplex)* The germs that—as with the gonococci—are capable of provoking urethritis are numerous. Various irritations may cause it, as by syringe treatment in gonorrhea. If a man has intercourse with a woman suffering from abdominal inflammation with discharge the two causes may work together. In the woman, her own discharge may cause urethritis. Simple urethritis, however, is quite harmless. It is accompanied by a considerably smaller discharge than gonorrheal urethritis, and with less pus. The treatment will depend upon the nature of the underlying cause in each case.

632. *Intertrigo* There may appear a redness on the skin surfaces that are so located that evaporation cannot easily take place and where the chances of survival of various, otherwise harmless, fungi are therefore particularly good. In some cases suppuration may occur where two surfaces rub against each other, especially in persons who are amply provided with fatty tissue.

This ailment, called *intertrigo,* most often lodges in the folds between the thighs and the sex organs, particularly in women. Powdering with a special *fungus powder* may often suffice eventually to eradicate the complaint.

In infants the so-called diaper rash—*diaper dermatitis*—may appear on and near the genital organs. This ailment appears as red, smooth, sometimes mildly infected blotches, often with yeast fungi. The majority of cases are due to the child having been lying for a rather long time with a closed, wet diaper.

633. Prurigo Vulvae Itching of the vulva is termed *prurigo vulvae*. This most uncomfortable condition may appear in conjunction with various complaints, particularly such as are accompanied by suppuration, like intertrigo or by discharge. It is sometimes associated with hypersensitivity, for instance in connection with liquor. The condition frequently appears in connection with the menopause or in diabetics. The itching may often be almost unbearable, and unfortunately it often proves very hard to get rid of. The treatment must above all be adapted to the cause, taking the underlying cause into consideration.

634. Prurigo Gravidarum In pregnant women itching may spread all over the genital organs or appear in other parts of the body. This condition is called *prurigo gravidarum.* The itching is believed to be caused by the presence of an abnormal amount of waste material in the pregnant woman's blood.

635. The Welander Sore The so-called Welander sore sometimes appears in girls and young women who normally would not have experienced intercourse. Its origin is unknown. The sore somewhat resembles a chancre. It heals in the course of a few weeks' application of compresses which have been saturated with a solution of chloride of lime.

636. Bartholinitis Gonorrhea is the most frequent cause for swelling of the greater vestibular mucous glands. However, this condition may also be due to many other causes; therefore, one cannot take it for granted that a woman has gonorrhea because she suffers from bartholinitis.

637. *Vaginitis* (*Colpitis, Elytritis*) Vaginitis is an inflammation of the vaginal mucous membrane. The causes are numerous and may be of a widely differing nature. For example, vaginitis may be caused, as a rule, by transmission of bacteria or rough treatment of the vagina, or the combination of both. Following the first intercourse, a so-called *defloration-colpitis* may occur. Using contraceptive devices, such as pessaries and condoms which have not been handled in a proper, sanitary manner, or introduction of some object for the purpose of masturbation, may cause vaginitis. The condition may also be caused by too frequent or unhygienically administered douches, or by diseases in the internal organs, particularly if they are accompanied by a discharge.

The disease often seems to be connected with malfunctioning of hormone production; in young girls there is frequently anemia present also. In elderly women it may appear as a so-called *colpitis senilis*, formerly called *elytritis vetularum*, caused by senile changes: the vagina shrinks, and small lesions may occur which easily become the focal points from where the disease spreads. It is often accompanied by a slightly bloody discharge. Otherwise the main symptom of vaginitis is an almost white discharge. It should be emphasized here that a woman may very well have a whitish discharge, so called *leucorrhea* (from the Greek word for white: *leukos*). Such a discharge does not indicate, however, that she has vaginitis, as this discharge may be the simple product of the glands in the walls of the cervical canal and of the small organisms normally present in the vagina. How vaginitis is treated depends upon what is found to be its cause.

638. *Inflammation of the Internal Female Genitals* (*Endometritis and Annexitis*) Annexitis or *salpingo-oophoritis* include both inflammation of the tubes (salpingitis) and inflammations of the ovaries. Inflammation of the mucous membrane of the uterus has already been described.

639. Constriction of the Foreskin (Phimosis) Phimosis must be treated by daily dilatation after having smeared the foreskin with vaseline. A special surgical operation is necessary only in very rare cases. What causes this ailment has already been described.

640. Paraphimosis (Spanish collar) The foreskin may be so tight that the glans of the penis swells to such proportions that the foreskin cannot be pulled down to cover it. The result of that condition is paraphimosis or Spanish collar. To relieve it, the doctor, after having administered a slight anesthetic, brings the tight foreskin down by special manipulation. This therapy may be applied if the condition has not lasted for more than twenty-four hours. If it is older than that, it will generally be necessary to apply compresses for some time until it becomes possible to pull the prepuce in place.

641. Inflammation of the Foreskin (Balanitis) Balanitis is a very frequent ailment. It occurs particularly in men with a narrow and tight foreskin, or who are deficient in cleanliness, often *because* of their tight foreskin. It may also occur in men who have intercourse with women suffering from pus-filled discharges.

The underlying causes are not yet quite clear; balanitis is probably due to the close coordination between different germs. Certain diseases, such as diabetes and gonorrhea, predispose a man to balanitis.

642. Gangrene of the Penis—Gangrenous Chancre Gangrene of the glans penis may sometimes occur in the form of a gangrenous chancre. It may occur independently or as a complication of some previously existing disease in the male sex organs, particularly balanitis. Similar conditions may arise in other spots too. In rare cases gangrenous chancre may be observed in women. The development of gangrene in the penis glans is favored by constriction of the prepuce, by herpes rash, and by lack of cleanliness.

Soon regular ulcers appear, their base covered with a dark scab, or perhaps secreting a very ill-smelling, dark brown substance. If the ulcers are not given proper attention, they may spread at a terrific rate, and in the course of a few days they may destroy great parts of the tissue. They may be cured, and, as a rule, are cured without surgery through treatment with sulfa drugs.

643. *Enlargement of the Prostate*   A special condition about the prostate gland must be mentioned. In older men whose production of semen—and, as a rule, also of sex hormones—is on the wane, the prostate gland has a tendency to grow larger, probably because certain gland cells around the urethra or in its walls reproduce themselves and swell the prostate. This condition may become so pronounced that the prostate will block the passage from the bladder into the urethra, partly or completely. An old man sometimes has trouble urinating. It is hard for him to get rid of the urine; he has to stand and wait for some time before it comes. When it finally comes it is often a very thin jet. Moreover, it is hard for him to empty the bladder completely. Enlargement of the prostate is by no means an uncommon ailment. It is estimated that no less than about 25 per cent of all old men are afflicted with it.

644. *Catheter Treatment of Enlarged Prostate*   It is hardly more than twenty years since the treatment most commonly applied to relieve this complaint was the following: Every time an old man felt the need of urinating he had to insert a long rubber tube (catheter) into the bladder and relieve himself through that. Afterwards he had to flush the urethra with a solution of nitrate of silver or some other disinfectant to prevent the risk of inflammation of the bladder (cystitis). Despite these precautions, cystitis, sometimes developing into nephro-cystitis involving the kidneys, caused the death of many old men suffering from enlarged prostates. Only few of the patients were able to insert the catheter themselves and use it. This brought to the initial risk of the treatment the added unpleasantness of the patient having to call upon his wife, a nurse or some other person to help him every time the catheter had to be used.

645. Surgical Treatment of Enlarged Prostate If the condition became too painful surgery might be applied. This was done by making an incision from below between the anus and the scrotum, or from above through the abdominal wall and the bladder, and removing the excessive gland tissue through the aperture. Nowadays surgeons use a considerably easier method. A thin metal tube, a *cystoscope* is inserted deeply into the bladder through the urethra. Though extremely thin this metal tube nevertheless contains several delicate instruments. At one end of the tube there is a tiny electric bulb to illuminate the interior of the bladder, and inside the tube, a telescope system that makes it possible to examine it. Through a couple of very thin tubes on both sides of the cystoscope the surgeon is able constantly to flush the bladder with clean water. Finally, the cystoscope contains a razor thin blade by means of which the operator can peel off small quantities of the superfluous glandular tissue. The peelings are washed away through the side tubes.

646. Hormone Treatment of Enlarged Prostate In recent years a new treatment for enlarged prostate has been introduced. It consists in injections of *androgenic* or especially estrogenic substances, which in many cases have brought such favorable results that surgery can be either completely avoided or, at least, postponed.

647. Inflammation of the Epididymis (*Epididymitis*) and Inflammation of the Testes (*Orchitis*) In connection with a simple urethritis a corresponding *epididymitis* may occur which, if it involves both the right and the left side, may result in sterility (Haxthausen). The epididymitis may also give rise to inflammation of the testis or testes (*orchitis*—derived from the Greek for testis: *orchis*). Most frequently, however, orchitis originates as a consequence of some local infection in the body far removed from the testicles, and the infection is transmitted to them by the blood stream. This may be the case, for instance, in pneumonia, scarlet fever, typhoid and para-typhoid fever, and genuine blood poisoning (sepsis); however, in all of these cases the ailment rarely spreads to such an extent that it brings about azoospermia.

Orchitis in connection with *mumps* (*parotitis epidemica*) is, however, a different matter. Many regard orchitis as a by-product of mumps too; but it would rather seem as if orchitis is a special form of mumps. In certain mumps epidemics the testes are affected in 25 to 30 per cent of the patients; in others, only 10 per cent are affected. But sometimes the testes are the *only* organs affected by mumps. Orchitis in conjunction with mumps, as a rule, occurs only in men past the age of puberty, rarely in boys, and usually not until six or ten days after the onset of the mumps. Generally only one testis is affected, the right one twice as often as the left, but the illness may also attack both testes simultaneously. Orchitis in connection with mumps can be completely cured in the majority of cases. The great significance of this illness as it affects the sex life of the patient, is that between 50 and 60 per cent of the cases result in azoospermia and if both testes are thus affected, sterility may result. In very rare instances the ovaries—which, in women, correspond to the testicles in men—may be affected.

648. *Tuberculosis of the Male Sex Organs* Tuberculosis may lodge primarily in the epididymis and in the testes, as a rule, because the disease has been carried by the blood stream from *foci* in the lungs, the glands, or the intestinal tube. Tuberculosis of the epididymis may, however, also occur in direct connection with tuberculosis of the prostate or the cystite in which case the infection has been transmitted by way of the *vas deferens*. Double epididymis-tuberculosis (in the right and the left side) in most cases will cause sterility (Haxthausen).

649. *Tuberculosis of the Female Sex Organs* Tuberculosis of the female sex organs is not uncommon. It exists in about 1 or 2 per cent of all women, but the symptoms that lead to its discovery do not always manifest themselves during the life of the victim. However, in comparison with other infections that affect the female sex organs, tuberculosis is rare. The general medical opinion is that genital tuberculosis in women is almost invariably due to tuberculosis in some other organ. However, it is not entirely excluded that the infection is due to direct external causes, such as neglect of taking proper precautions against contact with tubercular spit, or with feces or urine containing live tubercular bacillae. On the other hand, cases of genital tuberculosis supposed to be transmitted to women by intercourse can hardly stand up to a searching analysis of the diagnosis.

The disease may appear in all parts of the female genital organs, but very unevenly distributed. Twelve per cent of the cases of genital tuberculosis hit the *ovaries,* as a rule in connection with infection of the Fallopian tubes. Women with infected tubes represent 85 per cent of the total number of victims of female genital tuberculosis. The *uterus* is affected in about 50 per cent of all cases; the *vagina* rarely, and then mostly in children. The *vulva* too is but rarely the seat of a genital tuberculosis.

650. *Tumors in the Sex Organs* Both in men and in women the genital organs may be the seat of various tumors. They are often harmless, but such growths should always be closely examined, in order to make sure that they are not of a cancerous nature.

651. *Cancer of the Male Sex Organs* The most frequent form of cancer in the male sex organs is located in the *bladder neck gland.* Every third or fourth man above the age of forty suffers from this disease even though only about every eighth of these get any symptoms of the disease. Of the patients hospitalized because of faulty urination, about every fifth has cancer in the bladder neck gland. The treatment with estrogenics has shown astoundingly good results as an introductory treatment before an operation as is true for cases of prostate hypertherapy.

Cancer may also occur in the skin of the *scrotum,* for instance the so-called chimney-sweepers' cancer. Cancer of the penis occurs frequently in younger as well as, especially, in older men. Cancerous tumors may develop in the testicles also.

652. *Cancer of the Female Sex Organs* The *ovaries* may, as we have mentioned several times before, become the seat of cancerous tumors that have to be removed or eradicated by radium or by X-ray treatment. Cancerous tumors may appear in the *Fallopian tubes* too. But it is the *uterine cancer* that is the really great danger. This form of cancer is responsible for the death of many women annually. If the cancer lodges in the uterus proper, it is less dangerous than if it settles in the uterine neck. One of the important symptoms of a uterine cancer is *irregular bleeding*. That is the great reason why every woman, particularly after her menopause, must be extremely vigilant and ought to report any irregular bleeding. Unusually ample *discharge* that may be thin and mixed with blood and, to a certain extent, also *pains*, are symptoms that definitely should persuade a woman to consult a doctor and insist on a gynecological examination.

Many women have had to pay a very high price for the false modesty that too long prevented them from having such a gynecological examination. In very rare instances a cancerous tumor may develop in the vagina; if it does, it can happen at any age; vaginal tumors have been found even in little girls, but the post-menopause period is probably the age at which this form of cancer most frequently develops in women.

16

SEXUAL EDUCATION

Chapter 65: **TEACHING CHILDREN ABOUT SEX**

653. *The Sex Life of Children* One of the discoveries of modern psychology and biology is that at an amazingly early age children react sexually, or, at any rate, are often made to react sexually. This would refer, for instance, to the fact that infants may give evidence of seemingly pleasurable enjoyment by rubbing their genitals. This is particularly true of little girls. Furthermore, it is a fact that newborn infants of both sexes secrete considerable quantities of *estrin*, apparently having been transmitted to the infant through the blood stream of the mother. After birth this estrin is evacuated with the urine as being useless to the infant organism. In this connection we may consider menstruation in newborn baby girls. During childhood estrin again appears in the child's urine, but only in very small quantities, and many people, therefore, think that the widespread talk of *sexual* inhibitions—Oedipus complexes, etc.—are, to a great extent, products of the imagination. Kinsey reports that boys in the cradle have *erections*. *Orgasms* have been observed in boys from the age of five months and in a little girl of only four months. In a few cases *ejaculation* has been observed in apparently normal boys of eight years. The fact that a very essential part of the *sexual need*, or *contact need*, is decisively developed already from early childhood, has been dealt with in detail in the section on the passive sexual urge. On the whole, it is obvious that one will have to consider children's sex life as a far greater reality than previously has been maintained.

654. *What Does a Child Know About Sex?* When the child is two or three years old it usually discovers that there are two different types of persons, without, however, being clear in its own mind as to what the difference actually means. About the age of five the child will ask: "Where did I come from?" and when that question has been answered, it will ask: "How did I come out?"

Not until the child has reached the age between eight and eleven will it begin to show an interest in the father's part in procreation. For one thing, the child's mind has developed so far that the question comes naturally. Secondly, the child has personally encountered the subject while listening to the talk of other children and grownups. When the child is about twelve or thirteen, puberty occurs and it enters upon an entirely new physiological-sexual phase. To this new development is then added the vast complex of emotions that characterize puberty.

These observations are, furthermore, corroborated by Kinsey who determined that 57 per cent of the men he interviewed were able to recall sexual interest and *sexual play* with other children from before the stage of puberty. In some children such play began at a very early age and continued up to puberty; in most children it took place between the ages of eight and thirteen years. At the age of twelve years 38.8 per cent had participated in sexual play of some kind, 29.4 per cent in *homosexual play*, 22.7 per cent in sexual plays with the other sex, and 12.9 per cent in *intercourse play*. The initial age for sexual play with the other sex was on an average between the ages of eight and nine years, and when the children had reached the eighth form in school, 28 per cent of all boys had had intercourse.

655. *No Teaching of Sex During Puberty!* During puberty the biological side of sex life becomes quite difficult, not to say impossible for the adolescent to grasp as *objective information*, because in the mind of the growing child it will be inevitably linked with innumerable subjective ideas and notions.

After realistic consideration, hardly anyone, who has even an iota of understanding about the emotional life of boys and girls during puberty, could hold the opinion that the children should be burdened with lessons on sex in any shape or form during this period. Puberty in itself is so running over with sensational changes and events that all that is humanly possible should be done to make this period a quiet time for the development of body and soul. Such relative peace can serve to produce the best results and create the greatest harmony in the adolescents themselves.

It is best for the child to have its sex curiosity satisfied before the physical changes of puberty. Take notice, therefore, in regard to our subject, of the two extremely important age-groups following closely one upon the other: *Between eight and eleven the child spontaneously inquires about the part the father plays and may experiment on its own. However, when the child has reached the age of twelve it is usually too late to impart sexual enlightenment in the classroom, if one would avoid getting entangled in the problems of puberty.*

If, therefore, the child is to learn about the most *elementary* rules and laws for human propagation in a satisfactory manner, *before* the time when the question crops up from experience, the sex education must be presented to the children *at the very latest between the ages of eight and eleven*, in order to avoid tragic circumstances.

656. Why Is It Considered Difficult to Teach Children About Sex? Such a question is often brushed aside by pointing to two difficulties. First, there is the excuse that there are no suitable alternative terms for the slang terminology. Some parents are only acquainted with the vernacular themselves. This difficulty, however, is definitely an imaginary, or, at least only a temporary one. Most adults know, and those who have read this book would find it difficult to ignore, what words like penis, vulva, and vagina mean. And these are, of course, the terms that should be employed in teaching children about sex. It is due to the rather ridiculous shyness or modesty of parents that "penis" in many homes is called by a number of other words.

I taught my own children the correct terms at the very first opportunity that came for talking with them about these matters, and they found nothing unnatural or sensational in it.

The other alleged drawback is that *parents lack positive knowledge*. This, too, is nothing but a poor excuse. For knowledge can be acquired, and you who have read this book already know much more than you will ever need for teaching your young children about sex.

657. The Two Real Difficulties to Be Overcome The only genuine difficulties are these:

  a. *Parents cannot make up their minds* as to what—that is, *how much*—they should tell their children, and *at what age* the information should be given.

  b. There is one thing in particular that *parents dare not tell their own children*.

658. What Parents Dare Not Tell Their Own Children While the child is growing there is one particular word which both teachers and parents avoid. It is *taboo*, a detail of sex life that parents, no matter how willing they are to impart sex knowledge to their children, cannot bring themselves to describe.

That word is *intercourse*. Many parents tell their children about sex organs, pregnancy, development of the embryo, and birth, but they leave out this one thing, intercourse, never telling their children about it. It could be stated simply, like this: the penis is introduced into the vagina and something liquid, called seminal fluid, flows from the penis into the vagina and there are very tiny invisible living seeds, the sperms, in the seminal fluid. Each of these sperms has a little tail, and by lashing it back and forth it can swim. These sperms swim through the vagina right up into the stomach of the mother. Once there, they meet an egg which has been sitting there, waiting ever since the mother herself was a baby. Then, perhaps, this egg begins to grow, and grows into a real big baby.

The mention of this sexual union is what all parents avoid with some embarrassment. *Therefore*, to most youngsters, throughout their childhood, intercourse becomes something secret, veiled in mystery which neither father, mother, nor teacher *dares* talk about. Meanwhile, from more or less unfortunate sources the children obtain more or less correct information about this mystery. The children have a very limited opportunity of getting clear, candid, unadulterated, authoritative information, and therefore they seek it in other places.

The greatest incentive to obscene talk among children and, therefore, the most favorable soil for the breeding of future, perhaps habitual pornographers, must be said to be the obstinate silence of the teachers and parents. There appears to be only one effective remedy: the whole matter must be stripped of the "naughty" and "exciting" aspects by openly explaining about sex, including intercourse, *before* the children have had a chance to get wrong information. We certainly do not need to tell our children the details of all sexual abnormalities. Nor should we perpetuate any myth! There must be some solid middle ground —between the stork and Havelock Ellis—on which to build an effective program of sexual education.

659. *At What Age Should Children Learn About Intercourse?* . . . For me, it was very easy and a quite natural thing to tell my little girls about intercourse when they were three and five years old. They accepted the information with the same objectivity and in the same manner of taking things for granted—an established fact not calling for further reflection or comment—as when I told them that if I put tobacco in my pipe, put a match to it, and sucked, *smoke* would come from it. It did not occur to them to ask about all the details, as *how* the tobacco could change into smoke.

The essential thing is that children get authoritative information about intercourse *before* they themselves begin to show an interest in it, and *before* they connect it with something piquant or "naughty," or regard it as something especially exciting. It is necessary that they get this information before they are about seven or eight years old. It can be done only if the information is given them by their parents *before they enter school*—or, at the very latest, by a teacher in the first grade.

660. *Suggestions for Teaching Children About Sex* On the basis of the above proposal I would suggest the following for teaching children about sex.

In those homes where the parents feel they are capable of doing it (and in thirty to fifty years time that will be many), they will tell their preschool age children some basic facts about sex, including the mention of the word intercourse. Parents who are good teachers may be able to give their children such information without reference to any printed matter. Others may be guided by some book or pamphlet. The instructions should give elementary guidance in human procreation: anatomy and functions of male and female sex organs, intercourse, fecundation, pregnancy, and childbirth. Corresponding facts should be given about a few domestic animals (horses, dogs, and—last—birds) which children may have occasion to observe. The instruction book should be illustrated and contain a section with text for adults, inasmuch as the children would not be able to read. It may be quite a problem to write this text, but it *can* be done if the person who does it approaches it with a great simplicity and a pure mind.

661. *Sex Education at School*   Since it cannot be taken for granted that all children have received sufficient enlightenment in their homes before entering school, they should have the information mentioned above in the first grade. It could be given by the grade teacher in general lessons devoted to some other subject. In other words, the lesson should *not* be marked: Sex Information. These classes could be made required for all students, and boys and girls should not be separated when they are held.

In the final year of high school a physician should give extracurricular classes on sex. Here, the ethical side of sex matters could be emphasized and venereal diseases mentioned. Attendance at these lectures could be voluntary perhaps dependent upon the parents' decision. The lectures should be given to boys and girls separately. Every boy and girl, on leaving school, should receive a book containing the information given in the lectures.

Chapter 66: SEX EDUCATION OF ADULTS

662. *Adolescents*   Present-day youth leads a more free and independent life than ever before, and it is, therefore, of the very greatest importance that young people should have proper knowledge of sex life and its laws. No one really can prevent them from doing what they want to do. However, one can make sure that they *are aware* of what they do. From the tens of thousands of young men and women with whom my work has brought me into contact I have received innumerable confidences in the secrecy of the consultation room. Among other things these conversations often revealed a helpless ignorance which many a young man and many a young woman bitterly regretted.

663. *Parents*   Similarly, parents themselves should acquire such knowledge as will enable them to achieve a happy sex life; the best guidance for the young is a good example. And parents must overcome the unreasonable shyness which they sometimes feel with their own children, and give them clear and adequate information before it is too late.

664. *Training of Teachers and Physicians*   Sex hygiene should be an obligatory subject in all teachers' colleges. The minimum knowledge required of the *teachers* should at least equal that which the children learn before leaving school. Thus, through all grades, a teacher will be able to reply to the questions pupils may present to them. The physicians should take additional courses in child and youth psychology, sex psychology, sex ethics, and ordinary mental hygiene.

Chapter 67: SIGNIFICANCE OF SEXUAL EDUCATION

665. *One Must Be Matter-of-Fact*   In the preceding chapters I have presented as objectively as possible what physicians know and what they do not know, generally leaving it to the reader to draw his own conclusions. It is another matter, however, when the purely educational question comes up, where personal opinions are often sharply opposed to each other, and where it is up to the individual to take his stand on the many problems that arise in this connection.

666. *The Value of Sexual Education Should Not Be Underestimated* The bitter fanatics who try to circumvent sexual problems by silence are not prudent. Any person who has read this book will share this opinion. Think, again, of women's sexual neuroses; think of the spread and the dread of venereal disease, sterility in marriage, and the innumerable women who destroy life or health by attempted abortions. Think of the diseases caused by insufficient sexual hygiene, think of the unsuccessful marriages, the hardships of pregnancy, and the great problems of intercourse and birth control.

667. *But Sexual Education Alone Is Not Enough* In fact, it is a foregone conclusion that we should help our children and young people. A postwar Gallup poll disclosed that five out of six having an opinion consider it is a good thing to have information on sex available. However, this unavoidable, central question arises: HOW? The reply must be: By educating children to affectionate unselfishness and making them fully conscious of their responsibility. At the same time, however, they should be given information on sex life, its risks as well as its potentialities.

Therefore, let us definitely agree that education and direct warnings will never be enough; greater knowledge will not suffice to prevent all mishaps and people coming to grief in the difficult field of sex life. No matter what fine forces cooperate toward this goal, and no matter how happily and ably they often succeed in solving their task, they will never make all human beings good, affectionate, unselfish, or make them exercise self-restraint, or conscious of their responsibility, and charitable. That would only be possible by a universal change of character, heart, and mind in human beings.

For Product Safety Concerns and Information please contact our EU
representative GPSR@taylorandfrancis.com
Taylor & Francis Verlag GmbH, Kaufingerstraße 24, 80331 München, Germany

www.ingramcontent.com/pod-product-compliance
Lightning Source LLC
Chambersburg PA
CBHW071152300426
44113CB00009B/1178